D1233083

AUDIOMETRY:

Principles and Practices

AUDIOMETRY:
Principles and Practices

edited by
ARAM GLORIG, M.D.

*Director, Callier Hearing and
Speech Center, Dallas, Texas*

sponsored by the
AMERICAN ACADEMY OF OPHTHALMOLOGY
AND OTOLARYNGOLOGY

THE WILLIAMS & WILKINS COMPANY
Baltimore / 1965

First Edition, 1965
Reprinted, October, 1966
Reprinted, January, 1968
Reprinted, April, 1971

Made in the United States of America

Library of Congress Catalog Card Number 65-21120

Composed and Printed at the
Waverly Press, Inc.
Mt. Royal and Guilford Avenue
Baltimore, Md.   21202   U.S.A.

Contributors

William L. Benedict, M.D., L.L.D., Executive Secretary-Treasurer of the American Academy of Ophthalmology and Otolaryngology and Editor in Chief of the *Transactions*; Professor Emeritus of Ophthalmology, Mayo Graduate School of Medicine, and Emeritus Head of the Section on Ophthalmology, Mayo Clinic, University of Minnesota at Rochester.

Marion Downs, M.A., Director of Clinical Audiology, University of Colorado School of Medicine, Denver, Colorado.

Meyer S. Fox, M.D., Assistant Clinical Professor, Department of Otolaryngology, Marquette University Medical School; Chief, Ear, Nose and Throat Section at Milwaukee Children's Hospital; Attending Otolaryngologist, Mt. Sinai Hospital, Milwaukee, Wisconsin.

Aram Glorig, M.D., Director, Callier Hearing and Speech Center, Dallas, Texas; Clinical Professor of Otolaryngology; Southwestern Medical School, University of Texas.

William G. Hardy, Ph.D., Audiologist in Charge at the Johns Hopkins Hospital; Director of the Hearing and Speech Center, Associate Professor of Laryngology and Otolaryngology, the Johns Hopkins School of Medicine; Associate Professor of Environmental Medicine, School of Hygiene and Public Health, the Johns Hopkins University School of Medicine, Baltimore, Maryland.

J. Donald Harris, Ph.D., Director of Research, The C. W. Shilling Auditory Research Center, Inc., Groton, Connecticut.

Wallace S. High, M.A., Glendale College, Glendale, California.

K. M. Simonton, M.D., Professor on Otolaryngology, Head of the Section on Otolaryngology, Mayo Clinic and Mayo Graduate School of Medicine, University of Minnesota, Rochester, Minnesota.

Scott N. Reger, Ph.D., Research Professor of Otolaryngology, University of Iowa Hospitals, Iowa City, Iowa.

William B. Snow, B.S., E.E., Head, Electro-Acoustics Laboratory, The Bisset-Berman Corporation, Santa Monica, California.

Juergen Tonndorf, M.D., Professor of Otolaryngology, College of Physicians and Surgeons, Columbia University, New York, New York.

W. Dixon Ward, Ph.D., Associate Professor, Department of Otolaryngology, University of Minnesota, Minneapolis, Minnesota.

Foreword

Investigations of the fundamental problems in hearing have expanded tremendously in number and scope since the advent of the audiometer. On the side of pure science, modern audiometry has opened a number of avenues for investigation of sound—its nature, transmission, control, appreciation, and application in extensive commercial enterprises in human relations. Far beyond the human recognition of sound there are variations in volume, amplitude, frequency, and mixture of air waves that are detected by the audiometer, measured by special methods, and classified on a number of scales that are significant to a scientist and useful in explaining the human response to a natural phenomenon.

Another side to the development of the audiometer has to do with its application in the field of hearing in the everyday economy of human endeavor. It is only natural that those who are engaged in the study of defective hearing should make use of the information that is gleaned from scientific advances in the entire field of sound, including noise, acoustics, phonics, reception, and silence. Defective hearing has interested medical scientists, who for centuries have endeavored to aid the deaf. Medical groups have combined their efforts with lay groups to bring education to the hearing handicapped and to train them in the various skills of communication. The social and psychological aspects of disability due to hearing loss have stimulated public assistance in the development of professional teachers for the deaf and the maintenance of institutes of learning and training. The telegraph, the telephone, and subsequently introduced electronic means of communication via electric transmission of signals were born of research in the effort to aid the hard of hearing. Their contribution to the world's economy is incalculable.

The causes of hearing loss were primarily the goals of medical research. Study of the diseases of the ear broadened to such areas as heredity, climate, systemic disorders, infection, ear pathology, ageing, environment, and occupational disease. As a result of these studies, literally hundreds of suggested remedies, some medical and some surgical, have been assiduously applied with varying success. The wave of adenoidectomy and tonsillectomy may be cited as one of the prophylactic measures to reduce ear disease in childhood. Amplifying devices, ear protectors, and electronic aids were commonly used but could not entirely replace finger signs. An unanticipated aftermath was the legal recognition of occupational noise as a cause of noise-induced hearing loss and made it compensable as the

result of damage to the ear resulting in loss of enjoyment of the pleasures
of life and the ability to compete in the pursuit of a livelihood. This opened
the way for new tables of classification of hearing defects and the measurement of functional loss, whether it was directly or indirectly brought
about by circumstances beyond the control of the victim.

New comparable testing procedures yielding reproducible data for evaluation became essential, as the commonly used methods of hearing testing
were inadequate. Measurement of an individual hearing threshold level is
made only by means of an audiometer. To evaluate the readings of an
audiometer indicating loss in comparable terms, a base or zero level must
be agreed upon and the degree or amount of deviation expressed in a reproducible unit. The unit now in use is the decibel (dB). The "Hearing-
Threshold Level" is arbitrary. At the present time two such hearing-
threshold levels or zero base lines are in use. Some method of equating
audiometric data appears necessary. The adoption of an international
"Hearing-Threshold Level" is being urged. If generally adopted, the present confusion in estimating the degree of disability resulting from hearing
impairment will be lessened. Opportunities for activity in the hearing
field have recruited hundreds of technicians, particularly in statistical
studies, in public schools, industrial plants, occupational zones, and by
hearing aid dispensers. All must use some form of audiometer whether
they understand what they are doing or not; and there are at least three
common types of audiometers in use.

The American Academy of Ophthalmology and Otolaryngology became
actively associated with the American Association of Organizations for
the Deaf in 1921, with the appointment of the Committee on Problems
of the Hard of Hearing. A number of Academy members were prominently
identified with efforts to aid the hearing handicapped. The first chairman
of the committee, Dr. Horace Newhart, prepared exhibits and demonstrations in hearing testing in the public schools for the annual conventions
and later, with Dr. Scott Reger, wrote a brochure entitled, "Manual for
School Hearing Conservations Programs." In 1925 Dr. Newhart urged
the Council of the American Academy of Ophthalmology and Otolaryngology to advocate national legislation requiring routine examination
of all public school children. Year by year the committee was expanded
and after reorganization as the Committee on Conservation of Hearing, a
number of subcommittees were activated, each with a major objective.
Under the adroit leadership of Dr. Dean M. Lierle, of Iowa, the Committee
on the Conservation of Hearing has now become the recognized promoter
of hearing research. The Subcommittee on Noise in Industry was appointed
in about 1947, and a laboratory under the direction of Dr. Aram Glorig
has worked for several years in the field of noise-induced hearing loss as

an occupational disease. Many papers by the members of Dr. Glorig's staff have been published for the enlightenment of industrialists, public health officials, lawyers, doctors, nurses, and technicians.

The rapid advances in the construction and efficiency of commercial audiometers have posed new problems requiring new techniques. The audiometrist, whether he be otologist, audiologist, or technician, should be thoroughly familiar with the equipment in use and should be experienced in testing hearing. The aim of the Academy is to aid in the achievement of this objective, and this book is regarded as a valuable contribution to the educational endeavors of many unselfishly dedicated workers.

William M. Benedict, M.D.

Preface

The task of preparing this book on audiometry was undertaken at the request of the Committee on Conservation of Hearing of the American Academy of Ophthalmology and Otolaryngology. The Committee has long felt the need of such a book for practicing otolaryngologists, residents in otolaryngology, and participants in the Academy Home Study Courses.

The original task was undertaken to satisfy this need, but as preparations continued it became increasingly obvious that such a volume would be useful to audiologists in training, as well as those in practice; industrial physicians and nurses, pediatricians and general practitioners, special education teachers, psychologists, safety engineers, school audiometrists and hearing aid dealers.

Realizing my inadequacies to satisfy this broad and urgent need, I have attempted to gather into one volume the abilities of those highly specialized authors I believed would be second to none.

This book is not intended to satisfy an "ivory tower" reader. It is intended to present the most advanced thinking on audiometry in language acceptable to the neophyte as well as the master. I believe it fills a gap which exists in the present literature. I do not know of a single volume that offers relatively complete and authoritative information on the various facets of audiometry. I hope this book will serve to standardize audiometric techniques and promote a better understanding of a complex multidisciplined subject.

It is impossible to acknowledge fully my gratitude to my long-suffering fellow chapter authors. This has indeed been a labor of love.

Finally, my sincere thanks to my fellow Committee on Conservation of Hearing members for reviewing and criticizing the original manuscript.

Aram Glorig

Contents

1

Introduction to Audiometry

Aram Glorig, M.D., and Marion Downs, M.A.

The term "audiometry" originally meant only the measurement of the auditory threshold for pure tones. This restricted meaning was gradually extended as different techniques of auditory measurement were developed. The field of audiometry now embraces pure-tone audiometry, speech audiometry, screening audiometry, group audiometry, and, recently, automatic audiometry.

The electronic audiometer is the instrument commonly used to measure hearing. It is necessary when using the general term "audiometer" to specify which type of instrument is meant: a pure-tone audiometer, speech audiometer, screening audiometer, automatic audiometer, group audiometer, etc. The measurement technique and the type of audiometer to be used for testing hearing are dictated by the purpose for which the test is being made.

Audiometry may be divided into two broad sub-fields on the basis of the type of stimulus used to elicit auditory responses: pure-tone audiometry and speech audiometry. Pure-tone audiometry is used primarily to determine air-conduction and bone-conduction thresholds of hearing. These thresholds are necessary for diagnostic evaluations of hearing loss. Pure-tone air-conduction tests and pure-tone screening tests are also used extensively in industrial and school hearing conservation programs. Speech audiometry is used principally to obtain speech reception thresholds and speech discrimination scores for diagnostic purposes and to evaluate the performance of hearing aids.

ANATOMY OF THE EAR

The ear is the most complex of the many sensory organs. Its dynamic range of response is enormous. Sounds so faint that they might have been caused by the Brownian motion of molecules can be heard, and yet man can

1

also hear without distortion sounds that are a million million times more intense. Man also possesses the ability to distinguish some 300,000 tones of different frequency and/or intensity and to analyze complex sounds into their component parts.

Obviously the mechanism which is capable of such diversity is a delicate, complicated structure. The following discussion will be somewhat simplified to provide the reader with a general understanding of the various parts of the ear, and of the function of hearing. The attention of the reader is directed to the list of references at the end of this chapter for more detailed information.

The ear is divided into three parts: an external ear, a middle ear, and an internal ear (inner ear).

The External Ear

The external ear acts in much the same manner as a megaphone, serving as a conducting channel for sound. It is bounded distally by the auricle or pinna and proximally by the external layer of the drumhead or tympanic membrane; it consists of the auricle and the external auditory canal. This canal is about 25 mm. long and is S-shaped. The outer third of its length is directed inward, forward, and slightly upward; the center third inward and backward; the internal third inward, forward, and slightly downward. Because of these many changes in direction, the canal must be straightened by an upward and backward pull on the auricle before the drumhead is visible.

The Middle Ear

Anatomically the middle ear is bounded externally by the inner layer of the drumhead and medially by the mucous membrane which covers the bony wall just external to the inner ear. Within the middle ear cavity are the three ear bones or ossicles: the malleus, the incus, and the stapes; and two small muscles: the stapedius, which is attached to the stapes, and the tensor tympani, which inserts at the handle of the malleus.

The middle ear cavity presents five openings: the one covered by the drumhead, the opening to the auditory tube, the opening into the mastoid cavity, the oval window, and the round window.

The flattened bony footplate of the stapes fits the oval window and acts as a hinge, allowing the stapes to move in trapdoor fashion. The round window is very small, is located below and in front of the oval window, and is covered by a thin membrane resembling the drumhead.

The middle ear has three functions:

1. It transmits energy from the sound vibrations in the air column of the external auditory canal, by means of the drumhead and ossicular chain,

into the fluid contained within the cochlea. It is apparent from the degree of hearing loss that exists when the drumhead and ossicular chain are not present in an ear that vibrating air particles alone do not exert enough force on the oval window to transfer adequate amounts of acoustic energy to the cochlear fluid. The surface area of the drumhead plus the ossicular chain, however, with its attached muscles and ligaments, and the footplate of the stapes, all act as a complex impedance-matching device effecting an efficient transfer of acoustic energy from airborne sound waves to sound waves in the fluid medium of the inner ear.

2. It protects the inner ear from the shock of intense sounds of low frequencies by the reflexive action of the middle ear muscles. These muscles tense the drumhead and ossicular chain, thus reducing the amplitude of large vibrations. This statement is oversimplified, however: recent studies have revealed that we really do not know exactly how the middle ear acts with respect to its protective role.

3. It equalizes through the auditory tube the air pressure acting on both surfaces of the drumhead.

The Inner Ear

The inner ear is the source of the sense of hearing. It consists of two main parts: (1) The semicircular canals which contain one part of the body's mechanism of balance. (Since the semicircular canals have nothing to do with hearing, they will not be discussed here.) (2) The cochlea. The cochlea is essentially a system of spiral canals separated by membranes (Reissner's and basilar). These canals are the scala tympani, the scala vestibuli, and the scala media. One canal, the scala vestibuli, leads in a spiral from the oval window, doubles back on itself at its apex, the helicotrema, and spirals as the scala tympani to its termination at the round window.

Within this system is located the scala media, which is separated from the scala vestibuli by Reissner's membrane, and from the scala tympani by the basilar membrane. It is essentially a closed tube, triangular in cross section, and encloses the highly specialized end organ of hearing, the organ of Corti.

These canals contain fluid and function as a hydro-dynamic system. Being connected, the oval and round windows act in phase: an inward movement of the stapes at the oval window produces an outward movement at the round window. This reciprocal movement allows waves to travel back and forth in the fluid of the spiral canal. These waves produce a fluid wave in the enclosed membranous canal. The resulting wave-like movement sets up nerve impulses in the organ of Corti which are reported to the brain for interpretation.

The organ of Corti is a tremendously complex structure resting on the basilar membrane. It consists in part of a series of projecting hair cells: the outer hair cells lie in three parallel rows; the inner hair cells lie in a single row parallel to the outer rows and are divided from them by a tunnel-like structure.

Nerve fibers run from the hair cells out into the central core of the cochlea. There they join to form the auditory nerve and pass through a channel in the temporal bone to the base of the brain, where they synapse with fibers leading to the central hearing mechanism in the cortex.

THEORIES OF HEARING

The principal theories of hearing are the place theory, the frequency theory, and the volley theory.

Place Theory and Frequency Theory

The theory of hearing that accounts for frequency discrimination in terms of highly localized areas of response along the basilar membrane is called the "place" theory. Adherents of this theory believe that it is the exact place of stimulation of the organ of Corti which determines the pitch perceived.

Subscribers to the "frequency" theory, however, hold that the auditory nerve receives and transmits a pattern that corresponds in detail to the characteristics of the external sound stimuli. Thus, a frequency of 500 cycles per second (c/s) would cause the auditory nerve fibers to discharge at a rate of 500 times per second. There is some evidence to suggest, however, that the nerve fibers are incapable of discharging at a rate greater than approximately 1000 times per second; therefore, this theory does not explain high pitch discrimination.

The main difference between place and frequency theories of hearing is the presumed location of the sound analyzer in the auditory system. Place theories hold that the analysis of the frequency composition of the stimulus is made in the peripheral organ; frequency theories maintain that the higher centers alone or in combination with the peripheral organ are responsible for such analysis.

In general, frequency theories are inadequate in that they do not satisfactorily explain how, in the hearing process, sound is analyzed into its component frequencies; nor do they allow for the limited impulses characteristic of nerve tissue.

The Volley Theory

This theory combines elements of the place theory and frequency theory. It states that the frequency of the nerve impulses discharging in "volleys" explains the perception of pitch at the lower frequencies, and that the excitation along the basilar membrane accounts for the perception of pitch of the higher frequencies.

There is not complete agreement about the mechanism of analysis and pitch discrimination, but most of the modern theories are in accord as to the mechanism of the stimulation of the nerve impulse. In brief, the impulse is, or rather appears to be, initiated by the hair cell endings. When the basilar membrane moves, the hair cells bend. During this bending an electrical discharge is triggered in the body of the hair cell, and this discharge in turn initiates the nerve impulse. Much of our knowledge of these processes of hearing has come from studies by von Békésy, Davis, Rosenblith, Stevens, and Wever.

FROM ACOUMETER TO AUDIOMETER—90 YEARS OF PROGRESS

This book concerns itself with audiometry—a testing technique that is entirely dependent upon an instrument known for many years as the *audiometer*. How many years? Who named it? And above all, who was responsible for its introduction into the medical and scientific world? As we go about the business of audiometric testing, we casually accept the fine, complex instruments of today, forgetting the men and the vision that made them possible. This chapter reviews the achievements of those men and the origins of the instrument we use.

1875 to 1914. The Tuning-Fork Audiometer

The development of the audiometer, like many other scientific advancements, cannot be wholly attributed to any one man of genius. It has been said that inventions seem to invent themselves when the culture is ripe for them, and the audiometer is no exception. It could only have been developed when all the pieces of an acoustic and electronic jigsaw puzzle fell together at a point of time when medical needs demanded such an instrument.

The point of time that made the audiometer possible was the year 1875, when Alexander Graham Bell first introduced the electric telephone. Bell's utilization of electric circuitry in sound transmission and his use of appropriate transducers—the microphone and earphones—were essential to the production of pure tones. The field of otology had already played its role in this invention: Clarence J. Blake (1) professor of otology at Harvard Medical School, reported that he had communicated to Bell certain physiological investigations on hearing that he and the distinguished otologist Politzer had made, which were vital to the telephone's development.

The rapidity with which the principle of the telephone was applied to the problem of hearing tests indicates that the time was indeed ripe for the development of a hearing testing device. By January 1878, Arthur Hartmann (2), head of otolaryngology in a Berlin Hospital, reported that he had devised an "acoumeter" (in German, *Hormesser*), which utilized a telephone receiver for the purpose of testing hearing. The principles of this instrument were essentially the same as those that came to be used in every electric hearing testing instrument from 1878 until 1914: a tuning fork was placed in the primary circuit of an induction coil, interrupting the circuit at regular intervals. The interruptions induced an alternating current in the secondary circuit, of which the telephone receiver was a part. The receiver reproduced a tone corresponding to that of the vibrating tuning fork, regulated in intensity by a rheocord, or sliding inductance.

When we consider that the essence of these early devices was the "interruption" of the current by a tuning fork, it is little wonder that we still find the inappropriate term "interrupter switch" applied to the tone presentation switch on present day audiometers.

Although Politzer (3) spoke enthusiastically in 1883 about the potential usefulness of Hartmann's instrument to otology, neither Hartmann's acoumeter nor the several variations that followed in the next 35 years were ever in general clinical use by otologists. The early instruments were bulky and difficult to keep in running order. Moreover, they were limited in their diagnostic scope: only tuning forks with a frequency of 1000 c/s or less could be used effectively, and the output intensity had no psychophysical referent. Several otologists (3, 4) of the day, in commenting on the instrument, recognized that it told nothing about the hearing for speech and was therefore limited in diagnostic value.

However meaningless these testing instruments were to the otologist, researchers continued to report modifications and refinements of the "acoumeter." Before the end of the year 1878, three other reports, from Hungary (5), Russia (6), and Poland (7), had mentioned apparatuses similar to Hartmann's.

In 1879, D. E. Hughes (8) in England described an "induction balance" originally used to analyze metals, but applied with a tuning fork to the testing of hearing. He called this instrument an "electric sonometer," but it was this instrument that inspired the first use of the term "audiometer." Referring to Hughes' instrument, the English physician Richardson (9) wrote in 1879, ". . . the world of science in general, and the world of medicine in particular, is under a deep debt of gratitude to Prof. Hughes for his simple and beautiful instrument which I have christened the audimeter, or less accurately but more euphoniously, the audiometer."

Whether "audiometer" is actually more euphonious than "audimeter" is no longer pertinent; it is the name that has persisted. The term "acoumeter" died a lingering death: as late as 1922 a medical report (10) is found, referring to acoumeter testing and reported in terms of number of feet, as in spoken and whispered voice tests. However this correlation was made is not known.

During the years that followed Hartmann's and Hughes' instruments, other devices were reported which used the induction coil to transform an interrupted direct current into an alternating current for producing pure tones. Among these was that of General Korting (11) of Germany, who in 1879 presaged modern military audiometry by applying a modification of the acoumeter to malingering and recruiting problems in the German Army. Other names prominent in the investigation of this type of instrument were Hospitalier, 1879 (12); Preyer, 1879 (13); Boudet de Paris, 1882 (14); Baratoux, 1882 (15); Lacharriere, 1882 (16); Urbantschitsch, 1884 (17); Cozzolino, 1885 (18); Cheval, 1890 (19); Jacobson, 1885 (20); Seashore, 1899 (21); Gradenigo, 1907 (22); Tretop, 1908 (23); and Foy, 1916 (24). Seashore's contribution is particularly interesting to Americans because of his extensive contributions then and later, made at the University of Iowa. In his audiometer the secondary windings were arranged as a series of coils in which the number of turns varied in a logarithmic ratio. This gave variations in the loudness of the stimulus to correspond with the Weber-Fechner law. Seashore used the term "audiometer" for his instrument; this may have been the first introduction of the term into America.

None of these early variations was able to apply exact psychophysical measurements to the entire range of human hearing. In 1903, J. Loudon (25) lamented the fact that the science of acoustics had found no way to measure the "physiological intensity of pitch." This fact limited the clinical usefulness of the early audiometer, and few references are found describing its actual clinical use. One of the uses was indicated by Bunch (26), who reported that "McMillan used an audiometer (Seashore's 1899 instrument) in tests of children in the Chicago Public Schools." This brief statement is our only clue to what may have been the first school hearing conservation program.

1914 to 1919. The Electric Generator

All in all, the 35 years following the invention of the tuning fork audiometer were relatively barren of clinical application, but in 1914 A. Stefanini (27) of Italy constructed an instrument which made the modern audiometer possible. This was an electric generator producing an alternating current with a complete range of frequencies. An iron-toothed pendulum passed through an electromagnetic field, causing magnetic changes. An alternating current was thus produced in the generator with a frequency depending on the speed of the pendulum's passing through the field. The distance which the pendulum fell governed the speed, and thus the frequency, that was produced. This was an experimental instrument and was never applied clinically.

On the basis of Stefanini's principles, Lee W. Dean, head of the Department of Otolaryngology at the University of Iowa, and Cordia C. Bunch

(28), his research assistant, applied the electric generator to the first clinically useful "pitch range audiometer" in 1919. It was so called because it produced all the tones between 30 and 10,000 c/s—"pure enough for all practical purposes"—by means of a small alternating current generator driven by a variable speed motor. The intensity of the tones could be varied from below threshold of audibility up to the threshold of pain.

Dean and Bunch's audiometer was never produced commercially, but the two inventors published several articles describing the clinical application and interpretation of their audiometric tests in otologic practice. They called the charts they obtained from threshold measurements "hearing fields," which seems rather appropriate inasmuch as they described testing for "all tones." Such testing resulted in their finding the existence of complete or partial tonal gaps, which were viewed with satisfaction and some wonderment by the otologists of those times.

Cordia Bunch himself was perhaps the greatest stimulator of audiometry in our history; his *Clinical Audiometry*, written in 1943 (29), remains a classic in the field and is presently on its way to becoming a collector's item.

1921 to 1940.   The Vacuum Tube Audiometer

After Dean and Bunch's contribution, it remained only for the application of the vacuum tube to make audiometers commercially feasible. Such instruments were first reported in 1921 by independent investigators: Minton and Wilson (30), and Guttman (31). Their instruments utilized the vacuum tube to obtain oscillating electric currents of almost any frequency desired. Although never commercialized, their instruments were prototypes of future commercial audiometers.

The principles of the first commercial clinical audiometer were presented in 1922 by the otologist Fowler and the physicist Wegel (32), who reported on the use of the Western Electric 1A audiometer. This instrument had been developed by Wegel and his fellow physicist Harvey Fletcher (33) for the Bell Telephone Laboratories and the Western Electric Company, subsidiaries of the American Telephone and Telegraph Company. Dr. Fowler was the otologic consultant to the engineers developing the 1A. Fowler and Wegel named the chart that was obtained from the threshold measurements an "audiogram." They made the interesting statement: "The attenuator used is direct reading in logarithmic units and if the logarithmic relation between stimulus and sensation be assumed, it may be considered to read directly in units of sensation rather than stimulus." Thus began a slight fiction which has led to false assumptions concerning the relation of the decibel to just noticeable differences (JND) of loudness sensation. However, the innovation of the decibel scale as reported by Fowler and Wegel was a signal improvement in the recording of threshold intensity levels. Their audiogram was plotted on the logarithmic scale of intensity in terms of percentage of hearing. Percentage was calculated on the basis of the range of hearing, from minimum audible threshold to threshold of feeling. The 100 % line (normal hearing) was on the top abcissa; the 0 % (total loss) on the bottom; and the ordinate represented Bels. This audiogram looked not unlike ours today. The 100 % point representing the average normal hearing threshold was determined by a statistical study of normal ears which might well have been a model for Beasley's later survey of hearing for the Public Health Department. Fowler and Wegel describe some of the problems of this study as follows:

> As an indication of the order of magnitude of one of the skew errors (No. 5), the difference between random choice and otological choice of ears was examined, as well as could be done with the data without further tests. The "random choice" of subjects for test was made by simply choosing subjects who were not obviously "hard of hearing." The subjects were not ever asked if they experienced difficulty in hearing. Otological examinations were then made of all whose audiograms fell below the mean of the first choice or showed unusual variations. Most of the others were also examined and found to be normal. Eliminations were then made of all showing abnormalities. While this is not a perfect "otological choice," it is very close to it from the standpoint of the result. A "frequency of occurrence" plot of the resulting readings of sensitivity was made (including all pitches in one curve) and it was found that the skewness, if any, was imperceptible and that the "standard deviation" was .33 units (B1 = .0059, B2 = 3.15, number of observations = 710). A similar plot of the "random choice" data showed a decrease in the average sensitivity of .07 units, a standard deviation of .43 units and a quite perceptible skewness. While this cannot be said to be, in any sense, a determination of the error of abnormality present in a "random choice," it does show to what extent it is necessary to get a serviceable curve in terms of which to measure, normal or abnormal ears (32).

The statistical problems described here have a familiar ring even today, when we see the difficulties that have been involved in changing to an international standard for the reference level of audiometers.

An interesting sidelight of Fowler and Wegel's presentation of the paper describing their audiometer was a discussion by the great otologist and educator, Max Goldstein (32). It was reported that: "Dr. Goldstein said that while he was not unmindful of the scientific value of these charts, he was not ready to forsake older methods of testing for diagnostic purposes. These charts contributed to the diagnosis as does a temperature chart, but if one used the temperature chart to judge the necessity of mastoid operations, one would be handicapped." Goldstein's chief objection, however, was that the air-conduction tests were useless without knowledge of the bone conduction, which could be tested easily with the tuning fork. We shall see that only 2 years elapsed before this inadequacy was remedied.

The Western Electric 1A audiometer was never widely used because of its prohibitive price—for that day—of $1500. One of the original models of the 1A can be seen today in the Audiology Department of the Johns Hopkins Medical School, and it is reported to be in excellent operating condition.

A less expensive model, the Western Electric 2A, soon succeeded the 1A and found its way into general use by otologists. Unlike the 1A, which produced a sweep frequency output from 32 to 8192 c/s, the 2A presented only the octave frequencies from 64 to 8192 c/s. A further model, the 3A, used complex noise stimulus but never found favor among otologists. Many years later, in 1950, the German otologist B. Langenbeck (34) was to resume experiments with noise audiometry, using filtered bands of noise. He reported in 1962 on the successful use for diagnostic purposes of these critical band widths in conjunction with pure tones (35).

The use of a bone-conduction receiver in connection with the pure-tone audiometer was finally reported in 1924 by Jones and Knudsen (36). Their "audioamplifier" included not only air conduction and bone conduction but also a speech circuit. The bone-conduction receiver was described as follows:

> The ordinary circular diaphragm of the (telephone) receiver is replaced by a narrow strip of magnetic steel. This reduces to a very slight amount the sound energy radiated to the air. Attached to the center of this strip is an aluminum rod about seven inches long. The rod and strip diaphragm combined are designed to have a natural frequency of about 256 d.v. (double vibrations). Hence, the diaphragm will respond more vigorously when excited with a frequency of 256 d.v. than it will for any other frequency of excitation. The bone conduction measurements are then made at this frequency, although it is possible to make measurements using the same receiver, at frequencies of 128 d.v. and 512 d.v.

The presentation of this bone-conduction unit was very satisfying to Dr. Goldstein, who had previously been reluctant to approve the audiometer. Following Jones and Knudsen's paper (36), he commented, "I think we will reach the point of differentiation which will take the place of the Rinne and Weber tests, one of our sheet anchors. These are new departures, but I think the development of bone conduction differentiation will be very valuable". He went on to warn against accepting bone-conduction results as valid in the case of deaf children: ". . . the results he [Dr. Pohlman, an experimenter with bone conduction] obtained in bone-conduction tests with the telephone apparatus were the result of increased education of the sensitivity of tactile impression." And so even in 1924 Dr. Goldstein was aware of an error in interpreting bone-conduction test results—an error that has plagued otologists to this day.

Another unique feature of Jones and Knudsen's audiometer was a masking noise source. Their noise apparatus consisted of an ordinary electric buzzer. This produced an interrupted direct current in the coils of the telephone receiver, creating a loud noise in the receiver. Here is apparently the first recognition of the need to mask a good ear while testing the poorer one.

Jones and Knudsen's audioamplifier was later modified and produced by the Sonotone Corporation as the Sonotone Jones-Knudsen Model 1 audiometer. Coincident with the report of Jones and Knudsen in 1924, F. W. Kranz (37) also presented a vacuum tube instrument with which he had made many useful clinical observations.

Speech Reception Testing

The application of audiometric principles to the measurement of speech reception should be mentioned in any historical review, largely because of the importance of speech reception testing in the origins of hearing conservation programs. This application to speech testing was known in 1904, when Sohier-Bryant (38) presented a phonograph audiometer based on the Edison phonograph design. The speech signal was emitted through stethoscope tubes, with the intensity controlled by a valve. A later instrument developed by Professor Bristol (39) used an electric pick-up and a telephone receiver to transmit the recorded speech. The intensity was controlled by means of resistances.

In 1920 Seashore (40) presented his classic studies on the testing of musical ability. He utilized the phonograph to produce records which were discriminative of such factors as pitch, interval, intensity, and consonance.

The technique of recorded speech testing via phonograph reached its apogee in 1927, in the Western Electric 4A audiometer (41). This instrument was a spring-wound phonograph with an electric pick-up. Entire classes of school children could be tested because 20 to 40 earphones could be used to listen to the recording. Spoken numbers were presented by the records, attenuated in 3-dB steps down to 0 dB re normal threshold. The numbers were recorded by the subjects on special forms that could be quickly interpreted, and failure to respond within normal ranges were easily detected.

Two distinguished otologists, H. Newhart of Minneapolis and B. McFarlan of Philadelphia, were chiefly responsible for inspiring the widespread use of the Western Electric 4A in school hearing conservation programs. In 1927, McFarlan (41) described the examining of children at the Glen Mills School by himself and Dr. Fletcher, the originator of the 4A. This was probably the first use of the test, but it is known that by 1927 Newhart had inspired the use of the 4A in many Minnesota school systems. Later, S. Reger of Iowa joined Newhart in writing the classic "Manual for School Hearing Conservation Programs" (42), based on the 4A testing.

Very properly, with the inevitability of progress, the voice-test instrument was replaced in the late 1940's by the more discriminating pure-tone screening tests. However, the large number of children whose hearing problems were identified and treated through the use of the 4A audiometer is a testimonial to the instrument and the men who sponsored its use.

As mentioned before, Jones and Knudsen in 1924 incorporated speech reception testing into their audioamplifier. Not only did they obtain threshold for speech by using normative values, but they built into the instrument a series of high- and low-pass filters, by means of which the ideal selective amplification could be determined for a particular hearing loss. This kind of complementing of the audiogram seems to pre-date by many years its modern counterpart in hearing aids.

1940 to the Present

Otologists and educators gradually found audiometric testing with both pure tones and speech to be increasingly useful, and 1940 saw several commercial audiometers on the market. In the nature of our system of free competition, manufacturers made advancements that resulted in remarkably new and better features in audiometers, until today we see instruments of a complex nature never envisioned by the early workers. These advancements have been largely in the way of refinements of general principles and in the use of the circuitry for test variations. In addition, transistors are replacing vacuum tubes in many instruments.

One unique principle was introduced into audiometry in 1947 by the Nobel prize-winner, Dr. Georg von Békésy (43). This was the automatic, self-recording audiometer, in which the tone fluctuates around the threshold under the subject's control. Dr. von Békésy stated, "In audiometric measurements sounds should be avoided that are appreciably louder than threshold because they cause fatigue and make the determinations erroneous. . . . In the ideal audiometer the test tone is always close to the threshold" (44). Whether one subscribes to this theory or not, the von Békésy audiometer was a signal innovation which has led to many extremely useful diagnostic interpretations.

At the time of this writing, developments are being made in audiometers and in their use with analog computers which may some day make obsolete the tremendously complex instruments in use today. But even the instruments of the future would not be possible without the contributions of the men whose work we have here reviewed.

REFERENCES

1. Blake, C. J.: Vereinigte Staaten von Nord-Amerika; In *Geschichte der Ohreheilkunde*, edited by A. Politzer, Vol. 2, pp. 432–466. Ferdinand Enke, Stuttgart, 1913.

2. Hartmann, A.: Eine Neue Methode der Horprufung mit Hulfe Elektrischer Strome. Arch. Physiol., p. 155, 1878.
3. Politzer, A.: *Diseases of the Ear*, translated by J. P. Cassells, p. 188. Henry C. Lea's Sons and Co., Philadelphia, 1883.
4. Green, J. O.: Report by James J. Putnam, Secretary, Boston Society of Medical Sciences. Boston M. & Surg. J., *103:* 474, 1880.
5. Hoegyes, A.: Telephonic determination of hearing power. J. Med. Nat. Sci., *3:* 12, 1878.
6. Tarachanow, J.: Das Telephon als Anzeiger der Nerven und Muske Strome beim Menschen und den Thieren. St. Petersburger Medicinisch Wchnschr., *3:* 353, 1878.
7. Wodtke, A.: *Uber Horprufung mit besonderer Berucksichtigung der Methods mit Hulfe elektrischer Strome.* Inaugural Dissertation, Rostock, Poland, 1878.
8. Hughes, D. E.: On an induction-currents balance and experimental researches made therewith. Proc. Roy. Soc. Med., *29:* 56, 1879.
9. Richardson, B. W.: Some researches with Prof. Hughes' new instrument for the measurement of hearing: the audiometer. Proc. Roy. Soc. Med., *29:* 65, 1879.
10. Burton, F. A.: Aural exostosis. Tr. Am. Laryng. Rhin. & Otol. Soc., p. 201, 1922.
11. Korting, G. E.: Uber telephonische Horprufung. Deutsche mil.-ärztl. Ztschr., *7:* 337, 1879.
12. Hospitalier, E.: L'audiometre ou sonometre. Lumiere Electrique, *1:* 54, 1879.
13. Preyer, T. W.: Die akumetrische Verwendung des Bellschen Telephons. Transactions of the Society of Medicine & Natural Science, Jean, February, 1879.
14. Boudet de Paris: Determination de la sensibilite auditive. Ann. mal. oreille, *8:* 301, 1882.
15. Baratoux, J.: Audiometers. Rev. Mens. de laryngol. d'otol., No. 8, 1882.
16. Lacharriere, L.: Des moyens d'apprecier la sensibilite auditive—nouvel audiometre. Ann. mal. oreille, larynx organes connexes, *8:* 134, 1882.
17. Urbanschitsch, V.: *Lehrbuch der Ohrenheilkunde*, p. 409. Urban & Schwarzenberg, Berlin, 1884.
18. Cozzolino, V.: L'audiometro elettro-telefonica. Boll. Mallattie 'Orec., Gola e Naso, *3:* 85, 1885.
19. Cheval, V.: Electroacoumetre; nouvelle methode pour la recherche de la surdite dans les Consuls de melice et de revision, etc. Bull. Acad. Roy. Med. Belgique, *4:* 258, 1890.
20. Jacobson, L.: Ein neuer telephonischer apparat zur Untersuchung und Behandlung des Gehororgans. Deutsche med. Wchnschr., *11:* 908, 1885.
21. Seashore, C. E.: An audiometer. University of Iowa Studies in Psychology, No. 2, p. 158, University of Iowa Press, Iowa City, 1899.
22. Gradenigo, G.: Acoumetre telephonique du Prof. Stefanini. Arch. internat. laryng. otol. rhin., *24:* 500, 1907.
23. Tretop, d'A.: Acoumetrie Millimetric. Arch. internat. laryng. otol. rhin., *26:* 157, 1908.
24. Foy, R.: Examen des surdites de guerre. Proc. Nouv. d'Acoumetrie. La Presse Med., *24:* 595, 1916.
25. Loudon, J.: A century of progress in acoustics. Science, *14* (New series): 987, 1901.
26. Bunch, C. C.: The development of the audiometer. Laryngoscope, *51:* 1100, 1941.
27. Stefanini, A.: Alternatore Pendolare Electromagnetico. Il Nuovo cimento, Series VI, *7:* 261, 1914.

28. Dean, L. W., and Bunch, C. C.: The use of the pitch range audiometer in otology. Laryngoscope, *29:* 453, 1919.
29. Bunch, C. C.: *Clinical Audiometry.* C. V. Mosby Company, St. Louis, 1943.
30. Minton, J. P., and Wilson, J. G.: The sensitivity of normal and defective ears for tones at various frequencies. Proc. Inst. Med., Chicago, *3:* 157, 1921.
31. Guttman, J.: A new method of measuring hearing power by means of an electric acumeter. Laryngoscope, *31:* 960, 1921.
32. Fowler, E. P., and Wegel, R. L.: Audiometric methods and their applications, Tr. Am. Laryng. Rhin. & Otol. Soc., *28;* 96, 1922.
33. Fletcher, H., and Wegel, R. L.: The frequency sensitivity of normal ears. Physiol. Rev., *19:* 553, 1922.
34. Langenbeck, B.: Gerauschaudiometrische Diagnostik. Die Absolutauswertung Arch. Ohr.-Nas.-Kehlkopfh., *158:* 458, 1950.
35. Langenbeck, B.: Noise-audiometry. International Audiology, *1:* 224, 1962.
36. Jones, I. H., and Knudsen, V. O.: Functional tests of hearing. Tr. Am. Laryng. Rhin. & Otol. Soc., *30:* 120, 1924.
37. Kranz, F. W.: Some aspects of the problem of testing audition, and demonstration of a new portable apparatus. Tr. Am. Laryng. Rhin. & Otol. Soc., *30:* 140, 1924.
38. Bryant, W. S.: A phonographic acoumeter. Arch. Otol., *33:* 438, 1904.
39. McFarlan, D.: History of Audiometry. Arch. Otolaryng., *29:* 514, 1939.
40. Seashore, C. E.: University of Iowa Studies in Psychology, No. 36, Vols. 1 and 2, University of Iowa Press, Iowa City, 1920.
41. McFarlan, D.: The voice test of hearing. Arch. Otolaryng., *5:* 1, 1927.
42. Newhart, H., and Reger, S. N.: *Supplement to the Transactions of the American Academy of Ophthalmology and Otolaryngology.* Douglas Printing Company, Omaha, 1945.
43. von Békésy, G.: New audiometer. Acta Oto-Laryng., *35:* 411–422, 1947.
44. von Békésy, G.: *Experiments in Hearing,* translated and edited by E. G. Wever, McGraw-Hill Book Company, Inc., New York, 1960.

2

Introduction to Acoustics

Juergen Tonndorf, M.D.

Audiometry, the testing of hearing, makes use of various sounds as testing signals. These sounds may be relatively simple tones, produced by tuning forks or the earphone of an audiometer, or *speech*, which as an auditory "signal" is not so easily defined. It is, therefore, appropriate to begin a discussion of audiometry with a description of sound. The science of sound is called *acoustics* and is a branch of physics. Definitions in a physical science are laid down quite rigidly and unambiguously in mathematical terms. However, since the present text is written from an introductory point of view, no mathematics will be used throughout it. Those desiring a more rigorous treatment are referred to actual textbooks on acoustics.

Sound is a form of energy like light, electricity, heat, etc. The ear, man's receptor for sound, is so sensitive that it is able to detect very minute amounts of energy. Like all other forms of energy, sound when dissipated is eventually converted into heat. Since the energy levels of ordinary sounds are so minute, the amount of heat thus produced is extremely small and escapes detection by ordinary means. However, when sound is made very intense (too loud to be tolerated by the human ear) it can be made to overheat, and eventually kill, small fur-bearing animals. This heat is due to the absorption of sound energy by the furs of such animals.

Sound is generated by the motion of a body, for example, the vibrations of a tuning fork. This motion is then imparted to the surrounding medium, usually air. After traveling some distance, the sound energy strikes a receptor, e.g., the diaphragm of a microphone, which it sets into motion. The electrical events thus elicited in the microphone can be registered by a suitable instrument, a voltmeter, for instance. In a similar manner, when the sound strikes the ear, a chain of mechanical and neural events is elicited which eventually leads to cortical awareness, i.e., to hearing.

GENERATION, TRANSMISSION, AND RECEPTION OF SOUND

In the following, some of the events pertinent to the understanding of generation, transmission, and reception of sound will be described.

Periodic Motion—Simple Harmonic Motion

Let us first consider the motion of a generator which leads to the production of sound. Such motions may belong to either of two classes: (1) sustained (long lasting), or (2) transient (short lasting). "Sustained" motions are usually of a periodic character: an identical pattern of to-and-fro motion repeated over and over. Such "vibratory" displacement occurs in *time*, and, therefore, its pattern is difficult to visualize. The to-and-fro swinging of an ordinary pendulum may serve as an example of vibratory motion. The time pattern of this motion can be demonstrated by the simple arrangement shown in Figure 2.1. The pendulum traces its path by constantly dispensing a small amount of sand from its tip. This sand is made to fall upon a strip of paper which is moving at a uniform rate of speed perpendicular to the plane of the pendular swing. This way, a record is obtained, in the manner of a kymogram, of the vibratory displacement against time. (There are more advanced and more elegant ways of obtaining such records, but the basic principle just outlined is common to all of them.) Figure 2.2 shows a

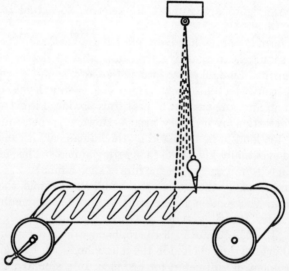

FIG. 2.1. Arrangement for tracing the sine-wave motion of a pendulum by adding a time axis.

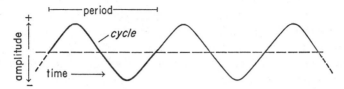

FIG. 2.2 Sinusoidal wave pattern: amplitude versus time

record (or a short piece of it) which might have been obtained in the way just described. The zero line (dashed in the figure) is that line which the pendulum would write when at rest. The actual displacement then occurs in two directions from the zero line which we shall call positive (upward on the paper) and negative (downward on the paper). With time, it forms a smooth and continuous outline which repeats itself in a "cyclic" manner. The particular form shown in Figure 2.2 is known as a *sinusoidal wave*. (This name derives from the fact that, because of its cyclic nature, it can be described mathematically by sine (or cosine) functions.) If the paper speed is known, the record of Figure 2.2 can be read in terms of time.

Period, Cycle, Frequency, and Amplitude. Several properties of a sine wave are apparent: (1) The *time duration* of one complete cycle is constant throughout the record. It is known as a *period*. Starting at the zero line, for example, it involves one positive excursion, crosses the zero line to take in one negative excursion, and finally returns back to the zero line. Such a count could be started at any other point along the curve; but in each case it must end precisely at an "equivalent" later point. (2) If one counts the number of such *cycles* as they occur per unit time (1 second), one obtains the *frequency* of the cyclic event. Frequency is, therefore, expressed as cycles per second (c/s). (3) The height of the excursion (in the positive or negative directions from the zero line) is a measure of the *amplitude* of displacement that the generator was executing when the record was taken. We must differentiate the *instantaneous* amplitude from the *maximal* and from the *root mean square* (*RMS*) amplitude. The instantaneous amplitude is that occurring at any given instant and may, therefore, vary between zero (at all zero crossings) and the maximal value (at all peaks of excursion). The maximal amplitude is that at the peak values only. The RMS amplitude is a statistical average of amplitude at *all* times. In the particular case of a sine wave, the RMS value is equal to the maximal amplitude divided by the square root of 2; i.e., it is approximately 0.707 times the maximal value. The RMS amplitude is of practical interest because it is registered by most measuring instruments, such as voltmeters used in noise level meters. These instruments do not react rapidly enough to follow each single excursion. Therefore, they register an average value. Furthermore, RMS values are important in power considerations. They represent the *effective* power values. This point is best illustrated by referring to electrical currents: The RMS value of a sine-wave (a.c.) current produces the same heating (power) in a resistor as an identical direct (d.c.) current.

Frequency may be high or low. The records of a high-frequency vibration would show the zero crossings narrowly spaced and those of a low-frequency vibration would show the crossings more widely spaced, provided both records were obtained at the same paper speed. Frequency is that property of sound which is most closely related to pitch.

Amplitude may be large or small. For a given sound, it is most closely linked to loudness. Because of the large range over which the human ear can differentiate loudness, the range of amplitude of audible sounds is in the order of more than 1:1 million; i.e., the range from the faintest sound an ear can barely detect to the loudest which can still be tolerated before pain is experienced in the ear. Frequency and amplitude are the two dimensions necessary for the definition of a sinusoidal event.

Phase. Sometimes the necessity arises of comparing two sinusoidal events of the same frequency (not necessarily of the same amplitude) as to their relative conditions at any given time. As shown in the two examples in Figure 2.3, one of the two events may be a little ahead in time of the other. For example, curve A of Figure 2.3a crosses the zero line earlier than does curve B. It is desirable in such cases to define these time differences precisely. They are referred to as differences in *phase*. It was already mentioned that the mathematical definition of periodic motion is derived from circular functions. Therefore, one can subdivide a cycle into 360° or fractions of 2π

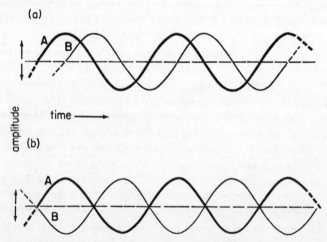

FIG. 2.3. Various phase relationships between two sinusoidal events of identical frequency. *a*, event A leads event B by a phase angle of 90° (¼); *b*, events A and B are of opposite phases.

($2\pi r$ being the circumference of a circle). In Figure 2.3a, for example, curve A is precisely 90° (or $\frac{1}{2}\pi$) ahead in phase of curve B. Conversely, curve B may be said to lag by 90° of phase behind curve A. In Figure 2.3b, the two curves differ by 180° (or 1π) from each other; they may also be said to be in *phase opposition* to each other. (Here the terms "lagging" and "leading" do not apply since the phase angles are equal in both directions.) If two events are synchronized so that their two time curves coincide, they are said to be *in phase*.

The concept of phase will permit us to discuss now the effect of two sinusoidal forces of the same frequency acting upon the same system. Since the electrical currents causing a sinusoidal displacement of the diaphragm of an earphone must themselves change sinusoidally with time, it is possible for *two* such (sinusoidal) vibratory forces to act upon the diaphragm at the same time. Obviously the diaphragm cannot execute simultaneously two motions in two different directions. Under such circumstances it will move in the direction of the resultant of the two forces. Graphically, such resultants are obtained by adding the displacements of both curves at consecutive points in time, paying attention to their positive or negative signs. Figure 2.4 shows several possible combinations: If both curves are in phase and of equal amplitude (Fig. 2.4a), the resultant will have exactly twice the amplitude of either of them alone, i.e., both events will reinforce each other at all times. If both curves are in exact phase opposition and again of equal amplitude (Fig. 2.4b), the resultant will be a straight line, i.e., complete cancellation will take place. However, when amplitudes are not exactly equal while two events are in phase opposition (Fig. 2.4c), only partial cancellation will result. Finally, when the phase angle is anywhere between

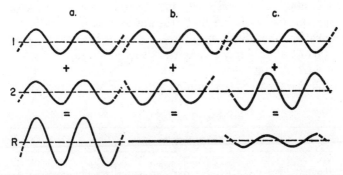

FIG. 2.4. Combined effect of two sine-wave components of identical frequency but in various phase relationships (*R*—resultant). *a*, in-phase relation, identical amplitude = cancellation of resultant amplitude; *b*, phase opposition, identical amplitude = cancellation of resultant amplitude; *c*, phase opposition, amplitudes not identical = partial cancellation of resultant amplitude.

the two extremes of 0° and 180°, partial reinforcement or partial cancellation will occur. The dividing line between reinforcement and cancellation is given by a phase angle of 120°. In all of these cases, except that of complete cancellation, the resultant is a sine wave of the same frequency as were the two primary wave motions. It may, however, differ from them in amplitude and/or in phase.

In all cases of Figure 2.4, the frequencies of both primary wave trains were identical to each other. However, when these frequencies are not identical, the resultant will not be a simple sine wave. Such a combination will lead (1) to complex waves or (2) to beats.

Complex Waves, Harmonic Spectrum

Complex waves will result when two or more different frequencies are sounded together. If they are related to each other by a ratio of whole numbers, e.g., as in 1:2, 1:3, 1:4, etc. but also as in 2:3, 2:5, 3:4, etc., they are said to be in *harmonic relationship* with each other. Table 2.1, listing such a series, containing four members, may serve to illustrate the various terminologies. Note the disagreement in the ordinal numbers denoting overtones, harmonics, and partials respectively. The term *overtone* derives from a none-too-good literal translation of the word *Obertone* used in the older German literature (e.g., Helmholtz). The terms *fundamental* and *basic frequency* as well as *harmonic* and *partial* are used almost interchangeably, although a partial must not necessarily be in harmonic relationship with the basic frequency. Under certain conditions, subharmonics may occur; in the example in Table 2.1, 50 c/s would be the first subharmonic.

As another example, the series 100, 300, 500, 700, ... c/s is obviously built upon the fundamental of 100 and consists of odd harmonics. The series of 200, 300, 400, ... c/s may be considered as that of the second, third, fourth, etc., partial with the first (the fundamental = 100 c/s) missing. Physiologically, the latter is an interesting series because the ear hears the pitch of 100 c/s, a phenomenon known as the case of supplying the "missing fundamental."

Two typical wave forms containing a first and second partial are given in

TABLE 2.1

Frequency	Musical Notation	Physical Notation
c/s		
100	Fundamental (1st harmonic)	Basic frequency (1st partial)
200	1st overtone (2nd harmonic)	2nd partial
300	2nd overtone (3rd harmonic)	3rd partial
400	3rd overtone (4th harmonic)	4th partial

a.   **b.**

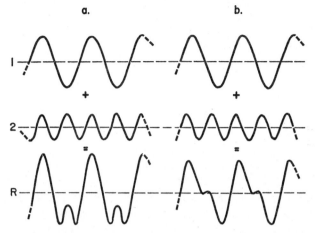

FIG. 2.5. Combined effect of two sine-wave events, one having twice the frequency of the other. The resultant (R) represents a complex wave form. Note the different wave forms (a and b) resulting from different phase relationships between the two primaries.

Figure 2.5. These figures indicate that the resultant wave form depends upon the phase relationship between the primary frequencies. It is easy to understand that combinations of more than two frequencies will produce rather complex patterns, and that, even for a given combination, the resulting wave form may look quite different, depending upon the phase relationships among partials.

Conversely, it is possible to analyze a given complex wave form and break it down into a series of sine waves of definite amplitude and phase relations. Such an analysis, known as a *Fourier analysis*, can be performed by means of either mathematics or suitable "wave analyzers." The point must be stressed that for a given wave form there is only one solution. Therefore, such an analysis is quite definite. By such an analysis one can determine the *spectrum* of a complex wave in much the same manner as one determines the spectral composition of light. The spectrum then furnishes a plot of frequency versus amplitude.

Of interest to engineers, for the purpose of testing electronic equipment, is a peculiarly shaped wave known as a *square wave* (Fig. 2.6). This wave contains an *infinite* series of odd harmonics, e.g., 100, 300, 500, 700, . . . c/s. Because of certain limitations in the generation of aerial sound, such wave forms cannot be realized too well in air. Also given in Figure 2.6 is the spectrum of a square wave. It consists of discrete lines and is, therefore, known as a line spectrum. All complex sounds have discrete-line spectra.

Sustained musical tones are actually complex sounds with the various

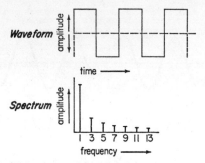

FIG. 2.6. Wave form and spectrum of a square wave

partials being in a harmonic relationship to each other. The lowest frequency of such a series, the fundamental, determines the pitch (even when it is absent as in the case of a "missing fundamental"). The number, distribution, and relative amplitudes of the various harmonics determine what is called the *quality* or timbre of the perceived tone. In general, the more harmonics a tone contains the fuller and richer it sounds. Pure tones consist of one (sine-wave) frequency only and have a peculiarly flat and dull sound. Audiometers are designed to produce pure tones. In general, it is more difficult to produce pure tones than complex tones.

Beats

It may be noted that the complex patterns of Figure 2.5 possess the same maximal amplitude for every cycle; i.e., a line connecting all amplitude peaks is perfectly straight. This is no longer so when the relationship between two frequencies occurring simultaneously is inharmonic, i.e., when their values do not form a ratio of whole numbers. The *beats* thus formed are characterized by a fluctuation (technically known as a modulation) in amplitude and sometimes also in frequency. Although beats will result from any inharmonic relationship, the present discussion will be limited to its simpler forms. Figure 2.7 shows a beat pattern resulting from the combination of two neighboring frequencies, such as 500 and 502 c/s, of equal amplitude. Because of the close relationship in frequency of the two primaries, such beats are known as *simple* beats or beats of *imperfect unison*. Moreover, when the primaries happen to be of equal amplitude (as they are in Fig. 2.7) such beats are known as *best* beats. The pattern of Figure 2.7 shows a sinusoidal amplitude modulation with time, the rate of which, the beat rate, is equal to the difference in frequency between the two primaries. In the above example the beat rate is 502 − 500 = 2 c/s. In the case of best beats, the two limits of the amplitude modulation are zero and maximal amplitude; the latter is twice the amplitude of the two primaries. The reason for the apparent amplitude modulation is easy

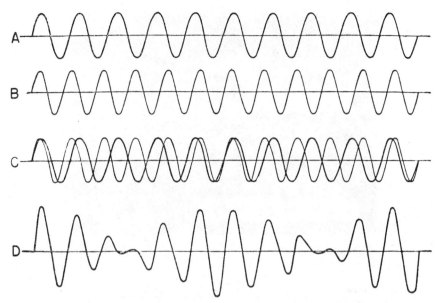

FIG. 2.7. A simple beat pattern (imperfect unison) formed by the combined effect of two sinusoidal events, not in harmonic relationship with each other. (*A* and *B*, primary frequencies; *C*, primaries superimposed; *D*, beat pattern.) Note that for the sake of illustration a frequency ratio of 5:6 between primaries has been chosen.

to understand. The phase between the two primaries is constantly changing, since the higher frequency completes one cycle faster than the other. Phases coincide when the resultant amplitude is maximal (simple addition) and oppose each other when the resultant amplitude is minimal (cancellation).

Some properties of the ear cause us actually to hear such beats as a surge in loudness when the beat rate is low, as a throbbing sensation when it is moderately fast, or as a roughness when it is still faster. However, we perceive neither of the two primary frequencies. Instead we hear their average, the so-called *intertone*.

Figure 2.8 shows one example of a complex beat pattern, between 50 and 104 c/s. Since 104 c/s is not quite the second harmonic over 50 c/s, such beats are generally known as *mistuned consonances*. The pattern of Figure 2.8 is decidedly more complex than that of a simple beat. It is also noted that the degree of modulation in Figure 2.8 is much lower than in the case of a simple beat although the two primaries contributing to the pattern in Figure 2.8 are again of equal amplitude. As a general rule, the degree of modulation and also the audibility of beats decline in the order of their complexity. Therefore, beats of imperfect unison are very noticeable, and beats of mistuned consonances are less prominent.

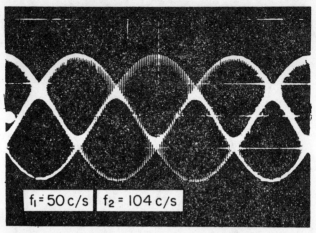

Fig. 2.8. Complex beat: mistuned consonance (primaries: 50 and 104 cycles per second (c/s).

Generation of Vibratory Motion

Events in mechanical systems are governed by forces. Most commonly, the force maintaining a vibratory event (after its initiation by an external force) is an elastic force. Elastic forces are inherent to mechanical structures and tend to restore their original shape after some deformation has taken place. Therefore, they also are referred to as restoring forces and in a given structure increase in proportion to the displacement (Hooke's law). However, this is only so within the elastic limits of a given material. For example, a steel spring is altered in shape permanently when extended beyond its elastic limits. Also, materials differ from each other by their "elastic modulus," a material constant. For instance, steel has a much stronger restoring force for a given displacement than does lead, which has almost none.

Another inherent property of mechanical bodies which comes into play during vibratory events is its mass: mass is known to display inertia; i.e., it opposes changes in speed. A body moving with a given velocity possesses momentum, the product of its mass and velocity. It continues moving until acted upon by an opposing force. Thus the momentum of a given body at any given time is proportional to its instantaneous velocity.

The vibrations of a tuning fork may serve to illustrate the interplay between the elastic and inertial properties in maintaining a given vibratory event. Tuning forks when set properly into vibrations execute simple harmonic motions in time. While the fork is at rest, all forces, by definition, are in a stable equilibrium. If some external force initially displaces the prongs from their resting position, an elastic counterforce is activated. When released, the prongs seek to restore their resting position under the effect of that force. The elastic force diminishes as the resting position is approached. However, as the moving prongs acquire velocity, their inherent inertia gives them momentum. In fact, velocity is highest, and momentum thus maximal, when the system reaches the resting position. Consequently, motion does not stop here but is carried beyond. As the displacement increases (with an opposite sign) the elastic force is activated once more (also with an opposite sign). It thus opposes the increase in displacement and consequently slows down the motion. Finally, the prongs are brought to a halt in their position of maximal displacement. Here the opposing elastic force is highest and the momentum is zero. Now the elastic force takes over again, and the prongs move once more toward (and through) their resting position.

It can be seen from this description that the elastic forces and the momentum must alter as sinusoidal functions of time. (The elastic force, for instance, is always proportional to displacement, which we know alters sinusoidally with time.) Moreover, the elastic force and the momentum interact in such a way that one of them is always maximal while the other is minimal. In a sinusoidal event, such a condition can exist only when the phase angle between both entities is 90° (Fig. 2.9a).

The velocity of a vibrating system decreases when the point of maximal displacement is approached. Since decreasing velocity means deceleration,

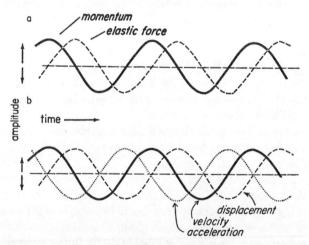

Fig. 2.9. a, phase relationship between the momentum and the elastic force of a sinusoidal event: the momentum leads the elastic force by a phase angle of 90°, both have sinusoidal wave forms but are not necessarily of equal amplitude as shown in the present example. b, phase relationship between the elastic force (displacement), the momentum (velocity), and the inertial force (acceleration) in sinusoidal motion; The elastic force lags behind the momentum by 90° of phase and is in phase opposition to the inertial force.

it follows that acceleration and displacement have opposite signs, and this holds true for all instances of a vibrating event. Consequently, if displacement varies sinusoidally with time, acceleration must do likewise, and the above condition is satisfied when, and only when, displacement and acceleration are in phase opposition to each other. Figure 2.9b then gives the phase relationships during sinusoidal motion of all three entities: displacement, velocity, and acceleration. It is to be noted that velocity leads the displacement by 90°. It is obvious from Figure 2.9b that there is an amplitude of displacement, one of velocity, and one of acceleration. They are not necessarily equal to each other as they are in the simplified example of Figure 2.9b. In speaking of amplitude one should therefore always make clear to which of the three entities one is referring.

That displacement, velocity, and acceleration have the same pattern is only true for simple sinusoidal events. In the case of square waves, for example, velocity is given by a pattern of alternate positive and negative spikes. In complex patterns, the velocity curve shows a phase shift between the component frequencies. The interested reader may try to derive these results on his own, starting from the displacement patterns given in Figure 2.5, a and b, respectively, and using the same type of reasoning as that employed in the preceding paragraph.

Natural Frequency—Resonance. A given tuning fork will always produce the same frequency. It is said to be tuned to a certain frequency and that frequency is considered its *natural frequency*. In order to affect the natural frequency, one must alter the mass or elastic properties of a given system. As to the effect of mass, tuning forks are again a good example. Some tuning forks are equipped with small weights which one can slide up and down their prongs. When these weights are put near the ends of the prongs (i.e., the vibrating masses are large), the natural frequency is lowered, and vice versa.

For elastic properties, we shall use a different example. The strings of a violin are tuned to different frequencies because of their individual tension. (Tension affects the elastic properties, i.e., stiffness.) Under high tension, strings produce high notes, and vice versa. Consequently, we have learned that stiffness is proportional to, and mass inversely related to, the natural frequency of a given vibratory system. More exactly, it is the square root of the ratio of stiffness to mass which determines the natural frequency. Since instruments like tuning forks vibrate easily in response to their own natural frequency or "resonate," this is also known as the point of *resonance*.

Damping. Figure 2.2 contained a slight inaccuracy which we shall now correct. The wave train with its uniform maximal amplitude has been said to represent a short section of a signal produced by a pendulum. This is not quite correct. The amplitude of vibrations of a pendulum or of a tuning fork, struck once, decreases gradually with time. This can be confirmed easily with the aid of large (low-frequency) tuning forks, since one can directly observe their relatively slow but large-amplitude vibrations. The force which opposes the vibrations is a frictional force, and its effect is called *damping*. No mechanical event can be completely free of friction. In vibrating tuning forks, for example, there is external friction by the surrounding air, but also internal friction within the metal itself. Friction is always evident during motion. Consequently, it is proportional to the velocity of vibrations and, according to Figure 2.9, it is, therefore, 90° ahead of the elastic force and lags 90° behind the inertial force.

Figure 2.10 shows some examples of *decremental* wave patterns under the effect of damping. When damping is low (as in tuning forks), the decrement is slow and vibrations, once initiated, last for a relatively long time. If damping is high, the decrement is steep and the event lasts only briefly. Under any condition of damping, the amplitude ratio between two consecutive cycles is the same anywhere along a decremental wave pattern. Since constant ratios can be expressed logarithmically, this type of decrement is referred to as a *logarithmic decrement*. Consequently, the amplitude ratio between two consecutive cycles of a decremental wave train can be used to express the degree of damping. The damping factor or decrement is the natural logarithm of this ratio.

Damping may actually become so high that a system when displaced will never be able to execute a single vibration, but it will gradually "creep" back to its resting position. The degree of damping at which this just occurs, i.e., at which vibrations just fail to materialize, is called *critical damping*. In excess of this limiting value, damping is said to be overcritical. Systems

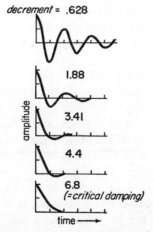

FIG. 2.10. Decremental wave patterns for various damping factors

which are that highly damped can never execute vibrations on their own
no matter how far they were originally displaced from their resting position.

Free Vibrations, Forced Vibrations, Narrow and Broad Tuning.
The vibrations of tuning forks, executed after the fork has been displaced
once, are a typical example of *free vibrations*. By definition, free vibrations
are displayed by structures on their own at their natural frequency, as
contrasted with forced vibrations. *Forced vibrations* are executed by a system when driven by an alternating force at any frequency (including its
natural frequency). This alternating force may represent a sinusoidal or a
complex event. When this alternating force is withdrawn, the system will
revert back to free vibrations, at its own natural frequency; the duration
of such "after-oscillation" depends upon the damping factor. Earphones
when driven by a sinusoidal electrical current are typical examples of forced
vibrations.

Tuning forks when subjected to forced vibrations respond poorly to frequencies remote from their natural frequencies. Hence, they are considered
narrowly tuned, i.e., to a narrow range of frequencies around their natural
frequency. By contrast, the diaphragm of an earphone is *broadly tuned;*
i.e., when driven by forced vibrations, earphones respond to a relatively
wide range of frequencies. When such a diaphragm is tapped so as to elicit
free vibrations, the response is very brief. Earphones are highly (but less
than critically) damped. For reasons which will be explained later, narrow
tuning is always associated with low damping and broad tuning with high
damping.

It is clear that a system which is broadly tuned is able to reproduce a
greater variety of signals than one narrowly tuned. Moreover, its high
damping reduces to a minimum free vibrations which otherwise might
occur as after-oscillations at the termination of forced vibrations. For these
two reasons an earphone is a better transducer (reproducer) of sound while
a tuning fork is a better generator. (Earphones must be driven by electrical
signals generated by other means.)

Transients. The point was made repeatedly in previous sections that
sine-wave signals are of long (theoretically of infinite) duration. The majority of sound signals encountered in practical situations are of limited
duration, some in the order of seconds, some others even in the order of
milliseconds ($\frac{1}{1000}$ sec.). The longer ones may be short sections of sine or
of complex waves. The shorter ones may not represent any periodic pattern
at all. Hence they are called *aperiodic signals*. (From the previous section it
should be clear that aperiodic signals can only be produced with some
degree of accuracy by systems which are quite heavily damped.) As a group,
all short-lasting signals are known as *transients*. Figure 2.11 shows some
examples of such transients. Without entering into a detailed discussion of

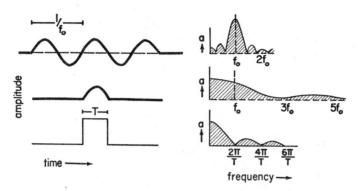

FIG. 2.11. Wave forms and spectra of some transients. Note that although spectra show nulls, usually at multiples of the natural frequency (f_0) or of the reciprocal time duration ($1/T$), these spectra represent continuous bands of frequencies.

their spectral composition, it is sufficient to state that transients are represented by continuous bands of frequencies of varying width. This is in sharp contrast to the discrete-line spectra of periodic signals (sine or complex waves). Even short sections of a sine-wave signal have continuous band spectra centered around the frequency corresponding to the period of the wave form. As a general rule, the longer the duration of a sine-wave signal, the narrower the frequency band. For practical purposes (as in audiometric testing), the section of a sinusoidal signal held for several seconds way be considered a pure tone. A very short-lasting section of a sinusoidal signal, however, is a broad-spectrum transient.

It is important to point out in this connection that any change in amplitude of a given sine-wave pattern represents a transient. Therefore, the beginning (change from zero to some other amplitude value) and the termination of a signal are accompanied by transients. The more sudden the transition in amplitude, the wider the spectral frequency band.

The equivalent of a transient, in terms of sensation, is a click. (The familiar "pops" and "frying noises" of the radio are practical examples.) Upon presentation of pure-tone signals, for rather obvious reasons, transients should be prevented. This can be accomplished (and is in commercial audiometers) by letting the signal amplitude increase and decrease in a gradual manner. By definition, the spectra of both transients thus become limited in width. They are deprived of their high-frequency components. Since the ear is more sensitive to high than to low frequencies, such transients become actually inaudible. This method, known as clickless switching, is specified by the *American Standards on Pure-Tone Audiometers*, the official guide for manufacturers, as follows: "After operation of the interrupter switch for 'tone on,' the time required for the acoustic output to reach a level within 1 dB of its final level shall not be less than 0.01 sec. or more than 0.5 sec." (This section is currently under consideration for revision. In addition to other changes it seems probable that the maximal duration of 0.5 sec. will be reduced to 0.2 sec.)

Transmission of Sound

The concept of forced vibrations introduces the question of how vibratory energy may be transmitted from a sound generator to the surrounding medium, or from one medium to another.

The prongs of a tuning fork in their to-and-fro motion move the surrounding air particles in a like manner. During their outward motion they push air particles closer together, creating a slight pressure increase, a "compression." During their inward motion, the air particles are allowed to expand from their compressed state, creating a slight pressure decrease, a "rarefaction." Air is an elastic medium. Therefore, the motion does not remain confined to the air particles in the immediate vicinity of the vibrating tuning fork. Each air particle moved by a vibratory event acts in turn as a source of vibration upon others, so that a wave-like disturbance is propagated through the air from the original source outward, not unlike the waves which travel away from the point of impact of a stone falling into water. There is one major difference: whereas upon the water surface particles appear to move up and down (transversally with respect to their direction of travel), sound waves in air are alternating sequences of compressions and rarefactions. Particles move in the same plane in which the wave motion propagates. Therefore, this particular mode is known as *longitudinal wave motion*. An example of genuine transversal waves is those of light. (Surface waves on water actually move transversally and longitudinally at the same time, so-called trochoidal wave motion.)

All previous figures have illustrated the *temporal* aspects of wave motion of a given structure. The propagation of a vibratory event through any medium occurs in *space*, thus adding a spatial aspect to the temporal one. (The motion of a single air particle along the pathways of propagating sound can again be described from the temporal standpoint alone and a record may be obtained like that of Figure 2.2.) Figure 2.12 gives a pattern of rarefactions and condensations representing, in a somewhat schematic manner, a small section along the pathway of a propagating sound wave. Shown together with this compressional pattern is a transversal-wave section which we immediately recognize as having a sinusoidal pattern. (The horizontal axis is now labeled "distance" instead of "time.") Comparison of the two modes of Figure 2.12 will show that compressions correspond to positive displacements and rarefactions to negative displacements in the transversal mode. For purposes of illustration, therefore, it is not essential which of the

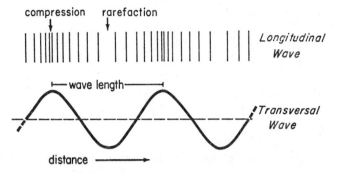

FIG. 2.12. Longitudinal and transversal wave forms of the same wave length

two modes is chosen. A transversal pattern is more easily drawn and recognized, and, therefore, it is preferred for representation of spatial as well as temporal patterns.

Propagation Velocity, Wave Length. When a vibratory event travels through a given medium, the velocity of such propagation can be measured. The speed of sound in air varies somewhat with temperature. At a temperature of 20°C (68°F) for example, this speed is 344 meters per sec. (1120 ft. per sec.). The speed differs for different media (again depending upon their elastic and inertial properties). In water (fresh water of 8°C) (46°F), it is roughly four times that in air, namely 1435 meters per sec. (4700 ft. per sec.). In steel, it is about 16 times that in air, namely 5000 meters per sec. (16,200 ft. per sec.).

Two pertinent statements may be made about the propagation of sound waves: (1) a given vibratory event when propagating never alters its frequency, and (2) within a given medium the propagation velocity is independent of frequency. It follows from these two statements that in a given situation the distance from crest to crest, the *wave length*, must be in a reciprocal relation to frequency as in

$$c = f \times \lambda$$

(c = propagation velocity, f = frequency, λ = wave length). By the same token, the wave length must alter in proportion to the change in propagation velocity in different media.

Sound Attenuation with Distance (Inverse-Square Law). A tuning fork radiates sound predominantly outward from both prongs within the plane of their movement. However, theoretically, we may think of a sound source which would radiate equally in all directions. Such a hypothetical sound source will aid us in the understanding of some further properties of sound fields. We shall further suppose that the medium in which sound is transmitted has uniform properties and is quite unlimited in all directions.

Such a condition is known as a *free field*. Disturbances which are created simultaneously at the source (e.g., a specific crest of a traveling wave caused by a sinusoidal event) will then propagate with the same velocity in all directions. Consequently, at any given time, each crest will form a spherical shell around the source (as do all of its predecessors and successors). Such a shell is known as a *wave front*. The distance from the source, i.e., the radius of the spherical shell, is proportional to the time lapsed since the movement was first generated.

The source, originally, imparted energy to the medium. This energy is spread thinner and thinner with the expansion of each wave front. In other words, the energy density is decreasing with distance from the source. Energy density is usually known as *intensity*, which is a common measure of sound. (Intensity is defined as the amount of energy flow per unit time through a unit area perpendicular to the direction of flow.) As intensity decreases in proportion to the growing area of the wave front, it is inversely related to the square of the distance, i.e., to the square of the radius of the wave front. (The latter relation obtains from the fact that the area of the wave front is a two-dimensional entity, whereas the distance is only a unidimensional one.) This *inverse-square* law still holds rather well even when the distribution does not occur in a strictly spherical manner.

Reflection of Sound, Standing Waves. So far we have hypothesized an unlimited medium, a condition which is rarely attained in actual practice. Everyone knows that sound "echoes" back when striking a hard surface. Under similar circumstances, such *reflections* (that is what echoes actually are) occur with other forms of radiating energy, notably light and surface waves. When sound is prevented from spreading beyond the reflecting boundaries, energy is retained within the original medium. Therefore, the inverse-square law does not hold within small enclosures, especially in view of a peculiar phenomenon known as *standing waves*.

When energy is reflected directly into the pathway of the incident waves, two sets of waves ought to be traveling in the same plane, only in opposite directions. As in other similar cases of superimposed wave motion described earlier, the actual motion must be the resultant of the two original ones. When in the present case (i.e., the interaction of incident and reflected waves) both trains happen to be alike in amplitude and are in phase opposition, the resultant is not a cancellation of amplitude but a *cessation of wave propagation*. In such standing waves, places which are of zero amplitude at all times, so-called *nodes*, alternate with places in which amplitudes constantly changes from maximal positive, through zero, to maximal negative displacements, so-called *antinodes*. The distance from one node to the next is one half wave length. There are two conditions necessary for the generation of standing waves: (1) that reflection be total (partial reflection will be described presently), and (2) that the length of the path of the incident wave be an integral multiple of one half wave length; this will assure out-of-phase relationship between incident and reflected waves. If these conditions are not met, partial standing waves will result; i.e., some wave travel remains superimposed upon a pattern of standing waves. (Condition 2, it should be noted, actually defines a state of resonance between the frequency of the incident sound and the space in which the standing waves take place.)

The amplitude of (complete) standing waves is twice that of the incident wave which follows from the principle of wave superposition. In narrow enclosures, therefore, the amplitude of certain frequencies (the half wave length of which happens to be an integral multiple of the length of the enclosure) varies considerably about the room. In some spots (at the antinodes) the displacement amplitude may be twice as high as expected from free-field measurement, whereas at others (nodes) it is minimal, i.e., close to or even equal to zero.

Defraction, Diffraction (Scattering), Absorption

Like other waves, sound waves are also *refracted* and *diffracted*, i.e., scattered. In this regard, the same laws apply as those pertinent to the case of light waves. Specifically, sound "bends" around small obstacles (as does light). The acoustical "shadow" cast by an obstacle depends upon the relation in size between the obstacle and the wave length of the incident waves. Therefore, low-frequency sounds (long wave lengths) are heard around corners.

In heavy fog, sound is diffused in a manner similar to light. Fog is a non-homogeneous medium, the air being interspersed with countless water droplets. Millions of interstitial boundaries are thus formed between which sound energy is reflected in a completely random manner. At each collision some small part of the energy is "absorbed" by the water droplet; the rest of it is reflected. The energy absorbed is finally converted into heat. Because of the countless number of such reflections occurring when a beam of sound is penetrating into a sound-absorbing material for some distance, the total absorption may soon become sizable. Hence the sound is attenuated. Because the size of droplets is closer to the wave length of high frequencies than to that of low ones, the effectiveness of absorption is inversely related to frequency.

Common materials which are effective sound absorbers are cotton and glass-fiber wool. Even clear air is not quite free of absorption. Air absorption depends upon temperature and humidity, increasing with both factors, although taken as a whole, the absorption of sound in clear air is not a very serious factor. Therefore, the inverse-square law still represents a good approximation of the decrease of sound intensity in a free-field situation.

Room Acoustics. It is by reflection on hard walls and by absorption in loose material that one can control the acoustic properties of a room. Reflective walls keep energy from spreading beyond the confinements of the room so that even low-intensity sounds are heard from one end to the other. However, this advantage is paid for by the fact that such rooms are highly "reverberant." That is, each signal causes multiple echoes which last for some time afterward and tend to obscure subsequent signals. Walls covered with absorptive materials "deaden" a room. There is little or no reverberation, but sound does not "carry" either, so that low-intensity sounds are lost in such rooms. Moreover, because of the stronger effect of absorption upon high frequencies, signals are deprived of their high-frequency components and sound muffled. For these reasons one must seek a compromise between reflection and absorption. This compromise depends somewhat upon the purpose of the room.

A transient sound introduced into a reverberant room decays only gradually, very much in the manner of a decremental wave form (Fig. 2.9). The reverberation time is used as a measure of such decay. It is arbitrarily set as the time taken for a given sound to become attenuated to one millionth of its original intensity value. Two seconds is a good average value for lecture rooms, concert halls, churches, etc. Reverberation interferes with the perception of speech. Hence, for lecture halls the optimal value is slightly shorter than 2 sec. For the appreciation of music, "brilliance," i.e., the carrying of high frequencies, is highly desirable. In concert halls, therefore, reverberation times are slightly longer than 2 sec.

Rooms in which audiometric tests are to be conducted must be reasonably quiet. Testing must be disturbed neither by sounds created within the room nor by those intruding from the outside. Such rooms are known as sound-treated rooms. The outside walls of such rooms consist of a heavy, hard-surfaced shell in order to keep out extraneous noises. The inside is lined with absorptive material to keep reverberation low. (The "acoustic tiles," even the metal-covered variety, which are commonly used in such construction, have good sound absorptive qualities.) In so-called anechoic rooms, reverberation is kept extremely low by an elaborate inside construction which practically prevents all reflection. Such rooms which approach free-field conditions are used for instrumental testing and calibration of microphones and loudspeakers as well as for auditory research on problems which require free-field conditions.

Filtering of Sound. In the preceding paragraphs, reference has been made repeatedly to the fact that sound absorption is frequency-selective. Such action is called *filtering*. Since low frequencies are "passed" through absorptive materials while high frequencies are "rejected," this is called low-pass filtering. High-pass, band-pass, and band-rejection filters are also used. The automotive muffler is an example of a mechano-acoustic filter of the low-pass type. All aerial sounds, when transported over large distances, lose their high frequency components because of absorption. A distant thunder has a low rumbling quality. It has lost its original sharp cracking quality which was due to its high frequency components. Today most filtering is done in electrical filter networks after conversion of sound into electrical signals.

Impedance. Reflection was seen to be a property of the boundaries between two different media. The secondary medium prevents the sound energy from entering and sends it back into the primary one. Such reflection must not necessarily be complete as can be easily demonstrated for the case of visible light. More often than not, it is only partial so that part of the incident energy is admitted into the secondary medium. Nor is reflection necessarily confined to hard surfaces. It occurs at any boundary between different media. Consequently, it must be the media themselves which differ from each other in some respect. This particular property of a given system (or medium) is called its *impedance*. Impedance may be defined as the opposition to the transmission of sound into (or onto) the system under consideration. Impedance is therefore the reciprocal of transmission.

Let us first consider the case of a medium such as a large air space. Its impedance is referred to as the characteristic impedance and it is independent of frequency, since large unbounded media do not have resonant properties. Particle velocity per sound pressure at a given point within a medium is a measure of transmission. Consequently, the impedance, its reciprocal, is given as the ratio of sound pressure to particle velocity. It may also be expressed as the product of the density of and the propagation velocity within the medium. The values of the propagation velocity in air, water, and steel were given above, and it is recalled that they increase in the order named. The density of these three materials increases also in the same order. From this follows that, of the three materials mentioned, steel has the highest impedance and air the lowest, while water has an intermediate value. Table 2.2 gives densities of, propagation velocities within, and characteristic impedances of these three materials. The unit of the characteristic impedance is the (mechanical) Ohm per square centimeter.

The impedances of vibrating structures (of a tuning fork, for example)

TABLE 2.2

Material	Density	Propagation Velocity	Characteristic Impedance
	$gm./cm.^3$	$cm./sec.$	$gm./cm.^2 sec.$
Air	0.00129	33,000	41.5
Water	1.00	144,000	144,000
Steel	7.85	500,000	3,940,000

or of moving surfaces (e.g., of the diaphragm of an earphone), the mechanical and acoustical impedances respectively, are similarly defined. However, since such structures possess resonant properties, their impedances vary with frequency and depend upon the inertial, elastic, and frictional properties of the system in a complex manner. (It may be mentioned in passing that limited amounts of air or fluid enclosed in a small space, for example the fluids of the inner ear, have resonant properties. Their impedances are therefore frequency-dependent.)

Middle-ear function has been discussed in the otological literature in terms of the (mechanical) middle-ear impedance. For this purpose, the middle ear was assumed to be a simple resonant system having three elements in series which represent its mass, elasticity, and friction (damping) respectively. Although this is a gross oversimplification, there is some merit in such a discussion for the understanding of resonant systems in general. A few simple equations, which are also found in some textbooks on otology, cannot be avoided in this discussion.

The effect of elasticity is proportional to the displacement, that of mass to acceleration, and that of friction to particle velocity. It is recalled from Figure 2.9 that these three entities—displacement, acceleration and particle velocity—are not in phase with each other. Therefore, the combined effect of mass, elasticity, and friction is not simply the sum of their individual effects. They must be combined in the manner indicated in Figure 2.4. Mass and elasticity are 180° out of phase. Therefore, their combined effect, the reactance, is their arithmetical difference (cf. Fig. 2.4, b and c). Since the resistance (R), the effect of friction, differs from the reactance (X) by 90°, their combined effect is given by vectorial summation (cf. Fig. 2.4a). Mathematically, the impedance (Z) can be written as

$$Z = \sqrt{R^2 + X^2} \qquad (1)$$

which is recognized as the solution for the hypotenuse of a right-angled triangle.

Of these two factors, the resistance (R) is frequency-independent. The reactance (X) depends upon frequency in the following manner. It is recalled that the natural frequency (the frequency at which a vibratory system may execute free vibrations) is proportional to the system's elastic properties and inversely related to its mass:

$$f_0 = \frac{1}{2\pi} \sqrt{\frac{E}{M}} \qquad (2)$$

Consequently, the reactance is related in an inverse manner to these two entities:

$$X = 2\pi f M - \frac{E}{2\pi f} \qquad (3)$$

(The minus sign is due to the 180° phase relationship just mentioned.) The complete equation of the mechanical impedance of a simple resonant system can thus be written

$$Z = \sqrt{R^2 + \left(2\pi f M - \frac{E}{2\pi f}\right)^2}$$ (4)

This equation can now be used to explain the resonant properties of such a system. The condition of resonance is given by substituting equation 2 in equation 3, which then becomes

$$X = \sqrt{EM} - \sqrt{EM} = 0,$$

indicating that at this frequency the inertia and elastic factors exactly balance each other. Therefore, impedance is minimal, being solely determined by resistance. At frequencies lower than the natural frequency, the reactance is mainly determined by elasticity, because of the reciprocal relationship of elasticity and frequency. Conversely, at frequencies higher than the natural frequency, mass becomes the dominant factor.

The impedance concept also affords a simple explanation of the relationship between tuning and damping. It has been stated that tuning is invariably associated with low damping and vice versa. Any deviation of the signal frequency from the natural frequency must produce an increase in the reactance (mass-dominated when $f > f_0$ and elasticity-dominated when $f < f_0$). If damping is low, the contribution of resistance to the total impedance is small so that the latter alters sharply with any alteration of the reactance. Consequently, the response falls off steeply on both sides of the resonance point and tuning is narrow. Conversely, when damping is high, the impedance is mainly determined by the resistance, and changes in the reactance have a lesser effect. Thus tuning is broad.

Figure 2.13 shows a series of frequency response curves for various damping values. A frequency response curve represents a plot of amplitude versus frequency for a constant signal level at all frequencies. It is thus the reciprocal of impedance. It is seen from Figure 2.13 that the response curve flattens as damping is increased, a fact which is in line with the explanations just given. However, when damping approaches its critical value, there is simply an attenuation with frequency which already attains noticeable values well below the resonant point. It is for this reason that all systems which are designed for a wide frequency response must be highly, but less than critically, damped.

How efficiently energy is transmitted from one system to another does not depend on the impedance of the receiving system alone. It is rather due to the ratio between the respective impedances. Transfer of vibratory energy is better the closer this ratio is to unity. In that case impedances are said to be matched. If very different from each other they are said to

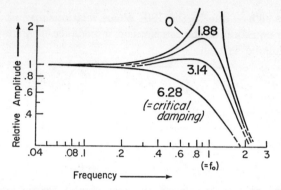

FIG. 2.13. Frequency response curves of a system under various degrees of damping (damping factors as indicated). It is noted that when damping is critical, the response curve slopes off before reaching the natural frequency (f_0). Therefore, systems with good frequency response are less than critically damped.

be mismatched. Transfer of energy is very inefficient in the latter case. A good measure of the impedance match is given by the ratio of reflected to transmitted energies, divided by the phase angle. If the impedance of one medium is known, that of the other can thus be measured. Based upon this principle, impedance-measuring devices have been built. The clinical usefulness of such instruments for the evaluation of middle-ear hearing losses by the assessment of the impedance of the middle ear has been demonstrated.

Sometimes impedances between two systems are badly mismatched and yet it may be desirable to transmit vibratory energy from one of these systems to the other. This can be accomplished by the interposition of an impedance-matching device. The middle ear is such a device. It has the task of providing impedance matching between the air in the ear canal (where impedance is low) and the fluids of the inner ear (where it is higher). If one or both systems have resonant properties, it is of course impossible to make the same impedance match for a wide range of frequencies. There will always be some frequencies at which the match is reasonably close and others at which it is less good.

Distortion. So far it has been assumed that a given system when transmitting vibratory energy reproduces the wave form of the incident sound in all details. However, this is not always the case. Structures and media may be limited in their response. The result is a *distortion* of the original wave pattern. Distortion may occur with respect to frequency, phase, and/or amplitude.

Frequency distortion is incurred when the secondary system cannot reproduce all frequencies with the same relative amplitude as does the primary system. In this sense, the relative loss of high-frequency components in low-pass filters is an example of frequency distortion.

Phase distortion is an unavoidable corollary of frequency distortion. Its effects are noted when the wave forms of complex sounds are altered in the sense of Figure 2.5. It used to be said that phase distortion would be of little consequence to the perception of sound. The ear was thought to be "phase-deaf." However, there is now some evidence that this is not quite correct.

Since transients are wave forms which represent frequency bands, it is understood that any limitation as to frequency and/or phase imposed by a given transmitting system must affect the wave form of such transients. (Such an occurrence is sometimes referred to as *transient distortion*.)

When electrical vibratory energy is conducted in (old-fashioned) telephone lines over large distances, low frequencies travel measurably faster than high ones. Thus it comes to a dissociation of signals, especially noticeable with speech signals. This time lag of high-frequency sounds causes the peculiar "birdies" one used to hear over long-distance telephone lines. Within the past decades this shortcoming has been eliminated by introducing proportional delays of low frequencies, thus preserving the original wave form.

Amplitude distortion is perhaps the most conspicuous of the three. It refers to the inability of a given system to reproduce the incident wave form properly. We must discuss separately its effect upon sine-wave and complex signals. The three examples of Figure 2.14 show some typical forms of amplitude distortion of a sine-wave signal: (a) asymmetry of the wave form; (b) half-wave rectification (which may be considered the extreme of a; and (c) bilateral peak clipping. These three distorted wave forms are no longer sinusoidal. When properly analyzed, they reveal themselves as complex waves. (The square wave of Figure 2.6 may serve as an example in this respect.) Thus amplitude distortion introduces new frequencies which had not been part of the original signal. Since these new frequencies are always harmonically related to the original frequency, this form of distortion is often referred to as *harmonic distortion*.

There is another way of looking upon harmonic distortion. Figure 2.14 illustrated the alteration of wave forms. Figure 2.15 gives what is known as the input-output function, showing the output of a sound-transmitting system, produced for any given input level. Note that both ordinates of Figure 2.15 are given in logarithmic values. Consequently, the 1:1 slope (45° angle) at the beginning of the curve (i.e., at low input values) means that for each increment of input there is a proportional increment of the output. (The output level, of course, may be higher (amplified) or lower (attenuated) than the input level. In these two cases, the curves run above (amplification) or below (attenuation) the 1:1 slope, but in either case are parallel to it.) In other words, the relationship between input and output is linear. From a certain point onward (x' in Fig. 2.15), output values cease to grow in proportion to the input, until finally (approximately at x'' in Fig. 2.15) a point is reached where further increments in input amplitude fail to produce any increment in output. The relationship has become non-linear. For this reason, amplitude distortion is also referred to as *non-linear distortion*.

Specifically, what has become non-linear in such a case is the relation-

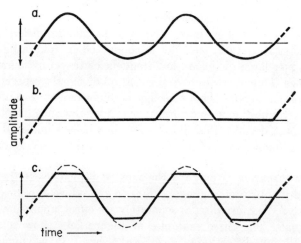

FIG. 2.14. Some common forms of amplitude distortion of a sinusoidal wave form: *a*, asymmetry; *b*, half-wave rectification; and *c*, bilateral peak clipping.

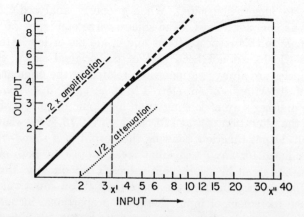

FIG. 2.15. Input-output function of a system limited to an output of 10 arbitrary units. Note that both ordinates are plotted in a log fashion. Short sections of curves for 2✕ amplification and ½ attenuation are also shown.

ship between the elastic force and the displacement. The limiting output value in Figure 2.14 represents the elastic limit of the system under consideration. The deviation from linearity at any given point of the input-output curve is a measure of the magnitude of distortion, i.e., the production of harmonics altering the wave form in the sense of Figure 2.14.

All mechanical systems possess an elastic limit. Hence they must eventually distort if driven high enough. If distortion is to be avoided (for instance in high-quality sound reproduction) the system must be operated within its linear range; i.e., input signals must never exceed the value marked x' in the example of Figure 2.15. Sound-reproducing systems also possess a lower limit which is given by their inherent noise. Signals which are lower than the noise level cannot be detected. The range between the (lower) limit of detection and the (upper) limit of linearity is known as the *dynamic range* of a given system.

When a composite signal consisting of at least two frequencies (not necessarily in harmonic relation) is transmitted through a system, giving rise to non-linear distortion, another set of new frequencies is generated. Suppose that the complex consists of frequencies f_1 and f_2. The new frequencies are known as combination tones: the so-called difference $(f_1 - f_2)$ and summation $(f_1 + f_2)$ tones. Between these first-order combination tones, the primary frequencies, and/or among themselves, second-, third-etc.-order summation and difference tones may be formed so that the end result is quite a complex of inharmonically related partials. This form is usually referred to as *intermodulation distortion*.

Although the ear is by no means free of all three types of distortion, hearing is quite sensitive to *extraneous distortion*, especially with respect to the reproduction of music in sound-reproducing systems. Considerable progress has been made within the past two decades in the development of distortion-free (so-called high fidelity) sound-reproducing equipment. The limitations of a given sound-transmitting or -receiving system can, therefore, be described in terms of its frequency and amplitude distortion. (Phase distortion follows necessarily from the former.) A measure of the frequency distortion is the frequency response curve of the system under consideration (cf. Fig. 2.13).

A useful measure of amplitude distortion (or the relative freedom thereof) is either the degree of harmonic distortion of single sinusoidal frequencies or the degree of intermodulation distortion between two specified frequencies. The information must include the output level at which the distortion was measured.

MEASUREMENT OF SOUND

Sound intensity was defined earlier as *energy density* or as the amount of energy flow per unit time through a unit area perpendicular to the direction of energy flow. Its unit measure is the watt per square centimeter. However, microphones, the common receivers of sound, do not measure sound intensity directly. Most microphones are sensitive to *sound pressure*. Sound pressure represents the excess of or deficit in pressure (in reference to the existing atmospheric pressure) produced during compression and rarefaction in a longitudinal-wave event. Since pressure is defined as force per area, sound pressure is given in dynes per square centimeter or in microbars. (One microbar equals 1 dyne per cm.^{2}) Sound pressure is linearly related to both the amplitude and the frequency of a given sinusoidal event. Sound intensity is proportional to the square of sound pressure.

For practical purposes, sound intensity and sound pressure data are frequently expressed in terms of decibels (dB). The decibel ($\frac{1}{10}$ of a Bel) was named in honor of Alexander Graham Bell. It expresses the logarithm of the ratio between two sound intensities, powers, or sound pressures; and it is also used for the expression of equivalent electrical measures such as power or voltage ratios. Since the ratio of two intensities, e.g., x' watts/cm.^{2} $\div$ x'' watts/cm.^{2} $= x'/x''$, is without a dimension, the decibel is a *dimensionless entity*, simply a number. Hence the symbol N_{dB} (number of decibels) is used.

$$N_{dB} = 10 \log \frac{I'}{I''}$$

$$\therefore 10 \log \frac{P'}{P''}$$

$$\therefore 20 \log \frac{p'}{p''}$$

where intensities (I) are given in watts per square centimeter, powers (P) in watts, and sound pressures (p) in dynes per square centimeter. The constant, 20, in the case of sound pressure ratios stems from the fact that intensity is proportional to the square of sound pressure. (An exponent behind a log sign is known to become a multiplier in front of it, e.g., $\log p^2 = 2 \log p$.)

The dB unit has several advantages. First of all, in many instances one is only interested in relative measures, i.e., how much higher or lower a certain measure is than another, so that the assessment of a ratio suffices. The attenuation of sound through the walls of a room, for example, is independent of the sound pressure outside the room; that is to say there is always a certain fraction of the sound energy which penetrates the wall whether the outside level is high or low. The use of logarithmic ratios also facilitates calculations. For example, when given in dB values

incident sound − transmitted sound = attenuated sound

Likewise given in dB values, the total attenuation (A) afforded by several walls (a', a'', a''', ...) is

$$A = a' + a'' + a''' \cdots$$

Furthermore, when one takes measurements at very different levels, instruments of different sensitivity must be employed. It is therefore virtually impossible to carry all of them through to the same decimal point. However, when the results are expressed as ratios, this is not really necessary. For example, the result of

$$\log \frac{9561.62}{9.56} = \log 1000.17 = 3.00007$$

is not significantly altered when one limits his measurements to the first three digits in both measurements:

$$\log \frac{9560}{9.56} = \log 1000 = 3.00$$

In the latter example, both measurements have been carried out with the same percentage accuracy, a task which in practice is relatively easy to realize. (In the present example, the accuracy happens to be to the 1% level).

If the ratio is larger than 1 (i.e., the first measurement results in a larger value than the second), the dB ratio is positive. For example,

$$10 \log \frac{10}{1} = (+)10 \text{ dB}$$

Conversely, when the ratio is smaller than 1, the resulting dB ratio is negative; e.g.,

$$10 \log \frac{1}{10} = -10 \text{ dB}$$

Attenuation is conveniently expressed in negative dB numbers, whereas amplification is given in positive numbers.

Some dB ratios which are frequently incurred are given in Table 2.3. This table serves also to indicate the difference between pressure ratios on the one hand and intensity and power ratios on the other. For example, the doubling of sound pressure produces an increment of 6 dB, whereas the doubling of intensity (or power) produces only an increment of 3 dB. More complete tables are available in many references and text books.

Under some circumstances, the results of measurements cannot be expressed in relative values. Suppose, for instance, that one wants to assess noise levels in various locations. It is not very meaningful when one finds that the noise level in location A is 20 dB higher than that in location

TABLE 2.3

Pressure	Intensity (Power) Ratio	dB
1.0	1.0	0
1.122	1.259	1
1.413	1.995	3
1.995	3.981	6
3.162	10.000	10
10.000	100.00	20
31.62	1,000.00	30
100.00	10,000.00	40
316.2	100,000.00	50
1,000.00	1,000,000.00	60

B when there is no information as to whether B is a very quiet or a noisy location. Moreover, when the level in location C is to be measured later on, location B may not be available for comparison anymore. Therefore, there is a need for a standard reference level to which all such measurements can be referred. For such a purpose, it is only necessary to assign a fixed value to the denominators in the above dB equations. For instance, one may determine all measurements of sound pressure levels in reference to 1 dyne per cm.^{2}, the centimeter-gram-second unit of sound pressure. (The term "level" is used whenever measurements are referred to an accepted standard. The abbreviation SPL stands for "sound pressure level.") The reference level of 1 dyne per cm.^{2} has in fact been used in the past. However, this level is already higher than that of conversational speech with the speaker and listener a few feet apart; and conversations are carried out at levels which are considerably higher than the threshold of hearing. Therefore, when it became possible with the advent of electronic amplification to extend the range of microphones to lower pressure levels, a revision of the reference level was indicated. It was then set by international agreement to 0.0002 dyne per cm.^{2}, a value which is reasonably close to the threshold of hearing at 1000 c/s for young, healthy adults. The corresponding reference value in terms of sound intensity is 10^{-16} watts per cm.^{2} ($= 10^{-10}$ micro-watts per cm.^{2}). The smallness of both sound pressure and sound intensity values serves once more to indicate the keen sensitivity of the sense of hearing.

Sound pressure levels are usually written as $\times$ dB SPL *re* 0.0002 dyne per cm.^{2}, or $\times$ dB *re* standard reference level.

The assignment of fixed values to the denominators of the dB equations facilitates the establishment of dB scales. For instance, there is a scale of sound pressure levels (in dB) which is illustrated by the examples of Table 2.4. Note that, because of the attenuation of sound with distance, SPL

TABLE 2.4
Some common examples of sound pressure levels

Near Source	dB	Environmental
Jet airplane during take-off (80 ft. from tail)	130	
		Boiler maker's shop
	120	
		Engine room of submarine (full speed)
Automatic punch press (3 ft.)	110	
		Inside DC-6 airliner
Annealing furnace (4 ft.)	100	
		Inside subway car
Heavy trucks (20 ft.)	90	Inside motor bus
	80	
Automobile (20 ft.)		Office with tabulating machines
	70	
Conventional speech (3 ft.)	60	
	50	Private business office
	40	
		Residential area at night
	30	
Whisper (5 ft.)	20	Motion-picture sound studio
	10	
Threshold of hearing 1000 c/s (young adults	0	

readings in free fields must always include the distance from the sound source at which the measurements have been taken.

If a scale transformation is desired, i.e., another reference level chosen, the conversion of one scale to the other is simply a matter of addition or subtraction of the dB ratio between the two reference values. For instance, the conversion factor from the old reference of 1 dyne per cm.^{2} to the new one of 0.0002 dyne per cm.^{2} is $+$ 74 dB, corresponding to a pressure ratio of 5000.

It should be clear to the reader that there is an important difference between a sound pressure scale in dynes per square centimeter and one in decibels. This is illustrated by the following table.

Scale 1 — 0 1 2 3 4 5 6 7 ⋯

Scale 2 — 0.1 1 10 100 1000 10000 ⋯

Scale 3 — −1 0 1 2 3 4 ⋯

The first is a *linear* scale (e.g., dyne/cm.²), and it is noted that there are constant *intervals* between each pair of successive members (one in scale 1). The second is a *geometric* scale where there are constant *ratios* between each two successive members (10 in scale 2). This difference must be kept in mind, although when a geometrical scale is expressed *logarithmically* (scale 3), the difference is no longer readily apparent. (The dB scale is of course of the same type as scale 3). Note the different significance of the zero value in scales 1 and 3. In the former, it implies an absolute limit, a "nothing." In the latter, it only stands for the reference value, whatever that happens to be. Ratio scales can be easily, and meaningfully, expanded into the domain of fractional values by means of negative logarithms.

It is in the nature of ratio scales that intervals get progressively larger with increasing values. Therefore, such scales may be said to emphasize intervals between small values and de-emphasize the intervals between large values. Note that an SPL of 20 dB stands for an increment of 0.0018 dyne per cm.², whereas the same ratio of 20 dB between 40 and 60 dB SPL stands for an increment of 0.18 dyne per cm.² This property of the dB scale turns out to be an added advantage. The human ear is more sensitive to sound pressure increments at low levels than at high levels, although it must be emphasized here that one decibel is not the smallest increment in sound pressure that the human ear can discriminate, as is still erroneously stated in some textbooks. Near threshold, the *difference limen* is equal to several dB (depending somewhat on frequency), whereas at higher levels it approaches a fraction of 1 dB.

SUGGESTED ADDITIONAL READINGS

1. American Standards Association Standards for Audiometers: (1) for general diagnostic purposes—Z24.5 (1951); (2) (pure tone) for screening purposes—Z24.12 (1952); (3) for speech audiometers—Z24.13 (1953). (Note: These specifications are currently being revised. The revised version, which is not expected to be in print for at least another year, will combine all three of the above separate standards.)
*2. Beranek, L. L.: *Acoustics*. McGraw-Hill Book Company, Inc., New York, 1954.
3. Van Bergeijk, W. A., Pierce, J. R., and David, E. E., Jr.: *Waves and the Ear*. Science Study Series, Anchor Books, Doubleday & Company, Inc., Garden City, N. Y., 1960.
*4. Colby, M. Y.: *Sound Waves and Acoustics*. Henry Holt & Company, Inc., New York, 1938.

*These items contain mathematical treatments and should be reserved for advanced readers.

5. Culver, C. A.: *Musical Acoustics*. Blakiston Division, McGraw-Hill Book Company, Inc.), New York, 1949.
6. Davis, H., and Silverman, S. R.: *Hearing and Deafness*, pp. 29–60. Holt, Rhinehart, and Winston, Inc., New York, 1960.
7. Pierce, J. R., and David, E. E., Jr.: *Man's World of Sound*. Doubleday & Company, Inc., New York, 1959.
*8. Randall, R. H.: *Introduction to Acoustics*. Addison-Wesley Press, Inc., Cambridge, Mass., 1951.
9. Stevens, S. S., and Davis, H.: *Hearing*, pp. 1–41. John Wiley & Sons, Inc., New York, 1938.
10. Wever, E. G., and Lawrence, L.: *Physiological Acoustics*, pp. 16–34. Princeton University Press, Princeton, 1954.
*11. Wood, A. B.: *A Textbook of Sound*. Bell & Sons, Ltd., London 1955.

3

Psychoacoustics

W. Dixon Ward, Ph.D.

We have seen in the second chapter that sounds may be specified in terms of the intensity, frequency, and phase of the vibrations. In the case of a pure tone, then, three numbers will completely describe the sound. Ordinary real-life sounds may be broken down mathematically into several sine waves, each of which is also uniquely specified by its intensity, frequency, and phase. In this chapter we shall consider the relation between these physical characteristics of sounds and the behavior of the individual who is exposed to them.

THE ABSOLUTE THRESHOLD

The concept most basic to audiometry, and to sensory psychology in general, is the *threshold*. In a broad sense, the threshold is the smallest change in the physical environment that elicits a differential response from the individual. However, in audiometry the unqualified term "threshold" usually denotes the "absolute" auditory threshold: the intensity at which a sound can just be distinguished from silence.

This absolute threshold is often thought of as a sharp line dividing the audible from the inaudible: if a sound is above a listener's threshold, he will respond; if it is below, he will not. As is often the case with simple views, this is too simple to be completely accurate. Whether or not a person responds to a particular sound depends not only on the intensity of the sound but also on many of the other conditions prevailing at the moment the sound is presented. Let us consider some of the variables that will affect the response even when we restrict the stimuli to pure tones generated by an audiometer, delivered to the ear of a listener by means of an earphone, in a completely quiet listening room.

48

The Stimulus

A major source of variability in threshold, if adequate control is not maintained, is the stimulus itself: the purity and duration of the tone. Tones lasting less than 200 msec. (⅕ sec.) have less chance of being heard than those lasting longer; the shorter the tone, the less likely its detection (1). A spuriously sensitive threshold response may be obtained if the tone is impure (contains more than one frequency), since the listener may be responding to some component other than the one the tester intends. Also, there should not be an audible click when the tone is turned on or off.

Frequency

The intensity required at the threshold of hearing is a minimum at frequencies from about 1000 to 4000 cycles per second (c/s), gradually increasing at higher and lower frequencies. Frequencies much above 20,000 c/s cannot be heard by man at any intensity, although some other animals can hear up to at least 80,000 c/s.

Method

The accepted clinical method for determining threshold will be described more fully in Chapter 5. However, a brief description is necessary here in order to emphasize that alternative methods may produce different results.

The approved clinical procedure employs the *method of limits* (combined method). The listener is first given a tone at a moderately high intensity. The intensity of succeeding tones is progressively lowered until the listener fails to respond. Then, beginning somewhere below this point, the intensity is raised by steps until the listener again responds, then once more lowered until there is no response, etc. Tones near threshold have a higher probability of being heard when the series is descending in intensity than when it is ascending. This dependence of response on the direction of the series, although a complicating factor in the clinical method, is not without its advantages, since it is the basis for the so-called Békésy method of determining threshold (2). In this technique (*modified method of limits*), the intensity is constantly either increased or decreased by an attenuator driven by a reversible motor that is controlled by the listener. He causes the intensity to decrease until the tone disappears, then to increase until he can hear it again, and so on. The changes in intensity thus produced are automatically recorded.

Another method, one used widely in the laboratory (and even in the clinic when you test your own hearing) is the *method of adjustment*. The listener adjusts the intensity of the tone so that he can "just barely hear it." This adjustment may be made directly, by means of a knob, or indirectly, using a motor. (If the apparatus for the Békésy method, above, had provisions for allowing the listener to stop the motor, this same apparatus could be used for the method of adjustment.)

A common variation of the standard clinical method (in which, it will be remembered, the listener simply indicates whether or not he heard *anything*) is one in which the listener is required to report more information about the signal. This is usually done by presenting zero, one, two, or three tone pulses in a given time period, and then asking the listener to write down the number of pulses heard. This is a method often used in group testing (3).

Each of these methods may give different values of threshold, even when all other conditions are held as nearly alike as possible.

Changes in Tester

For methods in which the responses of the listener are recorded mechanically, and threshold is calculated from these records, the behavior of the tester, once testing has begun, is relatively unimportant. However, if the clinical method is used, a certain amount of variability can be attributed to fluctuations in the *tester's* criterion for threshold: that is, the type and consistency of response he demands from the listener. Sometimes he may cross the listener's threshold three times, sometimes six. He may at one time regard a single positive response as sufficient to establish that a given intensity can be heard; at another time he may require three out of four. His expectations of what the threshold at a given frequency will turn out to be, based on what he has found at some other frequency, may also unconsciously influence his judgment. It has been shown that if the tester cannot see the audiometer dial, there will be fewer readings of "zero" recorded than when he can (4).

The Listener

Even if all the aforementioned conditions are held constant, a listener will sometimes respond to a given tone, sometimes not. These random fluctuations will determine the lower limit in variability of threshold that one can expect. Such things as breathing noises, heartbeats, attention, alertness, etc., are presumably responsible for this inherent variability.

In addition to this random variability, a systematic change in the probability of response as the testing progresses can sometimes be observed. This "learning" effect generally consists of a gradual improvement in sensitivity and, for some unknown reason, is greater at low than at high frequencies (5).

Changes in response can also be induced by changing the instructions to the listener. For example, the listener will more often report a tone if the instructions encourage reporting a tone when in doubt (i.e., when the listener has a "loose" criterion for tone) than when he is told to vote only when he is sure (a "strict" criterion) (6).

Session-to-Session Variability

So far the discussion has been limited to the uncertainty associated with thresholds on a given listener, made by a single tester, using a specific audiometer, at a single testing session. Relaxing any of these conditions, of course, increases the variability even more. Even when successive sessions follow each other within a matter of minutes, the variability between sessions will be greater than that within a single session provided that the phones are removed and replaced each time, because they will not be put back in exactly the same position on the ears (7). With days or weeks between successive tests, even such factors as the length of the listener's hair may provide additional variability by influencing the phone placement.

Audiometer Differences

If the sound intensity present at a listener's eardrum were actually measured at the time when the threshold was determined, the placement of the earphone would be irrelevant. However, routine measurements of this kind are completely impracticable. Instead, the audiometer is calibrated by measuring, and adjusting to a standard (this standard is discussed in the next section), the intensity developed by the earphone when coupled to a standard microphone by a 6-cc. coupler, a device whose volume is about that of an average ear canal. No account is taken of differences in headband tension and hardness of the earphone cushions, both of which, like phone placement, will affect the level actually produced at the eardrum. Different brands of audiometers may employ different types of earphones, and the difference between the intensity produced in the coupler and at the eardrum may not be the same for different phones. To top it all off, there are even two different types of 6-cc. coupler: one used by the National Bureau of Standards (NBS), the other favored by the Acoustical Society of America (ASA) (8). (In Europe, the accepted couplers have a volume of less than 6 cc.) All different couplers give different results at the higher frequencies, particularly at 6000 c/s and above (9).

An absolute threshold, then, is a function of many variables. It is, in any but a trivial sense, a broad, hazy area rather than a distinct point or line. The recorded threshold of a particular person depends on the earphone, the cushion, the headband, the duration and shape of the tone, the instructions to the listener, all aspects of the method of determining threshold, and the criteria adopted by the listener and by the tester.

Of course, many of these factors have such a slight effect that if one's concern is with a single patient, they require only perfunctory attention. After all, a 5- or 10-dB error in threshold would seldom alter a diagnosis. On the other hand, if one is ever to compare the hearing of two *groups* of people, or is trying to assess a *change* in a given individual's hearing, it is clearly necessary either (1) to make sure that all these conditions are identical during both tests, or (2) to determine the correction factor or factors to be applied to one set of data. (If possible, one should choose the first alternative, since this eliminates the chance of human error in applying correction factors in the wrong direction.)

HEARING LEVEL (HL)

In view of all this uncertainty, it is hardly surprising that when different investigators try to define "normal hearing" there is little chance that they will agree. In addition to the complicating factors just discussed, there is another difficulty inherent in the concept of "normality" itself: there are at least two ways of interpreting the word. One view regards "normal" as implying "adequate" or "non-pathological"; the other takes it to mean "typical" or "average." There would probably be much less confusion in this field if the word "normal" had never been applied to the set of somewhat arbitrary intensities corresponding to the zero settings of an audiometer dial. Perhaps we might have avoided the chaos that will prevail in the next few years, after the reference level is officially changed from the old to the new.

The present reference levels are based on average results of the 1935 United States Public Health Service surveys (10). For many reasons (e.g., the fact that the earphone was held to the ear by hand), these levels are definitely higher than those obtained later in more careful field studies of young people who were rigidly pre-selected in terms of socially adequate hearing (11, 12). Therefore, there has been much agitation to lower the reference levels for audiometers about 10 dB.

Line *A* in Figure 3.1 shows the present reference levels, give in terms of the sound pressure levels (SPL) (dB above 0.0002 dyne per cm.^{2}) generated in a 6-cc. coupler by a PDR-8 earphone in an MX-41/AR earmuff, as a function of frequency. Line *B* is the proposed new reference level. Since both *A* and *B* indicate levels generated in a coupler, they apply to earphone listening. Line *C* is yet another reference level; in this case, the curve is for "free-field" listening. This line represents measurements of average minimum audible levels made at the approximate position of the listener's uncovered ear in a situation where there are no echoes (13). No-

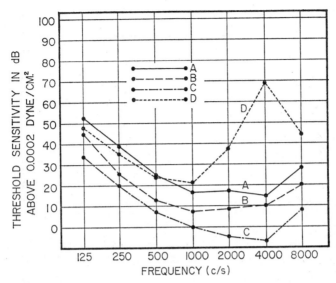

FIG. 3.1. Threshold sound pressure level as a function of frequency. Curves A and B are norms for earphone listening. Curve C applies to free-field measurements. Curve D is a typical example of the sensitivity of a particular ear of an industrial worker. (See text for details.)

tice that the curve passes through the 0-dB SPL line (i.e., 0.0002 dyne per cm.²) at 1000 c/s.

In order to avoid confusion among these reference levels, the best course would be to refer explicitly to the one being used, and to employ the phrase "normal hearing" only in a very broad sense, to indicate that the thresholds lie within some range of levels, as, for example, within 15 dB of the reference level concerned. This usage will be followed in the remainder of this chapter.

In Figure 3.1, since intensity increases in an *upward* direction, hearing that is less sensitive than the standard would be represented by a line lying above the reference. Line D shows the hearing one might measure in a person who has just come from an environment of high noise. However, it has become customary to plot audiograms as in Figure 3.2. Here the zero line, instead of being a fixed physical value, is the "standard hearing" curve of Figure 3.1, line A (straightened out, of course), and a *downward* deflection of the record indicates a higher threshold (lowered sensitivity, "worse" hearing). The ordinate here is "hearing level," abbreviated HL, which stands for "the number of dB less sensitive than standard hearing at the particular frequency concerned." Commercial audiometers are calibrated to read HL directly. Although the readings of the audiometer dial were formerly called "hearing loss" values, it is felt

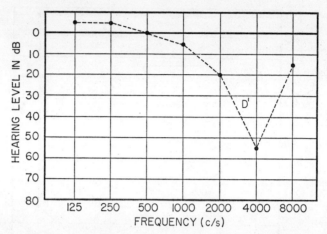

FIG. 3.2. Audiometric data presented in accepted clinical fashion. The zero line in this figure corresponds to line A in Fig. 3.1. The line marked D' represents the same sample audiogram (D) shown in Fig. 3.1.

that the term "loss" here somewhat overstates the case, so that "hearing level," a more neutral term, is now encouraged (14). The line D in Figure 3.2 is the sample threshold curve (D) of Figure 3.1 replotted in terms of HL. If the new proposed reference level (B in Fig. 3.1) had been used, this audiogram would have been about 10 dB lower on the chart, since hearing levels will all increase by nearly this amount if and when the change in reference is made.

ATTRIBUTES OF SOUND

Once it exceeds the absolute threshold, the characteristics of a sound may be described not only in terms of the intensity, frequency, and phase of its components, but also by its subjective effect on a listener: its perceived pitch, loudness, and timbre. This section will deal with the relation between these physical and psychological characteristics.

Let us first briefly define the main subjective attributes. The *loudness* of a tone is primarily, but not completely, determined by its intensity. *Pitch*, in a corresponding manner, is primarily a function of the frequency of the tone. A sound with high frequency (more rapid vibrations) is said to have a high pitch, and one with a low frequency (slower vibrations) a low pitch. Although some scholars have contended that it is "natural" that rapid vibrations be called "high" (advancing, for example, the argument that rapid frequencies come from on high, as the songs of birds and mosquitoes, as contrasted with low-frequency rumble of hooves on the ground), it seems just as likely that the choice was accidental and arbitrary. Finally, the *timbre* of a sound is largely dependent on its complexity, that is, on the particular sine waves into which it can be analyzed. Timbre is something of a "wastebasket" attribute: if two tones are judged to be "different," and yet have the same pitch and the same loudness, then they must differ in timbre. Other attributes, such as *volume* (15) and *density* (16), have been considered; however, these do not as yet have much relevance to audiometry. It is worth mentioning, though, that volume is not the same as loudness. The "volume control" on a radio is primarily a loudness control, although the "voluminousness" of sound, as well as its loudness, does increase with intensity.

Loudness

Loudness has received by far the lion's share of the attention devoted to tonal attributes. As a result, the scales of *loudness*, in *sones*, and *loudness level*, in *phons*, are firmly established as useful concepts. A third related concept, *sensation level*, should also be considered here in order to keep them all from becoming confused. Let us consider them in reverse order.

Sensation Level (SL) is the simplest of the three: the sensation level of a sound is the number of dB by which the intensity level of the sound exceeds the absolute threshold *of a particular ear* for that sound. It cannot be emphasized too strongly that SL is inextricably tied to the threshold of a single listener. A tone having a sound pressure level of 50 dB (i.e., 50 dB above 0.0002 dyne per cm.^{2}) will have an SL of 30 dB for a person whose threshold in the ear concerned for that tone is 20 dB SPL, but an SL of only 10 dB for an ear whose threshold is 40 dB SPL.

The Loudness Level of a Sound, in Phons, is numerically equal to the SPL of a 1000-c/s pure tone whose loudness is judged equal to that of the sound in question. So, in order to determine the loudness level of a given sound, one sets up a situation in which the observer can adjust the intensity of a 1000-c/s tone until he is satisfied that it is just as loud as the sound in question, when the two are heard alternately. For example, consider a noise having an intensity of 90 dB SPL. If the noise is judged equal in loudness to a 1000-c/s tone with an SPL of 84 dB, then the loudness level of the noise is 84 phons.

Loudness, in Sones, is more complicated. This scale is based not only on judgments of "equal" by listeners, but also on judgments of ratios and of equal appearing intervals. For example, the listeners may be asked to adjust a variable tone to sound just "twice as loud" as a fixed one. If the fixed tone has a loudness of N sones, then the loudness of the adjusted tone will be $2N$. Thus only a single arbitrary point need be fixed to define the loudness scale. The point originally adopted by the Standards Committee of the Acoustical Society of America was a 1000-c/s tone at a sensation level of 40 dB: this tone was defined as having a loudness of 1 sone

(17). The use of some value of sensation level instead of sound pressure level for the reference point avoided the paradox of assigning a loudness of 1 sone to an inaudible sound (as would be the case for a person whose threshold was 45 dB SPL, if the reference point were 40 dB SPL). The choice of 40 dB seems to be completely arbitrary; any other value of SL would serve equally well. Even 0 dB SL (i.e., a tone just at threshold) could conceivably serve as the arbitrary reference point. Just as all sounds below threshold must have zero loudness, so must any audible sound have a loudness that is finite, even though small. However, the difficulty of making judgments of comparative loudness using a 0-dB SL standard are obvious.

The usefulness of a scale that is unique to a single listener is, of course, severely limited. Therefore, it has recently been suggested that for practical applications, such as predicting the total loudness of a complex noise, the sone be defined as the loudness experienced by a "typical listener" when listening binaurally to a tone of 1000 c/s at 40 dB SPL (18). This defines a sort of average loudness function for listeners whose thresholds at all frequencies are all reasonably close to (within 10 or 15 dB of) the new reference threshold function mentioned in the preceding section (curve B in Fig. 3.1). Notice that the two definitions of the sone will agree if the listener's threshold at 1000 c/s happens to be 0.0002 dyne per cm.^{2}.

Equal-Loudness Contours. A set of equal loudness contours for pure tones derived from judgments made by a "typical listener" in a free field situation are given in Figure 3.3 (19). All points on a given contour have the indicated loudness level in phons (first number) and loudness in sones (in parentheses). In general, it can be seen that low frequencies are not as loud as high frequencies. Notice that at the extreme low frequencies, the curves are not 10 dB apart even though they are each separated by 10 phons. This implies that loudness grows more rapidly with intensity at these frequencies than at intermediate frequencies. Thus, at higher loudness levels, the curves are more nearly level.

You will notice that the loudnesses in sones of adjacent contours (separated by 10 phons) have a ratio of about 2:1 except at the lowest levels (20). This means that in the mid-frequencies, a sound 10 dB more intense than another will sound twice as loud, one 20 dB more intense will appear 4 times as loud, one 30 dB higher will appear 8 times as loud, etc. This simple average relation seems to hold for noises as well as pure tones (21).

Confusion of Levels. In view of the chaos that occurs all too often when intensity level, sound pressure level, sensation level, loudness level, and hearing level are confused, it seems worthwhile to distinguish them here once more, in hope that this may reduce the number of articles that state, for example, "The patients were exposed to a 3000-cycle tone at

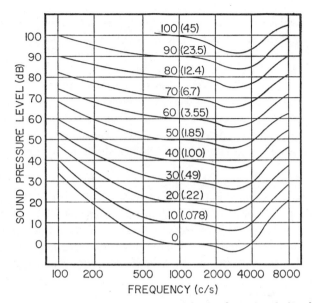

FIG. 3.3. Typical equal-loudness contours. The loudness level, in phons, of all points on a particular contour is given by the first parametric number. The corresponding loudness, in sones, is given in parentheses. The loudness of the lowest curve, which is supposed to represent threshold, has been deliberately omitted, since the loudness of threshold tones has not yet been determined satisfactorily.

80 dB for 3 minutes." All this sentence tells us about the intensity of the tone is that it probably sounded fairly loud to the average person.

"Intensity level" and "sound pressure level" are the only two of the preceding list that are in no way dependent on a listener. They simply indicate the relation, in dB, between the intensity of the sound in question and some reference intensity: *any* chosen reference in the case of intensity level, 0.0002 dyne per cm.² in the case of sound pressure level. When using intensity level, therefore, the reference point must be specified, but if the reference pressure is 0.0002 dyne per cm.² (0.0002 microbar), then by merely stating "x dB SPL" the reader will know that "x dB above 0.0002 dyne per cm.² " is meant.

Hearing Level, the dial reading on an audiometer, is only one step removed from the purely physical. The main difference is that here the reference pressure changes with frequency. Instead of being 0.0002 dyne per cm.², the reference pressure is several dB higher, the exact value depending on frequency as shown in Figure 3.1. Since these values are standardized, one need not state the particular reference level involved. For example, "x dB HL at 1000 c/s" means "x + 15 dB SPL," since the reference threshold for the particular earphone-and-muff combination commonly used in audiometers at 1000 c/s is 15 dB SPL. After the impending change in standards for audiometer calibration, however, it will be necessary to indicate whether the old or new calibration is being used.

Sensation Level (SL) is nearly like HL except that, instead of an arbitrary set of reference levels, the threshold of a particular ear is used. So "*x* dB SL" means *x* dB above each individual listener's threshold for the sound concerned. It should not be used to mean "*x* dB above the average threshold of a group of listeners": unless these listeners happen to have identical thresholds, a given tone will have a different SL for each member of the group.

Loudness Level is another function that, strictly speaking, should always be related to a single observer's judgment. Saying that a sound has a loudness level of *x* phons implies that the *particular* observer concerned would say that the sound appeared just as loud as a 1000 c/s tone at *x* dB SPL. However, there is enough agreement among normal-hearing people that for such observers the average contours represented in Figure 3.3 may safely be assumed to hold.

Pitch

As in the case of loudness, it is essential to keep distinct the several terms pertaining to pitch. The *frequency* of a pure tone, measured in cycles per second, is of course not dependent on any responses of a listener, nor is its *frequency level*. Frequency level, in octaves, is analogous to SPL, being simply the logarithm to the base 2 (instead of base 10 as in the case of the decibel) of the ratio of a given frequency to a standard frequency of 16.352 c/s (22). (The particular value of 16.352 was chosen for musical reasons.) Frequency level is a term that is seldom used in audiometry, since it is frequency that usually is measured, and conversion to frequency level would take too much time for the slight advantages involved.

Pitch Level is a term that corresponds to loudness level. This term is needed because pitch does vary slightly with intensity, and because some complex sounds may have a pitch that is completely different from any of the components of which they are constituted. The pitch level of a sound is numerically equal to the frequency of a 40-phon pure tone whose pitch is judged equal to that of the sound in question (23). No one has yet named the units in which pitch level should be expressed, and so the usual practice is just to leave it as c/s. Thus, a sound judged equal in pitch to a pure tone with a loudness level of 40 phons and a frequency of 2600 c/s is said to have a pitch level of 2600 c/s.

A scale of pitch corresponding to the sone scale of loudness has been developed using the same type of judgment: by setting the frequency so that the pitch sounds half (or twice, or some other ratio) as high. This scale of pitch has as its unit the *mel* (24); 1000 mels is the pitch of a pure tone of 40 dB SPL and 1000 c/s. (This does not imply that a pure tone of 40 dB SPL and 2000 c/s will have a pitch of 2000 mels; rather, this 2000-c/s tone would, for the typical listener, have a pitch of about 1900 mels.)

The pitch difference between two sounds may thus be expressed in mels. However, a difference may also be expressed in terms of the subjective musical scale possessed by everyone who can whistle or sing a tune without accompaniment. For example, the difference in pitch between two sounds whose pitch levels are 1000 and 1500 c/s can be expressed either as 410 mels or as about 7 semitones. Let us underscore the fact that these musical-pitch intervals are not completely dependent on the frequencies involved. The fact that two frequencies stand in a ratio of 2:1 (i.e., a physical octave) does not necessarily mean that the musical-pitch difference will be an octave: instead, even many normal observers will say that the pitch difference between, for example, tones whose frequencies are 2000 and 4000 c/s is only 11 semitones rather than 12 (23).

Equal-Pitch Contours. Equal-pitch contours for pure tones can be derived in the same fashion as equal-loudness contours. The frequency of one tone is adjusted until the pitch sounds the same as that of a second tone having a different intensity. In normal-hearing persons, these pitch changes associated with intensity differences are not very large. The difference in pitch between a tone just above threshold and one of the same frequency at 90 dB SPL is usually less than a semitone: that is, less than 6 % change in frequency is required to make the two tones sound equal in pitch, even at the extreme high and low frequencies (25). In the middle ranges, the pitch difference is even smaller. The direction of these slight pitch changes depends on frequency: as the intensity is raised, the pitch of low tones (below 1000 c/s) becomes lower while that of high tones (above 4000 c/s) becomes higher.

DIFFERENCE LIMENS (DL)

One measure of the relative efficiency of an observer's auditory system is his ability to distinguish (1) slight differences of frequency, intensity, or complexity between two separate signals, or (2) small changes in a single stimulus. The smallest difference or change detectable is called the *differential threshold*, or *difference limen* (DL). Difference limens provide an index of an individual's auditory *acuity*, in contrast to the absolute threshold, which is a measure of *sensitivity*. As in the case of the absolute threshold, the DL depends on the method used to measure it. Slight changes in a continuous tone are more easily perceived than are small differences in two tones presented successively (26). The DL also varies with the time between the tones to be compared (27) or with the time taken to change the continuous tone (28). Further, the more information one requires from the listener, the higher the DL. Thus if he must simply judge whether the second of a pair of stimuli is higher or lower than the first, he will be correct more often than if he must indicate whether the third of three stimuli is more like the first or the second (29).

The method used most often in determining DL is the second one cited above; that is, detection of slight changes in a sustained stimulus. A continuous tone is caused to change smoothly between two intensities, or between two frequencies, at a regular rate. The listener may indicate, by tapping or waving a hand, the rhythm of the changes, or he may only be required to say that the fluctuations are audible. The former, of course, is the more objective procedure.

DISTORTION AND AURAL OVERLOAD

Every vibrating system has its limit of linearity. That is, the system will faithfully follow the motion of the driving force only within a certain range. If this range is exceeded, the system is said to be *overloaded* and the signal is *distorted*. The hearing mechanism has this limit. When the input signal is a pure tone (a sine wave), overload will produce an output wave that looks more square-topped; some part of the system reaches its limit so that even with additional increases in pressure, the part in question cannot move further.

Such a distorted wave can be analyzed into several components: one having the original frequency of the input signal, the others being harmonics (multiples in frequency). For example, a distorted 350-c/s tone may be analyzed into several different components having the frequencies 350, 700, 1050, 1400, etc. To a certain extent, these frequencies become separated in the analysis performed by the auditory system. However, few persons can actually "hear out" harmonics from such a sound, even when the harmonics are quite strong. So if we are interested in determining the intensity of a pure tone of 350 c/s that just produces distortion in the ear, we must use what is known as a "probe" tone. In addition to the 350-c/s tone, a weaker 702-c/s tone is introduced. This 702-c/s probe tone will produce beats with the 700-c/s second harmonic of the 350-c/s primary tone. These 2-per-second beats will be most noticeable when the intensity of the probe tone is nearly the same as the "effective intensity" of the 700-c/s aural harmonic. By gradually lowering the intensities of both signals, one finds the lowest SPL of the primary tone that will give beats when the probe tone is much weaker than the primary. This SPL is the *aural overload point* for the ear in question at that frequency (30). It is emphasized that the probe must be considerably weaker (20 dB or more) than the primary, since if it is only about 10 dB weaker, beats are produced that are not caused by aural overload (31). As a matter of fact, accurate determination of the aural overload point demands precise attention to so many details by the audiometrist, and such concentration on the part of the patient, that the test is seldom used routinely. The average normal listener will be able to hear beats with the probe tone when the primary is only about 60 dB SPL and the probe about 30 (32).

Just where in the auditory system the aural harmonics are produced is not clear. There is good evidence, though, that the middle ear does not introduce distortion until the SPL reaches 90 or 100 dB. Somewhere in the inner ear, then, is the process responsible for this distortion (33).

MASKING

If two sounds are introduced into the ear simultaneously, the threshold for one or both may be higher than when heard separately. The number of dB by which the threshold is raised is the amount of *masking*. Masking is greater, as one might expect, when the masking tone and the masked tone are closer together in frequency, or when the masking tone (or noise) is higher in intensity.

Masking of pure tones by pure tones is complicated by the fact that, even at fairly low intensities, distortion products may arise (combination tones and envelope detection caused by nonlinearity somewhere in the system). These will indicate the presence of the masked tone even though the latter cannot actually be heard by itself (34). Therefore most practical instances of masking (both desired and otherwise) involve masking of a pure tone or speech by noise.

At moderate intensities of noise, the masking produced is linearly related to the sound pressure level in the range of frequencies immediately surrounding the masked tone, the so-called "critical band" of frequencies (35). For example, the masking of a 1000-c/s tone depends on the noise energy from 920 to 1080 c/s. If a certain noise in this range produces 10 dB of masking for a given listener, then increasing the noise by 30 dB will also increase the masking by 30 dB, i.e., to 40 dB.

It is important to realize that the amount of masking produced by a noise depends not only on the noise level but also on the threshold (in quiet) of the particular observer for the sound to be masked. This is because in a specific noise level, it is impossible to hear a tone below a certain minimal SPL. If the listener's threshold in quiet is already higher than this minimal SPL, there will be no masking. If it is lower, he will show masking equal to the difference between his threshold and the minimal SPL mentioned.

This fact implies that *it is not possible to correct audiometric data for undesired masking produced by environmental noise.* For example, suppose that a particular noise makes it impossible to hear tones below 30 dB

SPL at 500 c/s. Since standard audiometric zero (Fig. 3.1) at 500 c/s is about 25 dB SPL, this means that the weakest tone that could be heard would be 5 dB HL. Hence, all persons whose normal thresholds are -20, -15, -10, -5, or 0 dB HL will, in the noise, show masked thresholds of 5 dB HL, while those whose normal thresholds are 5 dB HL or higher will not be affected. Clearly, subtracting 5 dB from all masked thresholds would not get us back to the correct unmasked threshold, either for the group or for many of the individuals. If the person's indicated threshold were 5 dB HL, his true threshold might be *any* value lower than this.

The preceding discussion has neglected several sources of variability. There *are* individual differences, though not large, in the ability to hear a masked signal, even when the observers have the same thresholds. In ordinary audiometry, also, the fit of the ear cushion will affect the amount of noise that gets into the ear, so that the minimal sound that can be heard will vary from person to person. Thus, even in the example cited above, there will be a few ears that show 0 and even -5 dB HL. However, the conclusion that audiograms *cannot* be corrected for masking still holds.

Figure 3.4 shows the lowest HLs than can be measured in the presence of given room noise levels as measured with an octave-band filter (36).

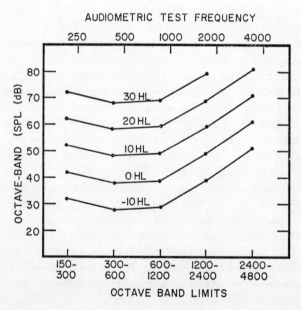

FIG. 3.4. Noise levels that must not be exceeded if hearing levels of the size indicated by the parameter are to be measured. The bottom abscissa indicates the frequency limits of the octave band of noise concerned; the top abscissa corresponds to the appropriate audiometric test frequency.

The average attenuation of room noise provided by standard (MX-41/AR) ear cushions has been taken into account in this graph. The abscissa shows frequency. Standard audiometric test frequencies are given along the top, and cutoff limits of the different octave bands are shown along the bottom of the graph. The ordinate shows the octave-band SPL that will just mask a pure tone at the HL indicated on each curve. Thus, for example, in a noise having 40 dB SPL in each octave band, the minimal measurable HLs will be about 0 dB for frequencies through 1000 c/s, −5 dB at 1500 c/s, and −10 dB at 2000 c/s. Masking at 3000 c/s and above will be negligible.

Masking is not always undesirable. Because of conduction around the head, a tone generated in one ear is only about 50 to 60 dB weaker in the other ear, even with the best seal of the earphone on the ear. So if one ear is more than 50 dB less sensitive than the other, a masking noise must be put into the more sensitive ear if a valid threshold measurement is to be obtained on the less sensitive ear. Some of the masking noises that have been used in this way are narrow bands of noise (a band with appropriate frequency characteristics for each test frequency), broad-band noise, and a buzz generated by distorting the 60-c/s line voltage. Narrow bands are the most efficient maskers for specific frequencies (that is, provide the most masking for the least energy), and the buzz is the least efficient (and the most annoying). The intensity of the masking noise should provide as much masking of the more sensitive ear as possible, but should not be so loud as to be uncomfortable or to produce a temporary threshold shift in the masked ear.

As the intensity of the masking noise is raised, even a narrow band of noise will begin to mask tones above it in frequency. This is ascribed to development, in the inner ear, of aural harmonics of the noise band. Eventually, at very high intensities of masking noise, it is found that even *lower* frequencies are masked (37). The cause of this phenomenon, termed "remote masking," seems to be principally distortion in the inner ear (38). However, recent research (39) has indicated that the auditory reflex may also be involved. The muscles of the middle ear contract in the presence of high-intensity sound, thereby affecting the transmission of low-frequency test tones not only in the ear to which the masking noise is presented but also in the contralateral ear. This effect constitutes another possible source of error in the use of masking of the better ear of an individual with a pronounced hearing loss in the other ear. If the masking noise has an over-all level of 90 dB SPL or more, some activation of the acoustic reflex will be produced. Therefore, unless the cause of the deficit in the poorer ear is such that the middle ear muscles have no effect (as, for example, in otosclerosis), a spuriously high hearing level may be measured.

Finally, there is also a phenomenon known as "central masking." Under certain conditions, a stimulus in one ear may raise the threshold of a tone in the other ear by up to 5 dB even though the level of the masking stimulus is so low that the change cannot be attributed to sound leaking around the head or to arousal of the acoustic reflex. This phenomenon is not clearly understood.

ATYPICAL HEARING PHENOMENA

Perstimulatory Fatigue

If a continuous tone is presented to a normal ear, its loudness decreases during the first few minutes of stimulation (40). This decrease is so gradual in the normal ear that one is generally not directly conscious of it, and so a special technique is needed to demonstrate the effect. Two tones are adjusted by the listener to give equal loudness: one tone, R, in the right ear; the other, L, in the left. Then one of the tones (say R) is turned off, and the other (L) is left on for several minutes. At the end of the time, R is again turned on. The listener will judge R to be much louder, and if instructed to set R to give the same loudness as L, will decrease the intensity level of R by as much as 30 dB. Turning off L for a few seconds nearly abolishes the effect.

In some ears the loudness of a tone initially well above threshold fades completely away after a few seconds or minutes. This condition seems to be generally associated with other abnormal auditory phenomena, although for the extremely high frequencies (above 12,000 c/s) even persons with relatively normal thresholds may show this effect. Although no one has named this effect, Albrecht was apparently the first to report it, according to Kobrak and associates (41).

No special apparatus is required to test for the Albrecht effect at the audiometric frequencies. After threshold has been determined in the usual way, the tone is presented either until the patient signals that it has disappeared, or until a set amount of time has elapsed. If he signals disappearance, the level is raised one step (5 dB) and the process is repeated, continuing until the tone is still heard at the end of the criterion time interval. Only recently has the Albrecht effect been studied in this country; in these first studies a criterion time of one minute has been used for "tone-decay" tests (42).

Temporary Threshold Shifts (TTS)

The decrease of sensitivity after exposure to acoustic stimulation has been called "auditory adaptation," "auditory fatigue," "acoustic trauma," and the more neutral "temporary threshold shift" (TTS). Except for the term acoustic trauma, which is commonly used to describe changes incurred by exposure to very high levels, the terms are usually used interchangeably, although a few investigators discriminate among them in order to indicate different types of exposure.

After-effects can be measured following any audible sound. However, after most sounds of everyday life, the effects are so slight and disappear so rapidly that they pose no problem for audiometry. On the other hand, industrial noise, gunfire, and severe blows to the head are sometimes able to produce TTS large enough to affect audiometric results.

In recent years much information has been amassed about TTS (43–45). The shift increases with exposure time in an exponential manner: that is, it grows swiftly at first, gradually becoming slower and slower. The recovery of TTS follows a similar course: fast recovery in the first few minutes after exposure, gradually slowing down. Measurable TTS enduring more than 2 min. after exposure can be observed only if the sound pressure level exceeds a certain minimal value. The TTS produced is directly proportional to the amount by which the noise exceeds the "base" SPL. For example, long exposure to a noise, at 85 dB SPL, having equal energy in each octave band (i.e., about 77 dB SPL in each octave band) will just barely avoid producing TTS. This means that 95 dB SPL (10 dB above the base SPL) will produce twice as much TTS as 90 dB SPL (5 dB above the base) and only half as much as 105 dB SPL, other things being equal.

The frequency range in which TTS occurs depends on the stimulus. In the case of broad-band noise (as in the example just preceding), the maximal TTS will be measured in the 3000- to 6000-c/s range. Pure tones and narrow bands of noise produce a maximal TTS at a frequency higher than that of the TTS-producing sound (from one half to one and one half octaves higher). The most "efficient" producer of TTS is thus a stimulus of about 3000 c/s.

If the exposures to noise are interrupted rather than continuous, the TTS is considerably smaller (46). That is, much more total energy can be tolerated if it is broken up into several exposures with interposed rest periods than if it is in a single continuous dose. An exposure of 30 min. to a continuous noise of 100 dB SPL will produce a TTS at 4000 c/s of about 20 dB in normal listeners. The same noise, if interrupted so that it is on for only half the time (1 min. on, 1 min. off) will produce only about 12 dB of TTS in an hour (i.e., the same total energy as ½ hr. of continuous exposure). To produce 20 dB of TTS with the interrupted noise requires 10 hours of exposure: that is, 10 times as much total energy.

If the TTS measured 2 min. after the noise ceases is less than about 40 dB, complete recovery can be expected in about 16 hours. Higher initial

TTSs may take much longer to disappear; in some laboratory experiments the course of recovery has been followed for several weeks (47). It requires no imagination to see that audiometry on men working in high noise levels presents a special problem. The men must be tested after a night's rest (or better yet, after a weekend away from the noise) in order to allow TTS to disappear. It is useless to test a man who has just come from high-intensity noise (unless you are studying TTS), since there is no accurate way of correcting the shifted thresholds of individuals to eliminate the TTS.

A group of men all working in the "same" noise will show widely varying degrees of TTS after a given time in the noise. Some of the differences can be ascribed to differences in exposure: perhaps one man was closer than another to a particular machine, took a longer "coffee break," etc. Another part of the variability can be correlated with differences in resting threshold: if an individual has a resting threshold of 40 dB HL, he will not show as much TTS as a normal observer.

Even with these factors accounted for, however, significant differences remain. The TTS produced by a carefully controlled exposure in two observers with nearly identical audiograms (or, for that matter, in the two ears of the same observer) can vary over a range of at least 2:1. Apparently there are internal differences that render some ears more susceptible than others to TTS.

Unfortunately, we do not yet know the relation between TTS and permanent loss of hearing. Are the people more resistant to TTS also more resistant to permanent damage? How much TTS can be tolerated without any permanent loss—indeed, is there any safe limit? It will probably be a long time before we are sure of the answers to these questions.

Recruitment

Recruitment is the term applied to an abnormally rapid growth of loudness that is sometimes associated with elevated thresholds. Persons with permanent tonal gaps (local regions of lowered sensitivity) (48) and those with Ménière's disease (49) usually show the phenomenon. Recruitment is also characteristic of the temporary losses induced by noise exposure. As an example of recruitment, if an ear with thresholds of 40 dB HL at 4000 c/s and 0 dB HL at 1000 c/s is tested by standard loudness-matching procedures, the results may show that by the time the intensity of the 4000-c/s tone is increased to 60 dB HL, the loudness is equal to that of the 1000-c/s tone also at 60 dB HL. Here, then, the loudness at 4000 c/s has grown in the 20-dB interval as much as that at 1000 c/s has grown in 60 dB.

Recruitment will not occur if the lowered sensitivity is due entirely to conductive impairment (lowered transmission through the middle ear due to such causes as inflammation, drum puncture, or otosclerosis). Therefore, tests for recruitment have been widely used as diagnostic tools for differentiating middle-ear pathology (which can often be repaired by surgery) from inner-ear or central involvement (which is not amenable to operative repair). However, conductive losses are characterized by approximately equal losses at all frequencies, and this clearly poses a problem. If the hearing level of a particular ear at 1000 c/s were as high as that at 4000 c/s, then loudness matching between two frequencies in this ear would not always detect recruitment; finding that loudness grows with level at the same rate at the two frequencies would only indicate either that neither frequency is recruiting (and hence the loss is conductive) or that they both are (in which case the loss is sensori-neural). If the listener's other ear had normal thresholds, it could be used for the reference loudness in loudness matching. But not very many cases of unilateral conductive deafness are found; besides, if one ear is normal, most people do not want to undergo an operation at all. As a last resort, one could, of course, determine the loudness function directly (by having the patient set the variable tone to be "half as loud," etc.); if less than 10 dB is needed for doubling the loudness, recruitment is indicated. However, these fractionation procedures are quite difficult, and many patients will display very little consistency.

Another measurement that is sometimes made to test for recruitment is to determine the difference limen for intensity. The reasoning here is that if loudness is growing at an abnormally fast rate, then the DL should be smaller. Although this argument rests on the postulate that loudness of a tone is proportional to the number of DLs between threshold and intensity concerned, there is good evidence that this assumption is not far wrong, generally, although there are exceptions. Of course, there are normally large individual differences among observers in the size of the DL, and so to avoid confusion the DL may be determined at two points, 10 and 40 dB SL; recruitment is indicated when the DL at 10 dB SL is much smaller than that at 40 dB SL (50). The presence of recruitment is sometimes indirectly indicated by an unusually small extent of the excursions of the record in a Békésy-type audiogram; however, this is not a very dependable relation.

Tinnitus

A ringing or buzzing in the ear is called *tinnitus*. Occasionally, in "objective tinnitus," this may be due to a spasm of middle-ear muscles; the tinnitus can be heard by another person merely by joining one of his ears to the one with tinnitus by means of a tube. Most tinnitus, however, originates in the inner ear or higher neural pathways. Despite many decades of speculation, we really have no idea what the physiological correlates of tinnitus may be.

A temporary tinnitus is not unusual for anyone, especially after exposure to noise or gunfire. Most people have heard a "spontaneous tinnitus": a ringing that begins suddenly while one is in a quiet place. At one time, it was thought that people who had experienced such spontaneous tinnitus were more susceptible to permanent damage from noise exposure than those who had not. However, subsequent studies have failed to confirm this. There *is* a good correlation between a permanent loss and reports of tinnitus following noise or gunfire (51), but this probably merely means that the more severe exposures are at the same time (1) more likely to produce tinnitus, and (2) more likely to produce permanent damage.

The pitch and timbre of a tinnitus may vary over wide limits: roaring, hissing, clicking, etc.; but no significance has yet been attached to such differences. In the tinnitus often associated with Ménière's syndrome, the loudness sometimes seems almost unbearable to the patient; yet when the patient is given an objective tone with which to match the loudness of the tinnitus, the result usually indicates that it is only as loud as a tone of 10 dB SL or so (52). Beats between a tinnitus and an objective tone of nearly the same pitch cannot be produced except in cases of objective tinnitus.

Diplacusis

Diplacusis means, literally, "double hearing." It is generally applied to *binaural diplacusis*, a condition in which a given tone, presented alternately to the right and left ears, is judged to have a different pitch in the two ears.

Slight amounts of diplacusis (1 to 6% difference) are to be found in observers with hearing that is otherwise normal. These are generally not noticed, however, since in normal life one does not hear the same frequency alternately in the two ears, and if the tone is presented to both ears simultaneously, only a single pitch is usually heard: a pitch lying somewhere between the pitches heard by the separate ears. Diplacusis is encountered clinically only when the pitch difference reaches a magnitude so great that the patient notices that certain frequencies sound "out of tune."

In the grosser examples of diplacusis associated with abnormal threshold in a single ear, it is found that the pitch of tones in the affected ear is shifted away from the area of increased HL, although the upward shifts are generally larger than the downward. This direction of shift probably holds for the small degrees of chronic diplacusis as well. Diplacusis is also found when an ear has been given a substantial temporary threshold shift (53).

If both ears are known to be abnormal, interpretation of pitch-matching tests will of course be difficult. For instance, if both ears are affected equally, the tests would show no right-left disparity in pitch. The only way such a shift in pitch could be detected would be to use the musical pitch relations mentioned previously (23). Given a reference tone whose frequency lies in the range of normal threshold for the ear, the patient would be required to set a continuously variable tone successively one octave, two octaves, etc., higher. The deviations of these settings from those of a normal observer (who can be expected to set the variable tone about 1 % higher than the physical octave) will provide an estimate of the disturbance of pitch. These tests are not often used, for several reasons: (1) a continuously variable oscillator must be employed; (2) the patient must be musical enough to make reliable judgments; (3) the adjustments are very time-consuming; and finally (4) the diagnostic significance of the pitch shifts that produce diplacusis has not yet been established.

A rarer form of diplacusis is *monaural diplacusis*, in which a single pure tone is heard as a group of tones or a noise (54). In the tonal variety, the additional tones are heard just above and below a particular frequency, called the idiofrequency (55). The pitches of these subjective tones are identical with those of the combination tones produced when a normal ear is presented with two tones: one at the frequency of the particular objective tone concerned, and the other at the idiofrequency. When certain objective tones are turned off, a decaying tone having the pitch of the idiofrequency can be heard. The Albrecht effect is sometimes observed in a narrowly circumscribed region near the idiofrequency: a tone well above threshold may become inaudible after only a few seconds, even though the same frequency may be heard indefinitely at both higher and lower intensities.

Monaural diplacusis may occur in ears in which absolute thresholds are quite within the normal limits. Its cause and significance are as yet not understood.

REFERENCES

1. Zwislocki, J.: Theory of temporal auditory summation. J. Acoust. Soc. America, *32:* 1046, 1960.
2. von Békésy, G.: A new audiometer. Acta oto-laryng., *35:* 411, 1947.
3. Webster, J. C., Himes, H. W., and Lichtenstein, M.: San Diego County fair hearing survey. J. Acoust. Soc. America, *22:* 473, 1950.
4. Westlake, G.: Reality of the zero reference line for pure tone testing. J. Speech & Hearing Disorders, *8:* 285, 1943.
5. Zwislocki, J., Maire, F., Feldman, A. S., and Rubin, H.: On the effect of practice and motivation of the threshold of audibility. J. Acoust. Soc. America, *30:* 254, 1958.
6. Stream, R. W., and McConnell, F.: A comparison of two methods of administration in Békésy-type audiometry. J. Auditory Res., *1:* 263, 1961.
7. Harris, J. D., and Myers, C. K.: Experiments on fluctuations of auditory acuity. J. Gen. Psychol., *50:* 87, 1954.

8. Burkhard, M. D., and Corliss, E. L. R.: The response of earphones in ears and couplers. J. Acoust. Soc. America, *26:* 679, 1954.
9. Morrical, K. C., Glaser, J. L., and Benson, R. W.: Interactions between microphones, couplers and earphones. J. Acoust. Soc. America, *21:* 190, 1949.
10. *National Health Survey (1935–1936): Preliminary Reports, Hearing Study Series,* Bulletins 1–7. U. S. Public Health Service, Washington, 1938.
11. Glorig, A., Quiggle, R., Wheeler, D. E., and Grings, W.: Determination of the normal hearing reference zero. J. Acoust. Soc. America, *28:* 1110, 1956.
12. Hinchcliffe, R.: The threshold of hearing of a random sample rural population Acta Oto-laryng., *50:* 411, 1959.
13. Sivian, L. J., and White, S. D.: On minimum audible sound fields. J. Acoust. Soc. America, *4:* 288, 1933.
14. Davis, H., Hoople, G. D., and Parrack, H. O.: The medical principles of monitoring audiometry. A. M. A. Arch. Indust. Hyg., *17:* 1, 1958.
15. Thomas, G. J.: Equal- volume judgments of tones. Am. J. Psychol., *62:* 182, 1949.
16. Stevens, S. S.: Tonal density. J. Exper. Psychol., *17:* 585, 1934.
17. *American Standard Acoustical Terminology,* Specification Z24.1 American Standards Association, New York, 1951.
18. Stevens, S. S.: Calculation of the loudness of complex noise. J. Acoust. Soc. America, *28:* 807, 1956.
19. Churcher, B. G., and King, A. J.: The performance of noise meters in terms of the primary standard. J. Inst. Elec. Engrs., *81:* 57, 1937.
20. Hellman, R. P., and Zwislocki, J.: Some factors affecting the estimation of loudness. J. Acoust. Soc. America, *33:* 687, 1961.
21. Stevens, S. S.: Procedure for calculating loudness: Mark VI. J. Acoust. Soc. America, *33:* 1577, 1961.
22. Young, R. W.: Terminology for logarithmic frequency units. J. Acoust. Soc. America, *11:* 134, 1939.
23. Ward, W. D.: Subjective Musical Pitch. J. Acoust. Soc. America, *26:* 369, 1954.
24. Stevens, S. S., and Volkmann, J.: The relation of pitch to frequency: a revised scale. Am. J. Psychol., *53:* 329, 1940.
25. Cohen, A.: Further investigation of the effects of intensity upon the pitch of pure tones. J. Acoust. Soc. America, *33:* 1363, 1961.
26. Montgomery, H. C.: Influence of experimental technique on the measurement of differential intensity sensitivity of the ear. J. Acoust. Soc. America, *7:* 39, 1935.
27. Pollack, I.: Intensity discrimination thresholds under several psychophysical procedures. J. Acoust. Soc. America, *26:* 1056, 1954.
28. Churcher, B. G., King, A. J., and Davies, H.: The minimum perceptible change of intensity of a pure tone. Phil. Mag., *18:* 927, 1934.
29. Rosenblith, W. A., and Stevens, K. N.: On the DL for frequency. J. Acoust. Soc. America, *25:* 980, 1953.
30. Lawrence, M.: Audiometric manifestations of inner ear physiology: the aural overload test. Tr. Am. Acad. Ophth., *62:* 104, 1958.
31. von Békésy, G.: Sensations on the skin similar to directional hearing, beats and harmonics of the ear. J. Acoust. Soc. America, *29:* 489, 1957.
32. Egan, J. P., and Klumpp, R. G.: The error due to masking in the measurement of aural harmonics by the method of best beats. J. Acoust. Soc. America, *23:* 275, 1951.
33. Wever, E. G., and Lawrence, M. *Physiological Acoustics,* Ch. 8 and 9. Princeton University Press, Princeton, 1954.

34. Wegel, R. L., and Lane, C. E.: The auditory masking of one pure tone by another and its probable relation to the dynamics of the ear. Physical. Rev., *23:* 266, 1924.

35. Greenwood, D. D.: Auditory masking and the critical band. J. Acoust. Soc. America, *33:* 484, 1961.

36. Cox, J. R., Jr.: How quiet must it be to measure normal hearing? Noise Control, *1 (1):* 25, 1955.

37. Bilger, R. C., and Hirsh, I. J. Masking of tones by bands of noise. J. Acoust. Soc. America, *28:* 623, 1956.

38. Deatherage, B. H., Davis, H., and Eldredge, D. H.: Physiological evidence for the masking of low frequencies by high. J. Acoust. Soc. America, *29:* 132, 1957.

39. Ward, W. D.: Suudies on the aural reflex. I. Contralateral remote masking as an indicator of reflex activity. J. Acoust. Soc. America, *33:* 1034, 1961.

40. Wright, H. N.: Measurement of perstimulatory auditory adaptation. J. Acoust. Soc. America, *32:* 1558, 1960.

41. Kobrak, H. G., Lindsay, J. R., and Perlman, H. B.: Experimental observations on the question of auditory fatigue. Laryngoscope, *51:* 798, 1941.

42. Carhart, R.: Clinical determination of abnormal auditory adaptation. Arch. Otolaryng., *65:* 32, 1957.

43. Ward, W. D., Glorig, A., and Sklar, D. L.: Dependence of temporary threshold shift at 4 KC on intensity and time. J. Acoust. Soc. America, *30:* 944, 1958.

44. Ward, W. D., Glorig, A., and Sklar, D. L.: Temporary threshold shift from octave-band noise: applications to damage-risk criteria. J. Acoust. Soc. America, *31:* 522, 1959.

45. Kylin, B.: Temporary threshold shift and auditory trauma following exposure to steady-state noise. Acta Otolaryng. *Suppl. 152*, 1960.

46. Ward, W. D., Glorig, A., and Sklar, D. L.: Temporary threshold shift produced by intermittent exposure to noise. J. Acoust. Soc. America, *31:* 791, 1959.

47. Ward, W. D.: Recovery from high values of temporary threshold shift. J. Acoust. Soc. America, *32:* 497, 1960.

48. Ward, W. D., Fleer, R. E., and Glorig, A.: Characteristics of hearing losses produced by gunfire and by steady noise. J. Auditory Res., *1:* 325, 1961.

49. Hallpike, C. S., and Hood, J. D. Observations upon the neurological mechanism of the loudness recruitment phenomenon. Acta Otolaryng., *50:* 472, 1959.

50. Jerger, J. F.: Differential intensity sensitivity in the ear with loudness recruitment. J. Speech & Hearing Disorders, *20:* 183, 1955.

51. Ward, W. D.: Hearing of naval aircraft maintenance personnel. J. Acoust. Soc. America, *29:* 1289, 1957.

52. Fowler, E. P.: Control of head noises, their illusion of loudness and timbre. Arch. Otolaryng., *37:* 391, 1943.

53. Davis, H., Morgan, C. T., Hawkins, J. E., Galambos, R., and Smith, F. W.: Temporary deafness following exposure to loud tones and noise. Acta Otolaryng. *Suppl. 88*, 1950.

54. Ward, W. D.: Tonal monaural diplacusis. J. Acoust. Soc. America, *27:* 365, 1955.

55. Flottorp, G.: Pure-tone tinnitus evoked by acoustic stimulation: the idiophone effect. Acta Otolaryng., *43:* 396, 1953.

4

Some Problems of Measurement and Methodology in Auditory Research

Wallace S. High, M.A.

Auditory research has become increasingly more sophisticated over the years. Today, the auditory research worker must have a broad background including knowledge of electronics, psychoacoustics, physiology, psychology, quantitative methods, and research methodology. This chapter deals with certain aspects of the latter two areas. The first section introduces some of the basic principles of measurement used in science and the second section discusses some selected problems encountered in auditory research. The material is presented with the assumption that the reader has preparation in elementary algebra and introductory statistics.

PRINCIPLES OF MEASUREMENT

Just what is meant by the term *measurement* and why is it important? Basically measurement is a quantitative description of events or objects, for example, the time it takes to run a mile, the height of a man, the tensile strength of a wire, the impedance of an electrical circuit, or the sensitivity of a person's hearing. The actual process of measurement is accomplished by assigning numerals to the object or events according to pre-established rules. *Numerals* are symbols which according to convention imply uniqueness or identity.*

---

*There is a problem associated with the term "numeral" in the definition of measurement. Numerals are sometimes taken to be only symbols or marks on a piece of paper. When we refer to the numerousness or the property of numerosity of things or events, we generally use the term "number." However, the term "numeral" is more than just an ink mark on paper; each numeral is distinct and different

72

Many advantages have been claimed for the measurement process, but most of them may be grouped under three headings. First, measurement enables us to describe objects or events with a high degree of objectivity. Objectivity as used here means interpersonal agreement and is essential for many scientific purposes. A second advantage of quantitative description is ease and accuracy of communication. The meaning of numerals does not suffer from the ambiguity that often plagues qualitative descriptions. But it is necessary to keep in mind the fact that the rules and operations by which numerals are assigned to objects or events constitute an integral part of their meaning. The third advantage of quantitative description is the ease with which numerical symbols can be manipulated. The kind of manipulations referred to here are arithmetic ones—addition, substraction, multiplication, and division. The kinds of permissible manipulations depend on the particular measurement scale one is dealing with.

The Nature of Mathematics

The practical usefulness of measurement rests upon a foundation of mathematics. There has been a good deal of misunderstanding about the fundamental nature of mathematics, and it has been the philosophers who have done the most to clarify the picture (1–4). First, it should be understood that mathematics is an invention (or more accurately, a series of inventions) and not a discovery. Mathematics is not to be considered a science in the same sense as physics, chemistry, biology, or geology. That is, mathematics is not based on empirical observation, nor does it seek to codify observed natural uniformities in the form of laws.

Mathematics is a logical system based upon *postulates*, statements assumed to be true without further need of proof. Postulates are useful because of the deductions or conclusions (known as theorems) which may be drawn from them. *Theorems* are implications of postulates. If the postulates are true, as they are assumed to be, then the theorems must also be true. The kind of truth involved here is a logical truth; it is not necessary to support postulates or theorems with empirical evidence.

A requirement of postulates is that they not be contradictory. If postulates do contradict one another, they must be modified, or one must give way to another. Postulates should also be independent. This means that we should not be able to derive one from another. Actually, a system based upon non-independent postulates would not necessarily be invalid; it would just lack the elegance of simplicity.

from every other one. Thus numerals may be used to identify or label objects or groups. When used this way, numerals clearly imply at least one property of numbers, namely uniqueness or identity. The formal properties of uniqueness will be given in a later section.

Since mathematics appears to be a kind of intellectual game, one might legitimately ask what it has to do with the observable realities of science or, more particularly, with auditory research. The answer is that on the basis of past experience we know that nature is sufficiently parallel with the structure of some mathematical and logical systems that we can accurately describe certain aspects of nature with numbers. The similarity between the structure of mathematical systems and the structure of nature is known as *isomorphism*. Parallelism or isomorphism makes mathematics a powerful tool for science. As long as numbers bear some meaningful relationship to empirical events, we can manipulate the numerical symbols to discover new relationships among the empirical events.

Numbers and Measurement

We have already mentioned the principle of isomorphism, the relationship of number systems to certain aspects of nature. According to this principle we may use numbers to describe things or events to the extent that the properties of numbers are similar to the properties of things.

Before proceeding we shall attempt to define more clearly what is meant by the term "number." While it is probably true that there is no single definition which applies to all numbers, there is a definition (attributed to Bertrand Russell) which describes rational numbers well. This definition says that a *number* is the class of all classes. What is meant is that objects can belong to a class because of their numerousness. That is, if we have three men, three houses, three dollar bills, or three of anything, they all belong to the class "three" because each class of objects shares the property of threeness. A simple test may be performed to see whether two classes belong to the same class. The test is to pair off elements of the two classes. If no elements are left over, the numerosity of each class is identical, and each class may have the same numeral assigned to it. A *numeral* is the symbol that represents a number, but as was noted before, numerals may be considered to possess at least one property of numbers, e.g., identity.

The three properties of numbers recognized (5–7) as most important for measurement are *identity*, *rank order*, and *additivity*. We will discuss these properties of numbers and will attempt to show how they might be demonstrated to be properties of some of the events we wish to measure.

Identity. The concept of identity is specified by three of the basic postulates of algebra:

Either $a = b$ or $a \neq b$.

If $a = b$, then $b = a$.

If $a = b$ and $b = c$, then $a = c$.

The first of these postulates says that two numbers, a and b, are the same or not the same. They cannot be both. The second postulate says that when a condition of equality exists between numbers their relation is symmetrical. The third postulate is a statement of transitivity. It says that since *both* a and c are equal to b, then a and c must be equal.

Rank Order. There are three formal assumptions for establishing rank order among a class of elements.

$$\text{If } a \neq b, \text{ then either } a < b \text{ or } b < a.$$

$$\text{If } a < b, \text{ then } b \not< a.$$

$$\text{If } a < b \text{ and } b < c, \text{ then } a < c.$$

The first statement is a requirement of connectedness among the elements. If there are two elements in a class that are not equal, then one of them must be larger than, older than, higher than, etc. the other. The second statement shows that the relationship is asymmetrical. Put another way, if we take the statement $a < b$ as true, we cannot reverse a and b and accept the statement $b < a$ as true also. The third postulate, having to do with rank order, states that the elements in a class must bear a *transitive* relationship to one another. If a is lighter than b, and b is lighter than c, then a must also be lighter than c. There are situations in which the relationship of transitivity is broken. When this happens, it is not possible to rank order all the elements in the class on a given attribute. For example, if A is the father of B and B is the father of C, it does not follow that A is the father of C.

Additivity. The concept of additivity implies that the operation of addition applied to a set of numbers will yield internally consistent results. To satisfy the condition of additivity there are four properties of numbers that must be satisfied.

$$\text{If } a = c \text{ and } b > 0, \text{ then } a + b > c.$$

$$a + b = b + a.$$

$$\text{If } a = c \text{ and } b = d, \text{ then } a + b = c + d.$$

$$(a + b) + c = a + (b + c).$$

The first postulate indicates the possibility of addition and implies that the addition of zero leaves the number invariant. The next postulate states that the order in which numbers are added does not change the result. The third postulate states that equal objects may be substituted for one another. The last postulate means that the order of combinations does not affect the result of addition.

If we are to assign numerals to events with any confidence that the principle of isomorphism will be satisfied, we should have some means of demonstrating (other than the use of intuition) that the events possess at least some of the properties of numbers. As indicated above, the properties of greatest concern are those of rank order and additivity. We can usually demonstrate rank order without much difficulty, but demonstrating the property of additivity is rarely accomplished easily.

Demonstration of Rank Order. Numerous examples are available to demonstrate the property of order in events and objects. The psychological correlates of many physical stimuli are derived on the basis of "ordering" judgments. A pure tone of frequency x is judged to have a higher pitch than one of frequency $x - 1$; a tone of intensity y is judged to have a greater loudness than a tone of intensity $y - 1$; or a tone of intensity p and frequency q is judged to have a greater density than a tone of intensity $p - 1$ and a frequency $q - 1$. These examples from psychophysics may lack the intuitive satisfaction of examples from physics. The hardness of stones may be ordered by a simple scratching operation. If stone A scratches stone B, stone B scratches stone C, and stone C scratches stone D, a rank order of the four stones is established on the attribute of hardness. The accuracy of the ranking for hardness is likely to be greater than is the ranking of the psychological variables mentioned above. In the latter case, reversals are sometimes found when an observer is called upon to repeat his judgments on different occasions. These reversals are not allowed to invalidate the ranking unless the judgments are entirely capricious. Reversals of judgments are ordinarily treated as measurement or scaling errors and are evaluated statistically. In general, an order relation is generated when elements in a class are equivalent in regard to the attribute in question and when it can be shown that class A has more something than class B, when class B has more something than class C, and so on.

Demonstration of Additivity. It is difficult to show the property of additivity empirically, even in the physical sciences. The most obvious cases where it is possible are those of length and weight. Suppose we had two sticks, a and b, and determined their lengths on a calibrated distance scale. If stick a measured 4 units and stick b measured 6 units, we would predict that their combined length would be 10 units. We could verify this prediction empirically by placing the two sticks end-to-end along the distance scale and observing visually that the combined length was equal to 10 units. A similar set of operations could be performed with weights if we had a calibrated scale. There are limitations to experimental proofs of the additivity of even weights and lengths. Sub-atomic distances and astronomical distances cannot be placed end-to-end in the same fashion as objects having moderate dimensions. Consequently, the demonstration of addition must rest on some other grounds.

In the case of psychological scales such as pitch, loudness, brightness, and so on, additivity cannot be demonstrated experimentally. A physicist might argue, therefore, that the properties of equal units could not be developed for psychological response scales because equal-unit properties are derived from the experimental demonstration of addition. This argument is not fatal, though, because there are other ways to obtain equal-unit scales.

Before attempting to show how an equal-unit scale might be developed without addition, we wish to emphasize that the meaning of numbers under any conditions of measurement is merely an expression of the set of operations one has performed in assigning the numbers to a scale. Thus meanings attached to scale units obtained through psychological-measurement operations will be different from the meanings attached to scale units developed from the fundamental measurement operations of addition. The common centile scale may be used to illustrate this point. A distribution of measurements in a sample might be obtained by rating the individuals on some attribute. The distribution of ratings could then be transformed into a centile scale by determining the proportion of individuals that fell below any given raw score. A raw score of 23, for example, would convert to a centile score of 70 if 70 % of the sample had scores below 23. The meaning associated with intervals on a centile scale is precise, but it is not the same meaning that is applied to numbers *per se*. The difference between centile scores of 70 and 90, for example, indicates that 20 % of the individuals in the sample have scores that fall within that range. Thus equal intervals on a centile scale refer to *equal proportions of individuals* rather than equal units of magnitude on the measured variable.

One approach to an equal-unit scale without empirical demonstration of addition is through the method of *equal sense distances*. The purpose of this method is to obtain a scale of psychological magnitude such that adjacent scale values are equally spaced. The distance between every pair of adjacent scale values on such a scale would be the psychological equivalent of every other pair. The basic procedure in developing an equal sense distance scale is to have an individual bisect an interval on the basis of observation. A pair of tones might be presented which differ only in intensity. A subject would be instructed to adjust the intensity of a third tone until its loudness appeared to divide the intervals between the standard tones into two psychologically equal magnitudes. Numerous adjustments would be made by all subjects in the sample, and an average intensity setting for the sample would be used to represent the mid-point of the interval. The remainder of the scale would be built up by having the subjects bisect the interval between other pairs of standard tones in a similar fashion. Details of this and similar methods can be found in Guilford (6, Chap. 9). Scales obtained by equal sense distance methods are of the equal-interval type (see below). As of the moment, no experimental operations have been found by which a meaningful zero point can be established with this type of scale. Thus the property of equal ratios cannot be assured.

We should recognize that all sciences operate under the limitations imposed by their present state of knowledge. Each science must be permitted to decide what kinds of evidence it will use for demonstrating the measurability of the phenomena which fall within its domain. Within a given science, some things can be measured with greater accuracy and completeness than others. It is important to realize that isomorphism between events and number systems is not required to be complete in order for us to make meaningful measurements. However, there must be at least a partial isomorphism because it is the corresponding empirical operations performed on events and objects which justifies our using a formal number system for describing relationships in the physical world.

Levels of Measurement

This section describes the four levels of measurement generally recognized in science. The classification has been worked out most clearly by Stevens (7, 8). The four levels differ in terms of their completeness and are distinguished on the basis of the rules governing the application of numbers to events. The higher levels of measurement are associated with more restrictive rules.

Nominal Scales. The nominal scale is the lowest in the hierarchy of measurement scales. At first glance it might seem that this level does not possess the properties we usually associate with the term measurement, since this scale is not graduated or serial. The nominal scale uses numbers to represent a class or category. Numbers are used here as names or labels for classes or to identify elements within a given class. Two rules govern the assignment of numbers to events at this level of measurement. First, all elements in a class must have the same number, and second, the same number must not be assigned to more than one class.

The three postulates relating to the concept of identity (see above) apply to the nominal scale. Elements are assigned to classes on the basis of their equality with respect to some attribute. Examples would be numbering members of an athletic team or assigning type numbers to electronic parts.

The classification of objects into classes is sometimes the source of some confusion. The fact that we may judge two objects "equal" implies their "identity." Identity is an ideal condition that may not be realized because of our limited powers of observation or discrimination. In some cases we may not wish to make as fine a discrimination between objects as we are capable of doing so as to keep the classes we have to deal with at a manageable number. As a consequence, the condition of identity is sometimes only approximated because of deficiencies in our methods of observation or because of practical considerations.

There are few kinds of statistical operations that can be used with the nominal scale. Frequency counts can be made of the cases in each category, the modal (most numerous) class can be determined, and the coefficient of contingency can be computed (the interdependency of classified attributes where the objects have been classified in two ways). These statistics can also be used with higher level scales.

Ordinal Scales. The numbers on an ordinal scale result from the process of rank ordering. The three postulates required for establishing rank order have been stated previously. Guilford (6, p. 13) regards rank ordering as classifying objects or things according to quantitative categories, where the classification is based on some property or quality of the things ranked. When discrimination among objects is complete, each category will contain only a single object. However, ranking may be accomplished even though our ability to discriminate among objects is less than perfect. In this case, the various categories may contain more than a single case; i.e., one or more objects may be assigned the same rank number. Ordinal scales carry no implication that the distances between successive categories are equal. When the intervals between ranks are equal, we are dealing with the next highest level of measurement scale.

A good deal of misinformation has been published on the matter of what statistics may be appropriately used with ordinal scales. This question is important because most of the scales used in the behavorial sciences are of this type. For describing or interpreting distributions of ranked objects, the statistics appropriate for nominal scales may be used as well as medians, centiles, and rank-order coefficients of correlation. None of these statistics require that intervals between scale points be equal. Some writers have reservations about the use of Spearman's rank-order correlation with ordinal scales. However, there is little evidence to support this view if ranking is complete and if consecutive integers have been assigned to consecutive categories. The major assumption of the rank-order coefficient is that the distances between the rank numbers be equal. Hence, consecutive integers must be used in the ranking (with appropriate evaluation of tied rankings). There is no implication that the ranked objects are equally spaced on an ideal scale. The resulting coefficient provides information only about the extent to which the sets of integers agree.

When the purpose of an investigation is to assess the significance of differences between groups, it is appropriate to compute means, standard deviations, and other "equal-interval" statistics on rank numbers. The powerful parametric significance tests such as the F and t tests can then be used to determine the probability that the rank numbers associated with the different groups have been drawn from the same population. The use of means and standard deviations for describing and making interpretative statements about ordinal scale data may also be justified under some conditions. We will discuss these points further in the section on "Recent Developments in Measurement Theory."

Interval Scales. An interval scale possesses the additional property of equal units. Distances on an interval scale that are numerically equal represent empirically equal distances or amounts. Examples of interval scales are the two temperature scales, Fahrenheit and centigrade. The important limitation of this kind of scale is that the zero point is fixed at some arbitrary position. For this reason it is not possible to say that some value on an interval scale is twice some other value or is some proportion of another value. A further implication of the arbitrary zero point of the interval scale is that the property of additivity is not realized. It is not meaningful to add numbers on an interval scale since the absolute value of the numbers as well as their sums will depend on where the zero point happens to be placed. Although the addition of interval-scale numbers is not meaningful, the difference between two interval-scale values can be added to the difference between another pair of scale values to obtain a total distance. The reason why differences on an interval scale are additive is that any point on an interval scale may be expressed in terms of a linear equation of the form $y = ax + b$. When a *difference* between points on the scale is determined, the additive constant b disappears through the process of subtraction.

Most statistics may be used with interval-scale measurements. These include the mean, standard deviation, and product-moment correlation coefficient as well as those statistics that are derived from or are dependent upon them. One statistic which should not be used with interval-scale measurements is the coefficient of variation, an absolute measure of variability, which in any event is not often used.

Various procedures are available for developing psychological scales having equal intervals, though it is rare that success is complete. Scaling methods based on equal sense distances have already been mentioned. However, scales based on these methods are sometimes in disagreement with scales based on other types of judgments. Even though equal-interval scales based on equal sense distances are subject to error, many investigators feel that the approximations involved are justified. If a set of data is internally consistent, it is always possible that its validity can be established with future research or at least that discrepancies with other sets of data can be resolved.

Ratio Scales. All of the postulates relating to identity, rank order, and additivity apply to ratio scales. The distinguishing feature of the ratio scale is that it possesses a genuine zero point which unambiguously represents zero amount of the thing measured by the scale. Because of the absolute zero point characteristic of this highest level of measurement, it is meaningful to equate ratios of numbers (the values of points) on the scale. Thus 4:3 is equal to 12:9; each of these ratios represents the same relationship between the things measured by the scale. All statistical operations are permissible with ratio scales.

Ratio scales can be constructed even though an experimental demonstration of additivity may not be possible. Observational operations are available for this purpose. The constant-sum method (9) and the method of fractionation (6, Chap. 9) are examples. Stevens' scale for loudness and mel scale for pitch were constructed using similar procedures (10, 11).

A point about ratio scales sometimes overlooked because of its obviousness is that the scale of numerousness is itself a ratio scale. This is the scale we use to enumerate objects—5 chickens, 10 dollars, 4 associate professors, etc. Mention is made of this point because ratio properties are sometimes mistakenly attributed to a measured function when the measurement involves enumeration of objects or events. A test score based on the sum of individual items is sometimes the subject of this misuse. A total score may be obtained by counting the number of items responded to correctly. So long as one deals only with the number of correct items, one is dealing with a ratio scale and all statistical operations are permissible. When the "number correct" is used to represent the standing of a person on the attribute measured by the test, the situation is different. The number correct no longer has ratio properties since it has been transferred to a second scale—the scale of ability or whatever is measured by the test. If the test is one of ability, then the test scores probably possess only ordinal properties. A score of zero on this kind of test rarely indicates a zero amount of ability. The equality of score units on ability tests or attitude scales is also open to question.

Transformations

In what ways can scale values be changed without reducing the accuracy of measurement? The answer to this question brings up the concept of invariance. Briefly, invariance means uniformity, dependability, or generality. Invariance of relationships between variables is what a scientist looks for. When a relationship is found, the next step is to determine the conditions under which the relationship holds true. A law or relationship that holds true under widely varying conditions is a highly valued one; it has a high degree of invariance or generality. Put another way, the scientist looks for transformations that will leave the relationship invariant. This same principle can be used to test the level of a measurement scale.

Nominal scales permit a great deal of latitude in this matter. Any transformation can be applied that does not change the classes or the elements within a class. Since nominal scales use numbers essentially for labeling purposes, it is evident that any substitution of numbers is possible as long as the postulates of identity are not violated. Any one-for-one substitution of numbers can be made.

All transformations that do not have an effect on the rank order of scale numbers may be applied to ordinal scales. Thus any monotonic transformation is permissible—that is, any transformation where the transformed values continuously increase or decrease. For each number on an ordinal scale we could add a constant, multiply by a constant, take the square root (or any other positive root), or take the logarithm without changing the rank order of scale values. Transformations that have maximums or minimums, such as quadratic functions, are ruled out.

Even greater restrictions apply to interval scales. Only linear transformations of the form $y = ax + b$ will leave an interval scale invariant. This requirement means that powers, roots, and logarithms may not be used. Examination of the general linear equation $y = ax + b$ reveals that both multiplication and addition of a constant are involved in linear transformations. Neither operation affects the equality of scale intervals. The addition of a constant changes the zero point of a scale, but this does not matter with an interval scale. As has been pointed out above, an interval scale does not have an absolute zero; its origin may be fixed at any convenient point.

Multiplication by a constant is the only transformation that can be made on a ratio scale without destroying its property of equal ratios. The only restriction is that the constant multiplier may not be zero.

Recent Developments in Measurement Theory

The preceding discussion is based primarily on the taxonomy of measurement scales proposed by Stevens (7). Since its publication, a number of articles have appeared which elaborate certain aspects of Stevens' work. Coombs (12), for example, recognizes some additional classes of scales that lie between Stevens' ordinal and interval scales. These need not concern us here except as a reminder that other classifications of measurement scales are possible. Anderson (13) in a different context quotes a remark by K. MacCorquodale that is appropriate here: "Measurement theory should be descriptive, not proscriptive, nor prescriptive."

The question of what kinds of statistics are appropriate for what levels of measurement has been the subject of some confusion. Senders (14) and Siegel (15) hold that inferential statistics such as the t and F test are inappropriately applied to ordinal scale data. They base their position on grounds that the operations of addition and multiplication used in computing t and F are not meaningful unless applied to scores that are "numerical," i.e., unless the scale intervals are equal. Burke (16) and Lord (17) have pointed out the error in this reasoning. They argue that the validity of a statistical inference is not dependent on the type of measuring scale used. Rather, a statistical test refers to distributions of numbers only; it has no knowledge of the empirical meaning of the scale numbers. Hence there is no reason why a t or F test may not be used to test the reliability of a difference between behaviors measured on an ordinal scale. There may be occasions when a rank-order or other distribution-free test is more powerful than the F test under conditions of ordinal measurement. However, the choice of significance test rests on statistical considerations rather than on the level of measurement scale. In Burke's words (16), ". . . the statistical technique begins and ends with the numbers and with statements about them. The psychological interpretation given to the experiment does take cognizance of the origin of the numbers but this is irrelevant for the statistical test as such."

Descriptive statistics which assume equal intervals (mean, standard deviation, product-moment correlation, etc.) may be justified for use with ordinal scale data under some conditions. Many ordinal scales used in experimental investigations may approach the condition of equal intervals, at least over part of the scale range. In such cases, the amount of error resulting from the use of "illegal" statistics is probably small enough to be tolerated. There is no question about the accuracy of results when any statistic is applied to a distribution of numbers *per se*. The point at issue is what the statistics tell us about the responses, traits, or attributes to which the scale numbers refer. To the extent that scale intervals depart from equality, conclusions about the measured trait which are based on equal interval statistics will be in error. The prudent investigator would be well advised to exercise caution in drawing conclusions when equal-interval statistics are used on ordinal data.

Some similar problems having to do with scale invariance have been pointed out by Anderson (13). Stevens (7, p. 24) observes that when one of the permissible transformations is made on a given scale, a statistic computed from the untransformed scale scores will remain invariant when the same transformation is made on the statistic. Anderson demonstrates that this ideal condition is not likely to hold up under the day-to-day working conditions of science. He cites examples showing that invariance of results cannot be guaranteed under some transformations of scale that may become necessary as knowledge accumulates in a given field. As knowledge advances, changes are made in the scales and experimental techniques for measuring a given phenomenon. A scale used by an investigator today may have a complicated relationship to the phenomenon he is studying. The next investigator may use a scale that has a different relationship to the same phenomenon. While Anderson agrees with Stevens that invariance of result is guaranteed by following the strictures pertaining to the use of permissible transformations, he argues convincingly that these kinds of considerations have little to do with the scale modifications an investigator is obliged to make in his work.

SOME SELECTED PROBLEMS IN RESEARCH

This section discusses some of the persistent problem areas of auditory research. (We do not mean to imply that other areas of science are free of the problems mentioned here; they are not.) The intention of the discussion is to point out some of the difficulties that face researchers and to aid the newcomer to evaluate the research reports he may read. The problems in conducting competent research are many. It has been necessary to select arbitrarily for discussion those problems which in our estimation seem most important.

Reliability

The basic purpose of research is to discover phenomena, the conditions that affect the phenomena, and the dependability or lawfulness of the conditions. One of the first things we must do when investigating a new area is to determine whether the phenomenon under investigation is a reliable one. If it is not, there is little point in carrying the investigation further. This obvious point is often overlooked or ignored by many investigators.

In audiology the dependent variable, the response under investigation, is identified and then an attempt is made to quantify the response. It is the reliability of this response measure with which we are most concerned. Science is only concerned with reproducible phenomena. If our measurements are not reliable, then we cannot reproduce them when we wish to. The scientific requirement for reproducibility, if rigorously observed, saves us from a lot of unnecessary and unfruitful work. For example, unidentified flying objects cannot be studied by the scientific method. They cannot be reproduced on demand, nor can the conditions that affect them be manipulated or controlled. We can speculate until doomsday on their origin and how they work, but we cannot study them with the methods of science until somebody catches one.

Much current work in audiology utilizes sophisticated electronic equipment. There seems to be an aura of precision about such equipment which may lead us to take its reliability for granted. Such faith is completely unjustified. Electronic equipment is continuously subject to breakdowns, and unlike the case with some mechanical equipment, the malfunctioning components are often hidden from view. Situations where responses appear to be inconsistent can often be traced to malfunctioning equipment. Not only can equipment problems produce unreliable responses in one experiment, but they can sometimes account for discrepancies in the results of different experiments. A number of such cases have been brought to our attention. Calibration and operating checks should be made a routine part of any experiment where electronic equipment is used.

A recent article by High, Glorig, and Nixon (18) lists some of the problems that must be faced if one is to obtain reliable measures of hearing sensitivity. The list, with some modifications, is presented below:

Physical Variables
    Improper placement of earphones
    Ambient noise levels in test room
    Equipment variables, such as accuracy of attenuator steps, type
        of earphone cushions, hum, noise, etc.
Physiological Variables
    Age and sex
    Pathology of the auditory organs
    General health of subject
    Temporary threshold shift
    Tinnitus and other head noises
Psychological Variables
    Motivation of subject
    Momentary fluctuations of attention
    Attitude toward the test situation
    Personality attributes
Intellectual Factors
    Comprehension of instructions
    Experience in test taking of any sort
Response Conditions
    Type of response required of subject, i.e., button pressing, finger
        raising, responding verbally, etc.
Methodological Variables
    Testing technique used
    Time interval between successive tests
    Instructions to subjects
    Order of presentation of test tones

Some of the variables listed are obviously more important than others, but in general, the more rigidly the experimental situation is controlled the more reliable the response measures will be. While failure to control any of the variables listed above may serve to reduce the reliability of a response measure, it should be pointed out that some of these variables may be the object of study in some experiments. Instructions might be systematically varied with different groups of subjects, for example. If the responses of the different groups were found to vary lawfully, then this variation would be treated as reliable variance instead of error.

Given some sort of reliability estimate for a set of response measures, the question arises as to what constitutes acceptable reliability. How large should a reliability estimate be before the response measures can be taken as useful indicators of behavior? Regretably, no precise answer can be given to this question. The numerical value of a reliability coefficient is affected by too many factors. A homogeneous population will yield lower coefficients than a heterogeneous population; the range of response-measure scores affects the magnitude of reliability coefficients; the type of reliability estimate used is another factor that influences the reliability coefficient— internal consistency estimates generally produce higher coefficients than do re-test estimates. These are but a few of the factors that confront the investigator in evaluating reliability estimates. Paper and pencil tests of ability, rating scales, and the like often show reliabilities of 0.90 or better, whereas certain types of psychophysical judgments may run no higher than 0.40. Such low figures might seem to be poor evidence of reliability, although it should be remembered that sampling problems, a narrow range of scores, and other conditions specific to a given experiment can make it all but impossible to achieve higher figures. In these situations, evidence of reliability can be supplemented with evidence from other experiments. When consistency or lawfulness of results is accumulated from one experiment to another, we begin to have confidence in the reliability of the response measures even though evidence from a single experiment is not convincing.

A further point about reliability that bears repetition is that an obtained reliability coefficient refers to a specific experimental situation and a specific population. Psychological-test publishers almost invariably report reliability coefficients with their tests. Many test users behave as though these reported values were *the* reliability coefficients associated with the test. Rather, the reported coefficients refer to reliability of the test with the particular sample used for standardization purposes and for the test-taking conditions in effect at the time. Actually, there is no such thing as *the* reliability of a test or, for that matter, of any response scale. As indicated above, there are many factors that affect reliability. It is up to each investigator to determine what the reliability is for his experimental situation and sample. It would be desirable if investigators would make it a common practice to make a determination of reliability when a new response measure is used or when a substantial change is made in old measures.

There have been a number of important developments in methods of estimating reliability that are better suited for the kinds of response measures encountered in experimental work than some of the traditional methods. These are mentioned because they have not yet found their way into many current textbooks on statistics. Hoyt and Krishnaiah (19) and Rajaratnam (20) have developed methods for estimating reliability based on analysis of variance procedures. They present formulas for treating different components of variance as error or true variance depending on the nature of the data at hand. Hoffman (21) has devised some procedures based on curve-fitting techniques. His methods are appropriate for situations where learning or practice effects result in systematic changes in magnitude of response measures over trials.

Validity

Validity deals with the extent to which a test score or response measure correlates with some practical criterion measure. Generally speaking, validity refers to what a score measures and what it predicts. A score is valid for predicting anything it correlates with (excluding itself; self-correlation is a problem of reliability). Questions of validity are beginning to receive some deserved attention in the fields of psychoacoustics and speech and hearing research. Before going further with this discussion, we will digress briefly into the realm of theory to establish the rationale of validity. For a more thorough background in this subject, the reader is referred to Guilford (6, Chap. 13).

Multiple-Factor Theory. The implications of validity can best be understood by relating it to multiple-factor theory. Factor theory accepts the proposition that the variance of any distribution of test scores or response measures may be broken into true and error components. The *variance* of a distribution is the square of its standard deviation and is symbolized σ^2. The true variance of a measure is that portion of its total variance that is reliable, and the error variance is the remaining variance attributed to random variation in the scores—errors of measurement, in other words. This relationship is expressed by the formula:

$$\sigma_t^2 = \sigma_\infty^2 + \sigma_e^2$$

where

$$\sigma_t^2 = \text{total variance}$$

$$\sigma_\infty^2 = \text{true variance}$$

$$\sigma_e^2 = \text{error variance}$$

The true and error components are conceived to be quantities measured on the same scale as the obtained score. The error component is a positive or negative increment that depends on the measurement conditions at the time a particular individual was tested. Some of the factors that can contribute to error were listed above in the section on reliability. Sometimes it is possible to identify sources of error, but usually they are unknown.

The true component of variance is of most importance in the matter of validity. Factor theory holds that this (the true) component of variance may be broken down further into additive components. These are *common-factor* variances plus one other component called *specific variance*. Common-factor variances are those components of the total variance that are shared by other measures. Specific variance is that component of a measure's true variance that is not shared by any other measure. One of the basic equations of factor theory shows these relationships:

$$\sigma_t^2 = \sigma_a^2 + \sigma_b^2 + \sigma_c^2 + \cdots + \sigma_q^2 + \sigma_s^2 + \sigma_e^2$$

where

$$\sigma_t^2 = \text{total variance of an obtained measure}$$

$$\sigma_a^2 + \sigma_b^2 + \sigma_c^2 + \cdots + \sigma_q^2 = \text{common factor variances (where there are } q \text{ common factors)}$$

$$\sigma_s^2 = \text{specific variance}$$

$$\sigma_e^2 = \text{error variance}$$

If each term in this equation is divided by the total variance, the resulting expression shows the proportion of variance contributed by each component to the total variance.

$$\frac{\sigma_t^2}{\sigma_t^2} = \frac{\sigma_a^2}{\sigma_t^2} + \frac{\sigma_b^2}{\sigma_t^2} + \frac{\sigma_c^2}{\sigma_t^2} + \cdots + \frac{\sigma_q^2}{\sigma_t^2} + \frac{\sigma_s^2}{\sigma_t^2} + \frac{\sigma_e^2}{\sigma_t^2}$$

Simplifying and substituting less complicated terms for the proportions, we have:

$$1.0 = a_x^2 + b_x^2 + c_x^2 + \cdots + q_x^2 + s_x^2 + \epsilon_x^2$$

where $a_x^2, b_x^2, \ldots q_x^2 = $ proportions of variance contributed to measure x by the common factors a through q, and s_x^2 and $\epsilon_x^2 = $ the proportions of variance contributed by the specific and error components. Now the reliability r_{xx} of test x can be shown as a sum of the proportions of true variance:

$$r_{xx} = a_x^2 + b_x^2 + c_x^2 + \cdots + q_x^2 + s_x^2 = 1 - \epsilon_x^2$$

The components of variance that have to do with a measure's validity are the common factor variances a through q. The sum of these variances is known as the *communality* of a test or measure. Communality is symbolized by h^2. In equation form:

$$h_x^2 = a_x^2 + b_x^2 + c_x^2 + \cdots + q_x^2$$

Stated another way, communality is the proportion of true variance less the proportion of specific variance. Expressed in the form of an equation:

$$h_x{}^2 = r_{xx} - s_x{}^2$$

We have made this excursion into factor theory to provide a framework for understanding correlation relationships between sets of measures. When a correlation is found between sets of scores, it is a consequence of the overlap between components of common variance in the two sets of scores. If the variance in test x is made up of common variance components a, b, and g, and test y is made up of common variance components b, c, and f, a correlation will be found between the scores for x and y. More important, all of the correlation can be attributed to the fact that both test x and test y share some variance in factor b. None of the correlation can be attributed to the variance components s^2 or ϵ^2, since according to the theory, one test does not share its specific variance with any other test, and error variance is the result of random variation which cannot correlate with anything. (We can see another reason here for keeping the error variance in response measures at a minimum—another way of saying that reliability should be high. The greater the error variance, the less will be the amount of common variance available for correlation with other measures.) In this example test x can be said to be valid for predicting test y. The converse of this statement is also true. The direction of prediction depends on the logic of the situation.

Criterion Measures. None of the foregoing discussion indicates how we could determine the number of common variance components present in a given measure, nor has it been shown how these components might be identified. Various factor-analysis methods and multi-dimensional scaling techniques are available for dealing with these problems, but they are beyond the scope of this chapter (22–25).

There is more to a carefully planned validation study than merely correlating two variables. Ordinarily when a research program is undertaken to discover the validity of one or more response measures, for example, different measures of speech discrimination, a criterion measure is selected against which to evaluate the predictors (the response measures). The criterion is an independent measure of the class of responses under investigation. It is usually regarded in a logical sense as the ultimate measure of, or at least as an approximation to, the thing we are interested in (26, pp. 120$\textit{ff}$.). In practice, the complete ultimate criterion is seldom if ever available for use, and it is necessary to settle for an intermediate or partial criterion.

The usefulness of a criterion measure depends upon its *relevance* to the responses we are studying. By relevance we mean that the components of common variance in the criterion measure must arise from the same sources that make for successful performance of the response under study. The determination of relevance must rest on rational grounds; there is no higher appeal. The excellence of the rational analysis depends on the investigator's experience and wisdom. Unfortunately, a more dependable basis for evaluating criterion measure relevance is not available.

Relevance is the fundamental requirement for criterion measures. It would be desirable for all the true variance in a criterion measure to be relevant, but it is essential that a substantial portion of it be relevant. When there is irrelevant variance in the criterion measure, it is possible for one or more predictor variables to correlate with the criterion on the basis of the irrelevant variance. Such a situation would lead an investigator to conclude that the predictors were valid when in fact the correlations arose because of a faulty criterion measure. Suppose that in the previous example of the correlation between tests x and y, test x was the predictor and y was the criterion. In the example, the correlation was due to the fact that both x and y shared variance in the common component b. However, if the common component b were irrelevant, it would then be erroneously concluded that test x was valid for predicting criterion y.

A recent example of a validation study is one by High, Fairbanks, and Glorig (27). The object of this study was to determine the validity of measures of hearing impairment for a criterion of hearing handicap. The criterion in this case was defined as any disadvantage in the activities of everyday life that resulted from impaired hearing. The measure of hearing handicap was a score obtained by otological patients on a self-rating scale whose items dealt with various situations where impairment of hearing was judged to put a person at a disadvantage. The predictor variables were a number of currently used tests of hearing impairment, speech threshold, speech discrimination, thresholds for pure tones, etc.

Three of the predictor variables showed substantial correlations with the criterion measure. It was anticipated that a weighted combination of these variables entered into a multiple regression equation would yield a higher correlation than any of the three predictors taken separately. As it turned out, this was not the case. The reason was that the correlations *among* the predictors were nearly as great as the correlations *between* each predictor and the criterion. The interpretation was that the three predictors correlated with the criterion because the *same* component of common variance was shared by the three predictors and by the criterion. Had the correlations among the three significant predictors been zero or near zero, it would have been possible to account for a much larger portion of the relevant variance in the criterion. If the data had turned out this way, each predictor would have correlated with the criterion because each would have shared a *different* component of common variance with the criterion than did the others.

The area of clinical audiology appears to be in need of research designed to establish the validity of many of the current tests of auditory function and, further, to identify the sources of variance that give rise to the responses elicited by the tests. At present, there is little agreement concerning the best methods of test administration or even what the test material should be. Practice varies widely from clinic to clinic on matters of live-voice versus recorded-voice testing, psychophysical method of establishing thresholds, type of stimulus words used, scoring methods, and so on. Indeed, there is insufficient information available on which to base decisions about the appropriateness of different test methods and materials. The development of ways to test hearing impairment has proceeded much faster than have ways to evaluate the tests. Better criterion measures of hearing handicap would be helpful. Good criteria of handicap would provide the basis for determining the effect of different kinds and amounts of hearing impairment (as currently measured) on an individual's everyday activities. Admittedly, criterion development in the area of hearing handicap is a difficult task. The amount of handicap experienced by persons with hearing difficulty is influenced by numerous factors such as age, sex, occupation, education, personality, and emotional status. However, research effort invested in this area should provide a worthwhile return.

Factor Analysis and Psychoacoustics

Factor-analytic studies on batteries of psychoacoustical tests, clinical hearing tests, and measures of hearing handicap (when they become available) would provide useful information on the nature of the functional properties of the auditory perceptual system. Many tests of hearing ability in use today appear superficially to measure distinctly different aspects of hearing function. Yet high correlations are often found between these measures, suggesting that some test behaviors may be mediated by common underlying processes. Factor analysis of such tests could be used to identify the underlying factors, and the results could be used as a guide for reducing the number of tests needed to measure the domain. Where tests are found to overlap in function, it is often possible to eliminate some of them without losing coverage of the domain we wish to measure. Knowledge of the underlying functional processes might also make it possible to devise new tests to measure the factors more efficiently. The main advantages to be realized would be the identification of important auditory skills, economy of measurement, and the promotion of laboratory research on the conditions and variables that affect the basic auditory abilities. The major practical difficulty standing in the way of factor-analytic studies of auditory tests is the enormous testing time required. Many psychoacoustic tests must be administered individually and require much elaborate and expensive laboratory equipment. In spite of the difficulties, factor-analytic studies would appear to have much to contribute to the field of audiology.

A few factor-analytic studies designed to reveal the primary auditory abilities have been carried out (28–31). A series of similar studies is under way in the Medical Research Laboratory under the direction of J. D. Harris (32, 33). These studies have unfortunately not received the attention they deserve.

Response- versus Stimulus-Oriented Research

The preceding discussion has indicated that factor analysis is used to infer the basic capacities or abilities of individuals from their responses to test situations. The stimuli for the responses are the tests, but the tests are not ordered along a single continuum as is the case in a laboratory investigation. In the laboratory, for example, different stimuli selected from the dimension of intensity may be chosen for study. In a factor-analytic study, the tests (stimuli) may not lie along a single dimension, at least in the first stages of investigation. The test are selected so as to cover all of the abilities the investigator thinks are important in the area he is studying. The dimensions are inferred from the correlations among responses given to the tests. The attention of the investigator in this kind of study is centered directly on the responses, and for this reason it is sometimes called *response-oriented research*.

Stimulus-oriented research deals with the effects of systematic manipulation of stimuli on responses. Changes in behavioral responses are observed as a stimulus is varied along a particular dimension. Although this description may not do justice to some of the sophisticated research designs used today, it does point out the essential distinction between two types of research. (For other classes of research involving organismic and environmental variables see Brown (34, pp. 13*ff.*).) The distinction is important for understanding how cause-effect relationships are generated. Response-oriented research seeks to discover reliable dimensions along which behavior varies, and relationships among various sorts of responses. Cause-and-effect relationships cannot be established on the basis of correlations between response measures. Stimulus-oriented research, though, can provide evidence for at least low-level cause-effect relationships. Consider the following example. A series of acoustic stimuli differing only in frequency is presented to an individual. If, on the basis of his auditory experience, the individual is able to order the stimuli reliably along the frequency dimension, we would be justified in naming the experience and in attributing its apparent cause to the frequency of the acoustical signal. It should be recognized that there are more immediate physiological mechanisms mediating the experience. One may wish to attribute the causal mechanism to the cochlea, the central nervous system, biochemical processes, or to some hypothetical construct that relates the stimuli to the responses. At the empirical level where the experimental operations were carried out, however, the manipulation of the stimulus may be viewed as a genuine cause of the experience. Chains of cause-effect relationships begin with empirical laws relating stimulus variables to response measures.

The preceding discussion should not be construed as an indictment of response-oriented research. Investigations of the relationships among responses are useful for identifying significant dimensions of behavior and for developing efficient means of measuring these dimensions. When these dimensions have been properly identified, stimulus-oriented research can be undertaken to determine the variables and conditions that affect them. It is tempting to attribute causal status to factors or dimensions that may emerge from a factor-analytic study. However, this kind of speculation is difficult to justify unless there is independent evidence to demonstrate that the standing of individuals with respect to a factor can be changed by manipulation of some stimulus or environmental variable. For example, if a factor-analytic study of psychoacoustical tests were to identify a factor such as complex pitch discrimination (33), it would have to be shown that training, nutritional considerations, administration of drugs, or noise exposure were capable of changing an individual's scores on the tests from which the factor was inferred before it could be asserted that the factor of complex pitch discrimination was the cause of the test performance.

Ex Post Facto Research

Ex post facto research has long been discredited as an adequate method for discovering cause-effect relationships. In spite of its failure to meet the necessary scientific standards, this method continues to be used, possibly because our national habit of record keeping provides such an abundance of data. The idea behind ex post facto research is to select on the basis of existing records two or more groups of subjects which were supposedly equivalent at some time in the past but which were subsequently subjected to different "treatments" through the course of events. The investigator then makes some measurements on the subjects. If differences are found, they are attributed to the different "treatments." Much of the evidence relating cigarette smoking to lung cancer is based on this kind of study. While cigarette smoking may indeed be involved in a chain of cause-effect relationships leading to the development of cancer, it is all but impossible to establish the connection by ex post facto research. The reason is simply that there is no way to determine whether the smokers and non-smokers in ex post facto studies were selected randomly from the same population. Random selection means that each subject will have an equal chance of being assigned to any group.

Some investigators try to get around the problem of random selection in ex post facto research by matching subjects in the various groups on variables thought to be correlated with the experimental response. The purpose of matching is the same as for random assignment of subjects, i.e., to obtain equivalent groups. Matching is accomplished by selecting individuals for each group who are equal with respect to age, sex, intelligence, experience, or whatever variables are related to the response measure. For matching to be effective, it is essential for the matching variables to be related to the response that is measured following introduction of the experimental treatment. Nothing is accomplished by matching on variables that have nothing to do with the response measure. It is incumbent on the investigator to demonstrate the relevance of his matching variables. Merely assuming relevance is not sufficient. If the matching variables are in fact not relevant, one is left with the assumption that the groups are random. Such an assumption is hardly tenable, since the inevitable loss of subjects during matching tends to introduce a bias. Other problems of matched group experiments are discussed by Underwood (35).

The requirement for equivalent groups in ex post facto studies is unlikely to be overcome by matching procedures. No matter how many variables are matched, there is always the possibility that the groups may differ on other relevant variables which cause differences to arise in the response measure. Ex post facto studies may provide evidence for predicting responses on the basis of the "experimental treatment," but it is not possible to establish causal relationships from this kind of study.

In experimental studies that attempt to establish causal relationships between some environmental or stimulus variable and a class of responses, the usual procedure is to treat two or more groups of subjects differently. The object of these studies is to arrive at conclusions based on the effects of the different treatments on the groups. For the conclusions to be sound, it is necessary for the various groups to be equivalent with respect to relevant abilities, skills, and experiences, *except* for the treatments deliberately introduced by the investigator. If the groups are not equivalent, it should be clear that the logical basis for attributing response differences to experimental treatments is destroyed. The obtained results might well be a consequence of differences in abilities or experiences among subject groups not under control of the investigator. Failure to appreciate this principle is responsible for a surprising number of research errors.

The best way to obtain equivalent groups is to assign subjects randomly to the various groups. There are two common procedures for subject selection. One is to select subjects for each group randomly from a common population. The other is to assign the available subjects randomly to different groups without regard to the population from which they came.

The reasoning behind random selection is that statistically significant ability or experience differences among groups selected this way are unlikely to occur. The probability of a difference occurring at random can be determined with the mathematics of sampling theory. This is a statistical issue and is treated in many textbooks. Note that random selection is no guarantee against biases entering into the composition of the groups. However, it does make the probability of a large bias very small.

The problems of designing and carrying out a competent piece of research are many, subtle, and sometimes controversial. For the reader who wishes to pursue the topic further, two books are especially commended, one dealing with the methodology of research (36) and the other with psychometric methods (6).

REFERENCES

1. Campbell, N. R.: Symposium: measurement and its importance for philosophy. Aristotelian Soc. Suppl., Vol. 17, 1938.
2. Russell, B.: *Introduction to Mathematical Philosophy*, Ed. 2. The Macmillian Company, New York, 1920.
3. Russell, B. *The Principles of Mathematics*. W. W. Norton & Company, Inc., New York, 1937.
4. Young, J. W.: *Lectures on the Fundamental Concepts of Algebra and Geometry*. The Macmillian Company, New York, 1911.
5. Comrey, A. L.: An operational approach to some problems in psychological measurement. Psychol. Rev., *57:* 217, 1950.
6. Guilford, J. P.: *Psychometric Methods*. McGraw-Hill Book Company, Inc., New York, 1954.
7. Stevens, S. S.: Mathematics, measurement, and psychophysics. In *Handbook of Experimental Psychology*, edited by S. S. Stevens. John Wiley & Sons, Inc., New York, 1951.
8. Stevens, S. S.: On the theory of scales of measurement. Science, *103:* 677, 1946.
9. Metfessel, M.: A proposal for quantitative reporting of comparative judgments. J. Psychol., *24:* 229, 1947.
10. Stevens, S. S.: A scale for the measurement of a psychological magnitude: loudness. Psychol. Rev., *43:* 405, 1936.
11. Stevens, S. S., and Volkmann, J.: The relation of pitch to frequency: a revised scale. Am. J. Psychol., *53:* 329, 1940.
12. Coombs, C. H.: A theory of psychological scaling. Bull. Eng. Res. Inst. Univ. Michigan, 1952.
13. Anderson, Norman H.: Scales and statistics: parametric and nonparametric. Psychol. Bull., *58:* 305, 1961.
14. Senders, V. L.: *Measurement and Statistics*. Oxford University Press, New York, 1958.
15. Siegel, S.: *Nonparametric Statistics*. McGraw-Hill Book Company, Inc., New York, 1956.

16. Burke, C. J.: Additive scales and statistics. Psychol. Rev., *60:* 73, 1953.
17. Lord, F. M.: On the statistical treatment of football numbers. Am. Psychologist, *8:* 750, 1953.
18. High, W. S., Glorig, A., and Nixon, J.: Estimating the reliability of auditory threshold measurements. J. Auditory Res., *4:* 247, 1961.
19. Hoyt, C., and Krishnaiah, P. R.: Estimation of test reliability by analysis of variance technique. J. Exper. Educ., *28:* 257, 1960.
20. Rajaratnam, N.: Reliability formulas for independent decision data when reliability data are matched. Psychometrika, *25:* 261, 1960.
21. Hoffman, P. J.: Test reliability and practice effects. Psychometrika, *28:* 273, 1963.
22. Attneave, F.: Dimensions of similarity. Am. J. Psychol., *57:* 245, 1950.
23. Harman, H. H.: *Modern Factor Analysis.* University of Chicago Press, Chicago, 1960.
24. Thurstone, L. L.: *Multiple Factor Analysis.* University of Chicago Press, Chicago, 1947.
25. Torgerson, W. S.: *A Theoretical and Empirical Investigation of Multidimensional Scaling.* Educational Testing Service, Princeton, 1951.
26. Thorndike, R. L.: *Personnel Selection: Test and Measurement Techniques.* John Wiley & Sons, Inc., New York, 1949.
27. High, W. S., Fairbanks, G., and Glorig, A.: Scale for self-assessment of hearing handicap. J. Speech & Hearing Res., *29: 215, 1964.*
28. Drake, R. M.: Factorial analysis of music tests by the Spearman tetrad-difference technique. J. Musicol., *1:* 6, 1939.
29. Hanley, C. N.: Factorial analysis of speech perception. J. Speech & Hearing Disorders, *21:* 76, 1956.
30. Karlin, J. E.: Music ability. Psychometrika, *6:* 61, 1941.
31. Karlin, J. E.: A factorial study of auditory function. Psychometrika, *7:* 250, 1942.
32. Harris, J. D.: A search toward the primary auditory abilities. In ONR Decennial Symposium, *A Decade of Basic and Applied Science in the Navy,* pp. 244–254, 1957.
33. O'Hare, J. J., Harris, J. D., Ehmer, R. H., and Cohen, B. H.: Some primary auditory abilities in pitch and loudness. U. S. Med. Res. Lab. Rept. No. 316, Sept., 1959.
34. Brown, Judson S.: *The Motivation of Behavior.* McGraw-Hill Book Company, Inc., New York, 1961.
35. Underwood, B. J.: *Experimental Psychology.* Appleton-Century-Crofts, Inc., New York, 1949.
36. Underwood, B. J.: *Psychological Research.* Appleton-Century-Crofts, Inc., New York, 1957.

5

Audiometric Test Environment

William B. Snow, B.S., E.E.

An audiometric test environment must meet the noise-level requirements of the American Standards Association, have sufficient space to handle equipment for any type of test to be given, and permit adequate comfort for the subject.

NOISE

The degree of perfection achieved in meeting these specifications may vary according to local conditions, but the one factor which does not yield to compromise is noise. If the noise level is too high, audiometer test sounds will be masked, and a hearing loss will be reported, even in subjects with normal hearing. No amount of skill on the part of the audiometrist or cooperation on the part of the subject will eliminate this source of error. Consequently, obtaining adequate quiet is not a matter of convenience or feasibility. It is a necessity if meaningful hearing tests are to be made.

The key words are "adequate quiet." The definition of "adequate" depends upon the particular conditions of the test to be made. For example, if the open-ear hearing level of young adults is the desired objective, extremely low background noise levels must be achieved. But if the requirement is to be a reliable audiogram using standard audiometer earphones down to the zero hearing-level setting, a less stringent noise-level requirement is set. For a screening test at 2000, or 4000 cycles per second (c/s), 20-dB hearing level, additional noise can be allowed.

For several years, a committee of the Acoustical Society of America and the American Standards Association has been working on a set of specifications for noise levels in audiometry. The Standard has now been issued as the *American Standard Criteria for Background Noise in Audiometer Rooms, S3.1-1961*. Table 5.1 is adapted from this Standard. It shows the sound levels which will permit reliable testing for the conditions stated, and for measurement conditions which will be discussed later. This table is given only for illustrative purposes. The Standard itself should be consulted if an actual testing area is being set up.

Types of Noises

Broad-Band Noise. Broad-band noise results from a combination of many sound sources and is so called because energy is present over a wide range of frequencies. (This is the most common type found in locations where audiometry is usually done.) Those frequencies close to the specific one being tested cause the masking interference. In measuring noise for its interfering effect, it is necessary to divide the frequency range into bands that surround the test tones. With a broad-band noise, the actual width of the analysis bands is not critical as long as they contain the test tones. Usual analyses are made in octave, half-octave, or third-octave frequency bands.

Narrow-Band Noise. In addition to broad-band noise, audiometric noise problems involve narrow-band *noises* and *tones*. The energy of these *noises* is concentrated within a small frequency interval, or at a single frequency. When the narrow-band noise encompasses the test tone, interference is caused. If its frequency is remote from that of the test tone, however, higher ambient noise levels can be allowed. This type of noise must be measured with a narrow-band analyzer which will show its precise frequency and intensity. Examples of narrow-band noise are the screech from a machine part, or a burbling peanut whistle.

Table 5.1 shows a set of levels of much smaller magnitude in the last column representing the case of narrow-band noise. The actual masking energy at frequencies near the audiometer test tone is consistent for the two cases, however, and the numerical differences only reflect the differ-

TABLE 5.1

Maximum allowable sound pressure levels for no masking above the zero hearing level setting of a standard audiometer (decibels re 0.0002 microbar)

Audiometric Test Frequency	Octave Band Cut-off Frequency	Sound Pressure Level	Spectrum Level of Narrow-Band Sound*
c/s	*c/s*	*dB*	*dB*
125	75–150	40	21
250	150–300	40	18
500	300–600	40	15
1000	600–1200	40	12
2000	1200–2400	47	16
4000	2400–4800	57	23
8000	4800–10000	67	30

* Which has a center frequency which is nearly that of the test tone.

ences in frequency band width used in preparing the table. It is true that, on the basis of over-all sound level, a more stringent requirement is necessary for a narrow-band noise. All of its energy, concentrated near the test tone, cannot exceed the required masking level, whereas only a small region of a broad-band noise is held to this requirement.

Tones usually come from humming motors, electrical equipment, or machine gears. They have a peculiar property, that of causing negative interference. Through the phenomenon of beats, they can cause a lower threshold and actually give a hearing level reading that is false. Tones must, therefore, be treated even more critically than narrow-band sounds.

Vibration. Vibration alone does not cause interference with audiometry. It is, nevertheless, an important factor of environment. Vibrating walls, floors, or ceilings generate noise. A structure that is adequate to shield against airborne noise may be set into vibration, sufficient to cause interfering sound levels inside the building. The vibration of a subject's chair may also cause interference.

Measurement of Noise

Instrumental Measurements. Noise levels can be measured with a standard sound level meter and sound analyzer. The latter can be of the contiguous octave- or fractional octave-band type for broad-band noise, or of a tunable narrow-band type for that class of interference. Noise cannot be properly measured with a sound-level meter alone because this instrument does not give the necessary frequency analysis.

For those measurements, the microphone should be placed where the subject is to be. It is most important to measure the noise under the least favorable conditions, with all usual noise sources operating, and with street and corridor traffic, telephone bells, talking, etc., included. Air-conditioning equipment should be operating, and the people normally in the area should be working at their regular tasks. It is permissible to ignore infrequent sounds such as those of aircraft or trains unless they would occur while hearing measurements were being made.

The space will be satisfactory for audiometry (to zero hearing level) if the sound levels measured under these unfavorable conditions fall below those of Table 5.1.

Non-Instrumental Measurement (Adequate Listener). Another way of judging the effectiveness of an environment for audiometry is to employ an adequate listener. This is a person whose hearing level is known to be zero, or a minus value, at the test frequency under consideration, as measured with an audiometer. In this procedure, several adequate listeners are tested in the proposed audiometric area. If their audiograms show a significant deviation from their known thresholds, a quieter testing place should be located.

For tests of narrow-band noises and tones, the adequate listener is particularly useful. If, in the presence of interference, he is able to obtain at least a zero hearing level and, with the audiometer dial set at zero for each frequency, can satisfy himself that no beats are audible, the environment is probably satisfactory. If the audiometer is in the same room, he should be certain that no tone directly radiated by the audiometer is audible when he is wearing the earphones.

Adequate listeners should make tests to assure that low-frequency vibrations of the body do not introduce masking noise. With earphones on, each should rest his elbow on a table or chair arm, place his hand on his forehead, rest his head on the chair back, or assume any other appropriate testing position. If his threshold is raised by vibrational energy because of these bodily positions, they should not be allowed.

Repetition of Measurements. Noise-level measurements should be repeated frequently and periodically to eliminate the possibility of undetected increases in noise level. This is particularly true if there are significant changes in the activities or facilities surrounding the test site.

OBTAINING REQUIRED CONDITIONS

There are few locations which, without modification, are quiet enough for audiometry. The problem of attaining adequate quiet has four parts: (1) measuring the normal noise levels at maximum; (2) determining how much noise reduction is needed; (3) devising a method of obtaining this reduction; and (4) measuring the final noise level to see if it is satisfactorily low.

Steps 1 and 4 have been discussed in the preceding sections. The determination of how much noise reduction is needed (step 2) involves comparing the measured noise levels with those required (Table 5.1). This leaves for discussion the most important step in the problem: devising a method of obtaining this reduction.

Location. Frequently, a proposed space does not meet noise-level requirements, and modification of the area is necessary. Noise reduction is expensive, but in audiometry it can neither be dispensed with nor delayed. If *large* noise reductions are needed at the location chosen for testing, it may be necessary to consider an alternate location, or even to relocate the source of the noise. The inconvenience and expense of using an alternate location, or relocating the noise source, must be balanced against the cost of reducing the noise level of the chosen environment.

Acoustical Treatment. If the room proposed for audiometric tests has hard surfaces (plaster or wood walls and ceiling; wood, cement, linoleum, or asphalt tile floor; and little furniture), sound will be reflected because of the non-absorbent surfaces. The noise level can be reduced if these surfaces are covered by materials which absorb sound effectively and reduce the reflections. The amount of noise reduction obtainable in this way is between 5 and 10 dB.

Improvement of conditions is obtained by the use of acoustical tile on the ceiling, acoustical tile or heavy drapes on walls, and carpet on the floor. The last is especially important when others are in the room besides the subject. A 3- or 4-foot wainscoting below the tile on the walls is permissible to prevent marring. (A wainscoting of perforated hardboard backed by an absorbent blanket is both strong and acoustically effective.)

All audiometric testing rooms must receive heavy acoustical treatment. The noise reduction obtained in this way may be adequate in itself. Additional measures are usually required, however, but they are effective only to the extent that the testing space is already heavily absorbent.

Isolation. When greater noise reduction is required than can be obtained by acoustical treatment alone, sound isolation is employed. The testing space is separated from the outer surroundings by walls, and possibly by individual ceiling and floor isolated from the building. The characteristics of a sound isolator differ from those of a sound absorber. The sound isolator acts by reflecting most of the sound, and transmitting only a small part of it. An isolator is impervious, solid, and massive in relation to an absorber. For example, an open doorway represents the perfect absorber to the source room. All sound from the source room falling upon its area is "absorbed" because none is reflected. However, as an isolator to the receiving room, it has a zero value since all of the "absorbed sound" is transmitted directly through it. On the other hand, if the rooms were separated by 12 inches of armor plate, substantially all sound in the source room hitting the plate would be reflected back into the room, the plate would move very little, and almost no sound would be radiated from its opposite side into the receiving room. The isolation would be excellent.

Of course, the materials used as sound absorbers have some isolating value, and isolators have sound absorption. Practical problems are solved by the use of both. They may be combined, as in the wall panels used in prefabricated audiometric testing booths, or they may be installed separately. Both are present in successful installations, either by accident or design.

The sound isolation of walls increases slowly with weight. Doubling the weight adds only about 5 dB. Consequently, it is seldom justifiable to build walls thicker or heavier than the standard. High sound isolation is secured most economically by using double-wall construction with the two layers separated by an air space of 4 inches or more. With these double structures,

TABLE 5.2
Sample noise reduction values of common partitions

Construction	Section	Octave Band—c/s				
		150–300	300–600	600–1200	1200–2400	2400–4800
				dB		
2 x 4 studs, both sides ¼-in. plywood		20	25	29	33	35
2 x 4 studs, both sides ½-in. plaster-board		30	35	40	45	48
2 x 4 staggered studs, both sides metal lath and ¾-in. plaster		47	47	51	54	60
4-in. cinder block, one side plastered		33	38	43	48	53
4-in. concrete block, both sides plastered and 4-in. brick or concrete		41	46	51	56	61
8-in. brick		46	51	56	61	66
Two walls 4-in. cinder block, plastered on outside surfaces, spaced 4-in.		55	55	58	64	72

it is imperative to maintain complete separation except at the necessary supporting edges.

The construction of a sound-isolating enclosure where large reductions are necessary is not to be undertaken lightly. It requires a knowledge of materials and techniques, plus a meticulous attention to detail. (Information on this subject is impossible to summarize here, but is covered in detail in the publications of the additional reading list.) As an illustration of what may be expected, Table 5.2 gives data that have been measured on several wall constructions.

Special Considerations

Certain problems in noise level reduction occur so frequently in practice that they are considered "pitfalls," and care must be taken to give them careful consideration during design and construction.

Openings. The openings into a room are frequent sources of noise. Ordinary windows and doors are of lighter construction than walls and are hung loosely in their frames. Ventilation openings, clearances around pipes, and even electrical outlet boxes interconnecting two rooms are additional examples. If noise levels are too high in a room, these leakage sources should be investigated. Double windows can be employed; massive doors can be made to close on sealing strips; ducts can be treated acoustically or sound traps can be installed; and small openings can be sealed. No enclosure construction will be satisfactory unless the leakage paths are minimized. Here, again, it is not a matter of convenience. If the sound leakage is too great, the room will be unsuitable for audiometric testing.

Floors and Ceilings. The data of Table 5.2 apply to wall constructions for airborne noise. But a room is bounded also by floor and ceiling. It does no good to have superlative walls if noise enters through these horizontal surfaces, which are apt to be vibrating from intimate contact with machinery, building frame, or such impact sources as footsteps. It is an unfortunate fact that good isolation in floor and ceiling structures is hard to obtain. Therefore a crucial part of an audiometric test-room design is providing floor and ceiling surfaces that are in balance with the wall design.

Ventilation. Air in testing rooms must be piped in and exhausted through ventilating openings. It is possible, however, to preserve isolation despite these openings. To do so requires a very complex duct installation, the special problems of which must be solved in the process of room design.

Lighting. Some fluorescent lighting fixtures create high noise levels because of humming parts. It is possible to avoid this through the selection of quiet fluorescent units, or through the use of ordinary incandescent lights.

Supervision of Construction. Good design is essential, but it is not enough to ensure proper results. Unless the actual construction rigorously follows the plan, the expected noise reduction will not be obtained. Frequently the work is done by artisans who, unaware of the necessity for the special details of construction, do not follow the plans to the letter. Consequently, an unusual amount of supervision is necessary by someone who has authority to stop the work if it is not being done according to specifications. Inevitably, field decisions are necessary about unexpected situations, and the supervisor must be qualified to make these decisions according to sound acoustical principles.

Prefabricated Audiometric Rooms

When significant noise reduction is needed, the prefabricated audiometric room offers an extremely attractive solution. It is a special-purpose structure as carefully designed as the audiometer. The large engineering design cost is spread over a number of installations. Sizes and types are available for many situations and requirements, but all are made up from standardized parts. The rooms are quickly erected and are easily taken down and moved. The cost is fixed and is reasonable for the performance delivered. Probably the greatest single advantage of the prefabricated room is that the performance is standardized and consistent, and can be relied upon to be as expected. Because the manufacturer is delivering a complete package, he can guarantee a certain noise reduction. The new

TABLE 5.3

Sample noise reduction values of prefabricated audiometric rooms

Room	Octave Band—c/s						
	75–150	150–300	300–600	600–1200	1200–2400	2400–4800	4800–9600
	dB						
2-in. walls	18	25	35	41	46	48	46
4-in. walls	26	40	49	52	56	60	60

Standard specifies a method of measuring this performance. Thus the prefabricated room avoids all of the design problems and pitfalls of the locally built structure when performance requirements are severe.

Table 5.3 lists sample noise reductions for prefabricated audiometric test rooms of two "weights." Greater reductions can be obtained from double-walled units.

Noise Reduction Requirements

When the ambient noise levels have been measured in the chosen location, the required noise reduction can be determined.

Low Frequencies. Usually the requirements for noise reduction will be set by the lower frequencies. Table 5.1 showed that the octave-band levels allowed in the test space are lowest at these frequencies. This is because the earphone cushions provide relatively small noise shielding in this frequency range. Such shielding increases at higher frequencies.

Tables 5.2 and 5.3 have shown that the sound reduction of structures increases sharply at higher frequencies. Thus, added protection is afforded where higher levels are already allowable. Unfortunately, the characteristic ambient noise in a testing area is usually higher in the lower octave bands. Most isolation treatment gives less attenuation below 1000 c/s than above 1000 c/s, which is opposite to audiometric environmental needs.

Table 5.4 illustrates the resulting situation. Row *1* is repeated from Table 5.1, giving the allowed inside noise levels. Row *2*, from Table 5.3, gives the reduction of a prefabricated room with walls 2 inches thick. The sum, row *3*, is the noise level allowable outside the room. Row *4* shows a sample noise as it might exist where industrial audiometry is desired. This criterion is just met for 500 c/s in the 300- to 600-c/s band, but levels are much too high at 125 and 250 c/s. If these frequencies must be tested, an alternate site must be chosen.

Rows *5* and *6* indicate that a 4-inch room would be satisfactory at 250 c/s, but not at 125 c/s. In fact, obtaining 20-dB additional noise reduction

TABLE 5.4

Effects at low frequencies

Test Frequency (c/s)	125	250	500	1000	2000	4000
Octave Band (c/s)	75–150	150–300	300–600	600–1200	1200–2400	2400–4800
				dB		
1. Allowed band level (Table 5.1)	40	40	40	40	47	57
2. Reduction, 2-in. room (Table 5.3)	18	25	35	41	46	48
3. Allowable ambient level (Sum, 1 and 2)	58	65	75	81	93	105
4. Sample ambient noise level	86	80	75	70	67	64
5. Reduction, 4-in. room (Table 5.3)	26	40	49	52	56	60
6. Allowable ambient level (Sum, 1 and 5)	66	80	89	92	103	117

at this frequency would be complicated, and an alternate site would probably have to be found as an economical solution.

Note that at high frequencies both rooms give a considerable margin above the required noise reduction. This example brings home the real economic sense of excluding unnecessary low-frequency tests. Providing for them often will add considerably to the cost of the installation.

Safety Factors. The numbers in the preceding discussion are necessarily based upon averages, which means that in some situations the realized noise protection will be less than indicated. It is also a frequent occurrence that the real maximal external noise levels over a long period exceed those that could be observed during the measurements. It is prudent to be very conservative about selecting the noise-reduction requirements for audiometry. Allowing a safety factor of 10 to 15 dB in selecting the isolation method to be used is recommended.

Space and Comfort Requirements

In designing the audiometric test area, consideration must be given to equating the area available with the equipment to be included, and with the comfort of the persons using the room. In some instances, when new construction is being undertaken, this problem can be solved in the initial stages of design. When existent space is being converted or special provisions are being made, some adjustments are inevitable. Certain principles, however, hold for any type of audiometric testing environment:

1. The layout of the testing area should be such that the tester can see

the subject easily to note reactions and signals, and the subject can see the tester (if necessary). Under no circumstances however, should the subject be able to observe the tester's manipulation of the audiometer. False clues obtained in this way can invalidate the test, even though the subject uses the visual clues unintentionally.

2. The work area of the audiometrist should be planned to permit the use of equipment with a minimal amount of moving around and confusion, particularly if the audiometrist and the subject are in the same room.

3. The room must be acoustically "dead" to give the subject a feeling of being tested in an appropriate place. This condition is obtained by acoustical treatment, draperies, carpeting, and upholstered furniture. These are also necessary for efficient reduction of noise.

4. Ventilation and lighting are extremely important. An adequate supply of fresh air at a comfortable temperature and humidity should be supplied. If the test booth is occupied only occasionally and for short periods, a system of giving a thorough airing between testings may be found adequate. For relatively steady testing, a continuous air supply should be furnished. The placement of lights and the amount of light should be pleasant for the subject, and adequate for good viewing by the tester. "Noiseless" lighting is required and has been discussed previously in this chapter.

5. Comfortable chairs should be furnished for the audiometrist and the person being tested. Attention should be paid to the construction and condition of the furniture so there are no squeaks when the person adjusts his position.

Group Audiometry. If a test is to be administered to a group, the above discussion on comfort applies, but the specifications for the work area will differ. It is desirable for the tester to have a general view of the group. To reduce mutual distractions between subjects, it is also desirable to provide as much visual and acoustical isolation as possible for them. The floor should be carpeted to reduce foot-scuffling and chair-scraping noises. Partial cubicles of drapes or acoustically absorbent panels between subjects are recommended. At the minimum, the room must be arranged so that the subjects cannot observe each other's responses.

SUGGESTED ADDITIONAL READINGS

1. Beranek, L. L.: *Acoustics*. McGraw-Hill Book Company, Inc., New York, 1954.
2. Burris-Meyer, H., and Goodfriend, L.: *Acoustics for the Architect*. Reinhold Publishing Company, New York, 1951.
3. Cullum, D. G. W.: *The Practical Application of Acoustic Principles*. Spon Ltd., London, 1949.
4. Harris, C. M. (Editor): *Handbook of Noise Control*. McGraw-Hill Book Company, Inc., New York, 1957.

5. Knudsen, V. O., and Harris, C. M.: *Acoustical Designing in Architecture*. John Wiley & Sons, Inc., New York, 1950.
6. *Sound Insulation of Wall, Floor and Door Constructions*. National Bureau of Standards, Building Materials and Structures Report 144 (1955), with Supplement (1956), United States Government Printing Office, Washington.
7. *Industrial Noise Manual*. American Industrial Hygiene Association, 14125 Prevost, Detroit 27, Michigan, April, 1958.

6

Pure-Tone Audiometry

Scott N. Reger, Ph.D.

In this chapter "pure-tone audiometry" is discussed in relation to otological practice. From this viewpoint pure-tone measurements are employed principally to: (1) *assist* in making the diagnosis of auditory pathology (including malingering and psychogenic aberrations); (2) ascertain the type and severity of the impairment in relation to suitability for rehabilitative middle ear surgery (tympanoplasty or stapedioplasty); (3) periodically check the progress of auditory sensitivity following surgery or medication; and (4) serve as a guide in the selection of rehabilitative procedures for patients with handicapping irreversible hearing impairments.

It cannot be stated too often or too emphatically that the results of the hearing tests alone usually have limited diagnostic value. The principal diagnostic role of the functional hearing tests is restricted to anatomic localization of the pathology associated with the hearing involvement. For example, the results of the hearing tests on a given patient may indicate that the pathology responsible for the impairment is confined to the tympanic (or middle ear) structures. It must be recognized clearly that the phrase "tympanic impairment" or "tympanic pathology" does not designate a diagnosis but an anatomic site in the auditory system. The diagnosis usually can be made only after evaluation of the ear history and physical examination in relation to the results of the hearing tests. A patient with tympanic pathology, based on the results of the hearing tests, will be diagnosed as having otosclerosis, otitis media, eustachian salpingitis, or some other type of tympanic disease, ascertained by the history and physical examination. This concept of the anatomic-localization implications of the functional hearing tests is developed elsewhere in more detail by Reger and Kos (1).

Both the pure-tone and speech tests make indispensable contributions to the anatomic localization of certain auditory pathologies, such as "central" impairment. Frequently, the quantitative relationships between the hearing levels for pure tones and the speech-reception threshold and articulation measures provide the significant localization clues. For example, if a patient has normal sensitivity for air-conducted pure tones but experiences difficulty in understanding speech, it may be assumed that his peripheral auditory mechanism possesses normal function.

Pure tones are uniquely suited for making threshold sensitivity measurements for the following reasons: (1) a pure tone is the simplest type of auditory stimulus. It can be described adequately in terms of its frequency and intensity, each of which can be controlled with a high degree of accuracy. The listener's task is correspondingly simple. He indicates only when he does and does not hear the tone. Usually he is not requested to describe any of its properties or to attach meaning to it. Unfortunately, most speech sounds are rather complex. And the frequency and intensity composition of speech sounds vary rapidly from instant to instant within most words. In addition, the listener usually is required to prove that he recognizes the speech stimuli by pronouncing or writing them or by pointing to pictures of words that are presented acoustically to him. For these reasons, pure-tone stimuli are especially useful for obtaining sensitivity measurements on patients with limited speech discrimination ability, such as those with severe hearing impairments and those with central pathologies due to accidental brain damage or degeneration of brain cells with age (phonemic regression). (2) Some patients may have approximately normal responses to speech but at the same time have high-frequency defects which are of prognostic significance. Most of the essential speech sounds are included within a frequency range of about 300 to 3000 cycles per second (c/s). Consequently, high-intensity-level occupational noise or toxins may produce considerable permanent damage to hearing at 4000 or 6000 c/s before the injury is apparent and before the injury can be detected by presently available speech tests. Pure-tone measurements at 4000 and 6000 c/s constitute a more sensitive monitor of the cumulative effect of noise on the ear than speech tests. (3) Changes in threshold sensitivity associated with various middle ear surgical procedures can be evaluated more precisely with the pure-tone than the speech tests. For example, the high-frequency sensitivity of some patients may be worse (decreased) after certain types of middle ear surgery than before the surgery. The relative merits of different surgical and prosthetic techniques can be evaluated in more detail at different frequency levels with the pure tone than with other kinds of measurement.

Certain *supra-threshold* reactions to special pure-tone tests also possess significant anatomic localization value. Among these reactions are the following: (1) diplacusis; (2) recruitment; (3) pathological temporary threshold drift; (4) changes in loudness associated with occlusion; (5) tone quality; and (6) middle ear impedance.

The principal limitation of the pure-tone tests is their inadequacy to predict ability to understand speech in certain types of mediotympanic pathologies with as much accuracy as does the direct measurement of speech perception.

THRESHOLD TESTS

Pure-Tone Air-Conduction (AC) Threshold Audiometry

The term "threshold" commonly refers to a place or point of entering or beginning. From the audiological point of view, the threshold of audibility is a statistically determined minimal intensity on the stimulus scale which is just barely adequate to elicit a response.

The auditory threshold is not an invariable fixed intensity above which sound is always heard and below which sound is never heard. The sensitivity of the auditory mechanism in an individual person is in a continuous state of flux, varying with interactions between certain psychological, physiological, and physical factors. (The more significant of these will be identified later.) The threshold may be regarded as an intensity range or zone of auditory uncertainty a few dB wide, within which sound stimuli at or near the statistically determined threshold sometimes are perceived and sometimes not perceived. (See Chapter 3.)

Method of Limits—Laboratory Technique. The procedure of choice for measurement of threshold sensitivity with a high degree of accuracy usually is the classical psychophysical *method of limits* (also called the method of minimal changes). This technique necessitates the use of a gain control over an intensity range sufficiently great to permit stimuli to be presented definitely above and below the listener's threshold. The intensity steps of the gain control should be smaller than the listener's difference limen for intensity. Step gain controls 1 dB in intensity, or even stepless controls (those having continuously variable intensity), are suitable. (A gain control is an intensity or volume control with the numerical markings on its dial correlated with its output so that increasing intensity is indicated by progressively larger numbers, such as the hearing level controls on most clinical audiometers. The reverse is the case with attenuators, in which the larger the number on the indicator dial, the lower the intensity of the output of the attenuator.)

In the following description of the method of limits, it is assumed that the gain control has an intensity range of 30 dB or more in 1-dB or smaller steps, and that the test tone is presented to the subject in an earphone. It also is assumed that the tests are conducted in a suitable noise-free environment. The subject is requested to indicate with a pre-arranged signal whenever and as long as he can hear the tone. The tones will be presented as pulses, from $\frac{1}{2}$ to 2 sec. in duration. Silent intervals between tones usually extend from $\frac{1}{2}$ to 5 sec.

Initially, the tone is presented above the threshold and then decreased in intensity from audibility to inaudibility in 1-dB steps or decrements until it can no longer be heard or detected (descending series). The minimal intensity setting of the gain control at which the tone is perceived is noted by the experimenter. The intensity is then increased from inaudibility to audibility in 1-dB steps or increments until the tone is perceived (ascending series). The minimal intensity at which the tone in the increasing intensity series is heard also is noted.

An equal number of the decreasing intensity and of the increasing intensity series are presented to the subject, the exact number being determined in advance in the design of the experiment. The threshold of the subject is obtained by averaging the minimal intensity levels at which the tone is heard on the decreasing intensity and the increasing intensity series and then calculating the mid-point between these two intensity values.

Not unexpectedly, the average minimal level heard on the decreasing intensity series is lower than the minimal level heard on the increasing intensity series. The measurements usually show an overlapping or criss-crossing of the data obtained on the decreasing intensity and the increasing intensity series. For example, the average of the intensity settings on the decreasing intensity series might be at the 19-dB intensity level and at 25 dB on the increasing intensity series. The threshold value in this instance is the sound intensity produced by the earphone when the gain control is set at 22—the mid-point between 19 and 25.

If the above average intensity values coincided with the comparable averages obtained on a statistically adequate group of young adults who presented negative ear histories and negative physical ear examinations, the data could be used for audiometer calibration purposes. To do so, the above statistically determined threshold—a gain control setting of 22—would be assigned a value of zero hearing level. The sound intensity produced at this setting would be measured by means of physical instruments and expressed in units of sound pressure—dynes per square centimeter. This sound pressure then would be used as the zero hearing-level reference for the test tone in an artificial ear, which is used to measure the sound-pressure outputs from audiometer earphones.

Obviously, the laboratory or research application of the method of limits is an exacting, time-consuming technique. For clinical use, the procedure usually is modified considerably (sometimes beyond recognition).

Method of Limits—Clinical Technique. (This is also called combined method.)

Instructions to the Patient. The patient is informed that one ear will be tested at a time—the better ear first. He is told that he is to listen for several tone pulses, some of which will be comfortably loud and some very, very "soft." He is instructed to signal—raise a finger or a hand or push on a signal key—whenever and as long as the tone can be heard. It is important to emphasize to the patient that the signal is to be given as soon as the sound is heard and not released until the sound is no longer heard. This type of sustained signal response will enable the examiner to differentiate between patient responses to sustained test tones and spurious gain control contact noise or other type of transient noise. Tinnitus also is often the cause of continuous prolonged responses while the tone is off.

The examiner and the patient should be seated so that the examiner can watch the patient's hand and the side of his face. The patient must not be able to see the examiner manipulate the control dials of the audiometer. The examiner must be so familiar with his audiometer and testing procedure that his attention is focused on the patient's responses rather than on the operation of the instrument.

Before placing the earphones over the patient's ears, make certain that the audiometer tone-interrupter key is in the "off" position and the hearing level dial is set at a low intensity level. The earphones should be fitted with a fairly strong spring-tension headband and earphone cushions which permit a firm but comfortable fit over the auricles and against the sides of the head. Tightly fitting earphone cushions attenuate room noise several dB and ensure close or tight acoustic coupling to the tympanic membrane, which is absolutely necessary to obtain accurate threshold measurements at the lower frequency levels. (The degree of coupling is a less important factor at frequency levels above about 1000 c/s.) Eyeglasses with large heavy temple pieces should be removed during the test so that the cushions will fit more snugly against the sides of the head.

Present the 1000-c/s tone first to the "better" ear in the following manner. While the tone interrupter is in the "off" position, set the frequency-selector dial at 1000 c/s and the hearing level dial at the 40-dB position. Then turn the tone interrupter to the "on" position. If the patient responds to the tone, turn it off and set the hearing level dial at 30 dB and turn on the tone at this level. If the patient responds, turn the tone off and set the hearing level at 20 dB and turn the tone on again, and so on, in successive 10-dB lower hearing levels until the patient fails to respond. If the patient does not respond at the 20-dB hearing level, increase the level to 25 dB. If the patient responds when the tone is turned on at the 25-dB level, decrease the hearing level in 5-dB steps until the patient no longer responds. Then increase the hearing level in 5-dB steps until a new response is obtained.

The threshold will be the lowest intensity or hearing level at which the patient responds two or three times out of three trials, two or more times out of four trials, or three or more times out of five trials on an increasing intensity series. Three increasing intensity trials will be sufficient to obtain a clinically reliable threshold if the patient makes consistent responses. If the patient makes frequent wrong responses because of tinnitus or for other reasons, a greater number of trials will be necessary before the examiner can form a reliable estimate of the threshold sensitivity.

If the patient does not respond at the 40-dB hearing level, turn the tone off, set the hearing level at 60 dB, and turn the tone on. If the patient still does not respond, increase the hearing level in 10-dB steps until a response is obtained. As soon as a response is obtained, decrease the hearing level in 5-dB steps until the tone is no longer heard. Then increase the hearing level of the tone in 5-dB steps until a uniform response is obtained on two or more increasing intensity series as described in the preceding paragraph. The threshold value recorded on the audiogram is the minimal hearing level at which the patient consistently responds to half or more of the pulse presentations on a given increasing intensity series.

This attenuated version of the method of limits is favored by many competent examiners. Carhart and Jerger (2) give a detailed analysis of this modification, plus an evaluation of other variations of the procedure.

If the patient's responses become somewhat erratic as the test progresses, it is advisable to present the tone again at a 10-dB higher level than his "apparent" threshold to refresh his memory of the nature of the test tone. Experienced examiners vary the duration of the tone presentation, and of the silent intervals between tones, to avoid a rhythmical "on-off" pattern which will induce the listener to make incorrect anticipatory responses. Randomized tone durations of ½ to 2 sec. and silent intervals of ½ to 5 sec. are recommended.

Some examiners prefer to obtain the threshold by means of the *decreasing-intensity* series. In this approach the tone is presented 10 or 15 dB above the patient's apparent threshold and then decreased in 5-dB steps until the patient stops responding. The lowest hearing level at which the patient responds is noted. The tone is then presented 10 dB above this level and again decreased in 5-dB steps until response ceases. The recorded threshold is the minimal identical hearing level at which the patient responds to the tone on one half or more of three or more separate decreasing intensity series.

Many examiners prefer to average the minimal hearing levels of the responses as the tone is (1) decreased from audibility to inaudibility and (2) increased from inaudibility to audibility. If this approach is used, the *decreasing-intensity* series should be presented first, followed by the *increasing-intensity* series, and so on alternately until a minimum of at least four threshold crossings have been completed. (An equal number of de-creasing- and increasing-intensity series should be presented.) The recorded threshold is the intensity value midway between the averages of the de-creasing-intensity series and the averages of the increasing-intensity series.

It is apparent that this procedure is identical to the classical psycho-physical *method of limits*. However, a 5-dB intensity step is considerably larger than that recommended for use in this approach. As a matter of fact, a 5-dB intensity step is so large that little or no significant difference in threshold measurements results from testing by means of the increasing-intensity series, the decreasing-intensity series, or the combined decreasing-and increasing-intensity series.

Many clinical pure-tone audiometers are equipped with stepless or continuously variable intensity-gain controls. (In some of these controls there are small discrete intensity increments which are below the intensity difference limen. For practical purposes they may be regarded as stepless.) Such audiometer hearing-level dials usually are marked in 5-dB step in-tervals. The examiner using this type of instrument has a choice between presenting the tones at the 5-dB intervals as indicated or presenting the tones at intensities between the 5-dB step markings.

The stepless type of control must be manipulated with caution. At first thought it seems logical and advantageous, while using such a control, to decrease the intensity gradually from audibility to inaudibility without interrupting the tone. This approach usually is responsible for inaccurate threshold values. The patient may be responding to tinnitus long after the tone has been decreased below his true threshold. A significant amount of adaptation may occur if the tone is sustained above the threshold for a few seconds. On the stepless increasing-intensity series, the patient may not become aware of the tone until it is several dB above his threshold value for that of an interrupted tone, as a result of the "on effect" associated with the sudden presentation of an interrupted tone. Variations in the velocity (decibels per second) with which the stepless control is rotated also introduces an additional variable which is difficult to control manually.

If the examiner wishes to obtain a threshold measurement at intensity levels between the 5-dB dial markings, it is recommended that the in-tensity of the tone be altered in 1- or 2-dB intervals, and that the tone be turned on and off with the tone-interrupter key as described above.

It also is advisable to turn the tone off before changing the setting of the hearing level dial to minimize contact noise transients originating in the control. This is essential while testing patients with severe impairments for high-frequency tones but who have normal or near-normal sensitivity for low frequencies.

Most examiners start the test at 1000 c/s. The hearing levels are next measured at 2000, 3000, 4000, and 8000 c/s in the order named. Then the measurement is repeated at 1000 c/s (if the first measurement was below normal) and extended to the successively lower test frequencies. (The threshold for 1000 c/s may be at a 5- to 10-dB lower intensity when the test is repeated at this frequency.)

Some examiners prefer to test the sensitivity for the lower frequencies first. The best technique for a given examiner is the one in which he has the most confidence, based on his study of the different approaches and the results of his personal experience with them. However, it is comforting to have a rational reason or explanation for adherence to a certain procedure.

Modification of technique is necessary if the patient is unable to follow the response instructions because of age or short memory span, or for another reason. The following modification is recommended for testing such individuals: remove an earphone-cushion assembly from the headband and hold it in the hand. With the tone "on" at the 40-dB hearing level, ask, "Can you hear a sound?" and then position the earphone tightly over the auricle and against the side of the head. If the patient indicates "yes," the earphone is removed, the intensity of the test tone attenuated, and the earphone again positioned as before. The tone-presentation sequence described earlier can be used. The question, "Can you hear it now?" can be asked just before the earphone is held in place. To counteract the suggestibility of children, it is necessary to avoid an "on-off" alternating sequence and to ask, "You can't hear it now, can you?" when the tone is presented at an occasional above threshold intensity level.

If the auditory sensitivity is normal at 1000 c/s, it can be assumed with a high degree of confidence that the hearing is normal for lower frequencies, especially in those patients with negative ear histories and negative physical examinations. However, normal response at 1000 c/s does not form a reliable basis for predicting the sensitivity at higher frequency levels. This characteristic of the auditory threshold is described by Glorig and House (3) and by Hanley and Gaddie (4).

Pure-Tone AC Masking Procedures. Threshold measurements on patients with unilateral hearing impairments present special problems. The examiner must be certain during the testing procedure that high intensity level sounds presented to the defective ear are not perceived in the "better" ear—the non-test ear. To avoid this source of error, a masking noise is used over the non-test ear while obtaining the measurements in order to make certain that the test tones are perceived only in the ear which is being tested.

The intensity calibration of masking noises in terms of *effective masking* possesses certain serious limitations. The amount of masking indicated on the noise-gain control dial assumes that the noise is applied to a normal ear.

The dial reading therefore is incorrect when the noise is applied to a "better" ear with a significant hearing impairment. Also the indicated amount of effective masking is misleading while making bone-conduction (BC) measurements. This is due to the fact that the effective masking concept compensates for the AC shadow curve (approximately 50 dB), whereas the BC shadow curve is so small it is insignificant. Also, placement of a masking-noise earphone over a normal middle ear increases the BC sensitivity in such an ear by several dB, especially at frequency levels below 2000 c/s. Unfortunately, the effective masking level indicated on the dial can be relied on only while making AC measurements on unilateral impairments.

In the present discussion it is assumed that the intensity control of the masking noise is calibrated in 5- or 10-dB steps above the zero hearing level of the masking noise. If this is not the case, it is possible to estimate the hearing levels of the masking noise by comparing and balancing the loudness levels of the noise with the loudness of the audiometer's 1000-c/s tone at various hearing levels for this tone. A masking noise equal in loudness to a 1000-c/s tone at a hearing level of 60 dB permits a quantification of the level of the masking noise which is more meaningful than stating that the masking noise control dial was set at one half on, three fourths on, or at the three o'clock position, the eight o'clock position, etc. It is desirable that the maximal intensity of the masking noise reach a hearing level of at least 100 dB.

Most masking noises are exceedingly complex, containing a wide randomized frequency distribution so that the noise will ensure masking over the audiometric frequency range. One of the most effective masking noises is a thermal noise (also called white noise), which is generated by the random electron emission of specially designed electronic circuits.

It has been learned that the shift of threshold sensitivity for a given frequency due to masking results from the energy in the components of the noise which coincide and are immediately adjacent to that frequency. For example, if the threshold for a 1000-c/s tone has been shifted 50 dB by wide-band noise, the randomized frequency components in this noise from about 980 to 1020 c/s have been most instrumental in producing the shift. Since the noise components outside this narrow band contribute significantly to the over-all loudness of the noise without contributing much to its masking effectiveness, narrow-band masking noises are preferred for masking purposes. Broad-band masking noise must be presented at a decidedly higher intensity (and loudness) level than narrow-band noise to produce the same threshold shift, especially at the lower frequency levels. This is due to the fact that the normal ear is significantly less sensitive to frequencies below about 500 c/s than to frequencies from about 500 to 4000 c/s. Broad-band noise would be around 20 dB above the threshold before the 250-c/s components of the noise became audible and begin shifting the threshold at this frequency.

Unfortunately, narrow-band masking noises are considerably more expensive than other types of noises. Narrow-band masking noises usually are obtained by filtering broad-band noise or by means of tuned circuits. A separate narrow-band masking noise is required for each test frequency produced by the audiometer. Clinical studies evaluating the effectiveness of narrow-band noise have been made by Liden, Nilsson and Anderson (5) and by Rittmanic (6).

As stated earlier, it is advisable to test the AC sensitivity of the better ear first in patients with noticeable differences in threshold sensitivity between ears. If the measurements on the defective ear indicate that the difference between the ears is as great as 40 dB or more, the possibility exists that the patient is hearing the tone in his good ear, in which case the responses obtained without masking are false and constitute a shadow curve. Considerable variation in the magnitudes of shadow curves has been noted.

Given a patient with normal threshold sensitivity in the right ear and an apparent loss of 50 dB in the left, the following masking procedure is recommended: (1) after testing the good ear, inform the patient that you must test the hearing in his worse ear while a loud noise is heard in his good ear and that he is to signal only while he hears the pure tone. Tell him the noise will have very little effect on his ability to hear the pure tone. (2) Before turning on the masking noise in the non-test ear, obtain a threshold at 1000 c/s without regard to the ear in which the tone is heard. This maneuver alerts the patient to the pitch of the tone for which he is to respond and gives the examiner a pure-tone unmasked base line against which to evaluate the effect of masking. This unmasked threshold should be recorded lightly on the audiogram blank. (3) Introduce a 50-dB hearing-level masking noise in the earphone over the normal ear and obtain the threshold for the test tone. A 50-dB hearing-level masking noise will induce a shift of about 25 dB in the normal ear. The exact value is partly a function of the type of masking noise used. The shift will be greater than 25 dB if a 50-dB hearing-level narrow-band masking noise is used. If the masked hearing level for the tone is increased only 5 or 10 dB (to the 55- or 60-dB hearing level in this particular patient), it may be concluded that this 55- or 60-dB value is not a shadow curve but the correct threshold value, which is the hearing level recorded on the audiogram. A notation should be made recording the level of the masking noise used while obtaining the measurement. (4) If presentation of the 50-dB hearing level masking noise shifts the apparent sensitivity of the ear under test by more than 25 dB, increase the masking noise to the 70-dB hearing level. If now the hearing level is shifted by another 20 dB, next present the masking noise at the 80-dB hearing level and so on until the pure-tone hearing level remains stabilized or is no longer heard. If the test tone is not heard at the 100-dB level (the maximal value on most clinical audiometers) when the masking noise is increased to high values, it may be assumed that the patient's hearing loss for the test tone is in excess of the 100-dB hearing level.

Most types of masking noises at the 80-dB hearing level provide sufficient masking to permit accurate AC measurements on patients with one normal ear and one non-functioning ear. It is well to keep in mind that when a broad-band masking noise and a pure tone are presented simultaneously to the same normal ear, the level of the masking noise must be increased to about the 20-dB hearing level before an appreciable shift in the pure-tone threshold results. This means that the first 20-dB increase above threshold of the masking noise produces very little masking or threshold shift of the pure tone. At higher intensity levels (above 20 dB), given dB increases in the level of the masking noise result in approximately equal increases in the amount of masking or threshold shift of the test tone—a linear relationship.

If a patient has a 30-dB AC loss in the right ear and an 80-dB loss in the left, it is obvious that a 50-dB hearing-level masking noise in the right ear would be only 20 dB above his threshold—which would not be a very effective masking noise level. When a patient presents a loss of 30 dB or more in his better ear and a difference of 40 dB or more between the ears, the initial presentation of the masking noise usually should start at the 60-dB level (which would be only 30 dB above the threshold of a patient with a 30-dB hearing impairment).

After obtaining the masked threshold of a given test tone in the worse ear, the masking noise should be turned off, and the procedure outlined above repeated for the next tone. Turning off the masking noise between presentations of the different test tones avoids undue annoyance and exposure to the masking noise. It will be noted that the procedure recommended above enables the examiner to learn when a sufficiently high-intensity level masking noise has been employed to ensure valid pure-tone measurements. When given dB increases in the intensity of the masking noise at high intensity levels fail to shift the pure-tone sensitivity by equal amounts, it may be assumed that a sufficiently high intensity level masking noise has been employed.

Recommended symbols for recording test results on the audiogram blank will be described later.

Pure-Tone AC Sources of Error. Among the factors which influence the reliability of pure-tone audiometer test results are the following: (1) the accuracy of the calibration of the audiometer; (2) the magnitude of the masking effect of ambient noise in the testing environment, which includes noise produced by the audiometrist, the patient, and any sound in the receiver resulting from operation of the audiometer other than the desired test tone; (3) failure to use effective masking to avoid shadow curves in unilateral hearing impairments; (4) position and pressure (coupling) of the sound reproducer in relation to the auricle or bones of the head; (5) physical conditions within the test room which influence body comfort, such as temperature, humidity, barometric pressure, altitude, and time of day; (6) age, intelligence, reaction time, and previous test experience of the patient; (7) physiological condition and mental attitude of the patient (alert, interested, relaxed, cooperative, drowsy, indifferent, lethargic, depressed, fatigued, tense, apprehensive, or antagonistic); (8) training, experience, insight, and personality of the audiometrist; (9) the complexity of the stimulus-presentation technique used in the determination of the auditory sensitivity; (10) ambiguity of response instructions to the patient; and (11) the use of complex recording methods.

Patients who experience tinnitus or auditory after-images, malingerers, and those with hysterical abnormalities present additional test difficulties. (See Chapters 3, 8, 10, and 11.)

Pure-Tone Bone-Conduction (BC) Threshold Audiometry

General Considerations. The response instructions and tone-presentation technique of AC threshold measurements are suitable for obtaining the BC threshold sensitivity measurements. The BC vibrator must make firm contact with the mastoid (or forehead) without touching the auricle. The loudness with which certain sounds are heard by BC will vary markedly as the pressure of the vibrator against the skull is varied from light to firm contact. However, when the pressure becomes sufficiently firm to ensure effective coupling of the vibrator to the skull, considerably greater additional pressure results in relatively small changes in the loudness. Unfortunately, most of the light, thin headbands supplied for use with audiometer BC vibrators do not hold the vibrator against the mastoid with sufficient pressure to ensure an effective transfer of vibrational energy to the skull. This deficiency can be improved by reinforcing the headband with a second one, or by having a mechanic construct a more rugged tension headband for use with the vibrator. The desired pressure is reached when additional pressure applied by a finger against the BC vibrator, which is in contact with the head, does not increase the loudness with which the sound is heard. This desired pressure is not at all painful to the patient. It is not advisable to permit the average patient to hold the vibrator against his skull since he probably would be unable to hold it against the same spot or with a constant pressure for the desired length of time. Holding the vibrator against the skull by hand also may introduce a certain amount of masking noise from muscle tremors and friction noise at the point of contact. Unfortunately, BC vibrator headbands which are adjustable to different size and shape heads, and which are equipped with pressure-indicating devices, are not commercially available at the present time. The use of such laboratory headbands in research studies permits repeat BC measurements on a given group of subjects which are approximately equal in accuracy to repeat AC measurements on the same group.

Sophisticated examiners always keep in mind the following facts about the hearing of sound by BC in order to obtain valid BC measurements and interpret them with clinical usefulness. (1) Individuals with normal AC also have normal BC. (2) Theoretically, it is impossible to have a greater dB loss for BC than for AC. However, an occasional patient (usually an elderly individual) is encountered who does appear to have greater losses for BC than for AC, particularly at frequencies below 1000 c/s. This interesting phenomenon is recognized clinically as disproportionately decreased BC. (3) The BC shadow curve has a value of only a few dB and may be zero or appear to have a negative value in certain instances. (4) Patients with unilateral tympanic pathologies usually lateralize BC sound to the involved ear. (5) Patients with unilateral cochlear or neural involvements usually lateralize BC sound to the better ear. (6) Patients with tympanic pathologies have impairments for AC sound but have normal BC sensitivity. (7) Patients with cochlear or neural pathologies have equal or identical AC and BC thresholds. (8) Patients with mixed or combined tympanic and medio-tympanic pathologies have losses for both AC and BC but greater losses for AC than for BC. (9) The maximal AC loss associated with normal BC is approximately 60 dB. This means that in the extreme cases with a 60-dB range between the AC and normal BC thresholds, masking noises above the 60-dB hearing level stimulate the ear by BC. This indicates that masking noises above such a patient's threshold will stimulate the BC thresholds in both ears at the same time owing to the nature of the BC shadow curve. In such patients the ear under test will be masked also, resulting in erroneous BC threshold sensitivity measurements. Zwislocki (7) and von Békésy (8) have shown that the interaural sound attenuation can be markedly increased by presenting sounds with the hearing-aid-type insert earphone or receiver.

The examiner must be aware of the possibility that patients with severe hearing losses for BC sound may respond to the vibrator with the vibration sense (pallesthesia) before the BC threshold is stimulated, thereby giving a false result. The vibration sense is much more sensitive to tones below 1000 c/s than to those at higher frequencies. If it is suspected that the patient is perceiving the tone as vibration and not sound, the vibrator should be held by the examiner with firm pressure, first against the mastoid (or forehead) and then against the styloid process of the radius bone (near the wrist). If identical sensations are experienced at both the mastoid and the distal end of the radius (or other bone away from the head), it is highly probable that the sensation perceived at the mastoid is that of vibration and not sound. A response of "vibration" or "feeling" can be indicated on the audiogram by recording "F" at the frequency and intensity level at which the "feeling" sensation occurs.

Before attempting to measure the BC sensitivity in either ear, it is usually advisable to perform the equivalent of the Weber bone-conduction lateralization test with the audiometer BC vibrator. *This is not a threshold test.* Position the vibrator by means of its headband in firm contact with the mid-line of the forehead, and tell the patient you wish to learn if he hears sounds through the bones of his head in one ear or both ears. Inform him in advance that he might hear sound only in the worse ear, only in the good ear, in both ears at the same time, or in the middle of his head or forehead. Present the tone at the desired frequency, and adjust the intensity until the patient hears the tone at a comfortable listening level. The examiner must make certain that the patient is hearing the tone at a comfortable listening level before asking him in which ear it is heard. At the bottom of the audiogram, record the ear in which each of the tones generated by the audiometer is heard (Fig. 6.1). The patient whose audiogram is shown in this figure had normal hearing in the right ear and an approximate AC loss of 30 dB over the audiometric frequency range in the left ear. The history and physical examination indicated otitis media in the left. To this patient's surprise, the 125-, 250-, 500-, and 1000-c/s tones were heard only in the affected ear and the 2000- and 4000-c/s tones were heard in the middle of his head. In such a patient, in which the history and physical examination are definitive, it is not necessary to use masking to obtain a clinically useful audiogram. It is not necessary to obtain BC threshold measurements on the right normal ear since it is axiomatic that BC sensitivity will be normal in the normal ear. If the patient has the same history and physical findings in each ear, presents approximately identical bilateral AC hearing levels in both ears, and does not lateralize the BC tones to either ear, then clinically useful BC thresholds can be obtained from each mastoid without the use of masking. The examiner must not overlook the possibility that the patient's report on lateralization sometimes might be in error. Fewer mistakes are made when adequate masking is used for every BC measurement.

Since the Rinne and Schwabach tuning-fork bone-conduction tests usually were made from the mastoid process, many examiners also place the BC vibrator in contact with the mastoid. At the present time, clinical

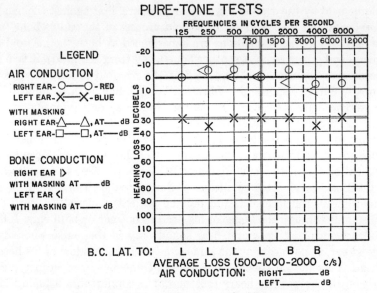

FIG. 6.1. BC lateralization of the Weber test

BC vibrators are calibrated for use at the mastoid without the presence of a masking noise over the opposite ear. No invalidating objections can be raised to the argument that BC measurements should be made with the vibrator contacting only the middle of the forehead, with an effective masking noise over the ear not under test. Several dB more power are required to stimulate the BC threshold from the forehead than from the mastoid. If this technique is adopted, the BC zero hearing level calibration should be determined with a specified masking noise level in the opposite ear. Naunton (9) and Studebaker (10) discuss the pros and cons of placing the vibrator against the middle of the forehead.

Pure-Tone BC Masking Procedures. As has been apparent, it is practically impossible to discuss BC audiometry without frequent reference to the use of masking. There is no good argument against the contention that BC measurements should be made only with a masking noise over the contralateral non-test ear. However, if an experienced examiner knows the patient's ear history, the results of the physical examination, and the AC thresholds, then certain BC measurements which are of clinical value can be made without the use of masking. This includes patients with unilateral tympanic pathologies who lateralize the audiometric Weber test to the involved ear, and patients with bilateral AC impairments who do not lateralize the BC stimuli to either ear. However, it is absolutely necessary to use masking over the better ear in patients with medio-tympanic pathologies while obtaining the BC sensitivity of the worse ear. The majority of the gross errors made in BC audiometry nearly always involve unilateral cochlear or neural pathologies.

To obtain a BC measurement with masking, it also is advisable first to obtain the BC threshold without masking. The purpose of this maneuver is to obtain an unmasked threshold against which to evaluate the effect of the masking noise. For illustrative purposes, assume a patient with a unilateral 40-dB AC hearing level in his left ear at 1000 c/s. Further assume that the ear history, physical examination, and the lateralization of the Weber test to the right ear suggest cochlear involvement in the affected ear. Position the vibrator in firm contact against the left mastoid (or forehead), and obtain a BC hearing level. This value may indicate normal BC sensitivity or even slightly increased BC, owing to the occlusion effect of the silent masking-noise receiver over the normal ear. (The occlusion effect is greater at the lower frequency levels. Occlusion will be discussed in more detail later.)

Now, present the masking noise to the right normal ear at the 50-dB hearing level and obtain a BC threshold for the 1000-c/s tone. Assume the tone is heard at the 25-dB level. This value varies significantly with the type of masking noise used and the magnitude of the occlusion shift. Next, present the masking noise at the 60-dB hearing level an so on at successively higher intensity levels until the threshold becomes stabilized— i.e., does not continue to shift significantly as the level of the noise is increased.

Experienced examiners know that apparent discrepancies of 10 to 15 dB (and sometimes larger) between AC and BC measurements can occur in patients with medio-tympanic pathologies. These differences occur as the result of certain errors and variables, plus possible distraction effects of the masking noise. Short cuts can be taken in regard to the original masking level. For example, in the detailed step-by-step masking procedure described above, the first presentation of the noise at the 50-dB hearing level could have been omitted and the noise first presented at the 70-dB level. However, it is usually advisable to condition patients to respond to low level pure tones in noise while the noise is at a comfortable listening level.

Over-masking rarely occurs while testing patients with medio-tympanic pathologies since such patients have equal threshold shifts for both AC and BC stimuli. The noise intensity level at which over-masking starts to occur while testing patients with tympanic pathologies becomes evident if the BC thresholds are obtained as the noise level is increased in successive 10-dB (or 15- or 20-dB) steps. Occasionally, a patient with tympanic pathology is encountered whose pure-tone threshold in the test ear is shifted significantly as the masking noise over the non-test ear is presented at high-intensity masking levels, which may result in over-masking. This masking dilemma is described in detail by Naunton (9).

Sources of Error in the Measurement of BC Sensitivity. BC measurements fall heir to practically all of the errors associated with AC tests, plus several other additional sources of variability.

1. The mass of the head; the thickness, density, and elasticity of the bones of the skull; and the thickness of the skin over the mastoid or forehead constitute uncontrollable variations from patient to patient.

2. A given sound pressure level (SPL) room noise may produce more masking and threshold shift for the BC than the AC pure-tone measurements, since the earphone cushions attenuate the room noise several dB, and BC tests usually are performed while the ears are uncovered. (The effect on BC sensitivity of covering or occluding the external auditory canal will be discussed later.)

3. Variations in pressure with which the BC vibrator is held against the skull while making measurements constitute another significant source of error. Patients with marked impairments of BC sensitivity may respond only to the vibration of the vibrator (pallesthesia) and not hear it as sound, especially at the lower frequencies. (These pressure and pallesthesia errors will be discussed more fully later.)

4. It is more difficult to obtain accurate instrumental checks on the calibration of BC vibrators than on earphones. Artificial ears for measuring the acoustic outputs from earphones are highly developed and are owned by many clinics. Artificial mastoids are few in type and number and are much more expensive than artificial ears.

5. Probably the greatest source of error in bone-conduction audiometry is due to the fact that a vibrating body in contact with any point on the head sets the entire skull in vibration. If the BC sensitivity is even slightly impaired, for example, in the left ear, the test tone may be heard only in the right (normal) ear, even though the vibrator is placed in contact with the left mastoid. The magnitude of the BC shadow curve differs so slightly from the BC threshold sensitivity in the opposite ear that a masking noise *must* be used over the ear with the better BC in order to obtain threshold measurements on an opposite ear with slightly worse BC sensitivity.

6. Presently available BC vibrators do not possess sufficient mass to permit an effective transfer of vibrational energy to the skull, especially below about 1500 c/s. The small hearing-aid type of BC vibrator, which weighs only an ounce or so, shakes the skull about as effectively as a mouse can shake a cat. The greatest need in clinical audiometry at the present time is an accurate, dependable, and efficient BC vibrator.

Special Tests

Rainville BC Test. Rainville (11) in 1955 described a new method for the determination of BC sensitivity which merits serious consideration. In this procedure the effect of a BC masking noise on the AC threshold is evaluated. The BC masking noise is produced by a BC vibrator in firm contact with the skull. Since the normal ear and patients with tympanic pathologies possess normal BC sensitivity, a given hearing-level BC masking noise will result in equal AC shifts in both the normal ear and the ear with tympanic pathology. If the patient has an impairment for BC sound, a given BC hearing-level masking noise will not produce as much AC theshold shift as in the normal ear or the ear with tympanic pathology. According to this technique, the amount of masking or the threshold shift of the AC pure tone produced by the BC masking noise is a function of the patient's BC sensitivity.

Evaluation, calibration, and modifications of the Rainville test are given by Lightfoot (12), Jerger and Tillman (13), Keys and Milburn (14), Palva and Palva (15) and Goldstein, Hayes, and Peterson (16).

Bing or Occlusion Test. Bing (17) in 1891 described a hearing test which possesses significant anatomic localization implications. He held a tuning fork of "medium pitch" against the skull (usually the mastoid of the ear being tested) which was vibrating with sufficient amplitude to be heard ("primary perception"). As soon as the patient stopped hearing the sound, the external auditory canal was occluded "moderately" by placing a finger gently in the orifice of the external acoustic meatus. If the sound then reappeared ("secondary perception"), it was concluded that the middle ear structures possessed normal function and the patient had "perception" deafness (Bing positive). However, if the sound did not reappear when the canal was occluded (Bing negative), the patient had some type of conductive deafness. (This test must not be confused with Bing's entotic test, which is described in *Dorland's Illustrated Medical Dictionary* as follows: "When words are not audible through an ear trumpet as ordinarily applied, but may be heard when spoken into a trumpet joined to a catheter in the eustachian tube, it is probable that there is a lesion of the incus or malleus." (18)).

The Bing test is so easy to administer, requires so little time to complete, necessitates the use of only the commonly available audiometric equipment, and reveals so much of value about the state of the mobility of the middle ear structures that its use, when indicated, is highly recommended.

The test is equally effective, if not more so, when performed by means of the audiometer BC vibrator instead of tuning forks. This approach permits the test to be conducted while the tone is perceived at a comfortable constant loudness level. The patient is requested to report if the tone is louder or remains unchanged when the ear canal is closed. The palm of the hand against the auricle, light pressure of the tragus against the orifice of the external acoustic meatus, or insertion of a finger gently into the meatus serve as convenient occlusion devices. If the tragus is pushed too firmly against the opening into the meatus or the finger inserted too tightly into the canal, a slight decrease in the loudness of the sound may occur in patients with normal middle ears because of increased air pressure against the drum.

The Bing test is especially valuable in the following clinical situations:

1. As is well known, patients with medio-tympanic impairments have the same hearing levels for both AC and BC sound. Often, however, patients are seen who have, e.g., 40-dB losses for AC and around 30-dB losses for BC. Does this difference indicate a mixed or combined pathology (which is predominantly medio-tympanic) or is this 10-dB difference an artifact, due to one or more of the sources of BC measurement error? To resolve this doubt, present a 500-c/s tone by bone conduction at a comfortable loudness, and alternately close and open the ear canal. If the sound is heard louder while the canal is occluded, the patient is free from middle ear pathology and the apparent difference between the AC and BC thresholds is an artifact. If, however, there is no change in the loudness with occlusion, middle ear pathology is present.

2. If the patient appears to have a BC loss greater than that which can be measured with the audiometer, sometimes the sound can be heard when the canal is occluded. For example, assume that the patient has a 70-db hearing loss for AC at 500 c/s but does not hear this frequency at the 60-dB BC hearing level—the maximal BC output of most audiometers. If the patient can hear this tone at the 60-dB BC hearing level when his ear canal is closed, the examiner can be certain that the patient's middle ear structures possess normal function.

3. Occasionally patients are seen with marked unilateral losses for BC sound who, in spite of a high intensity level masking noise over the non-test ear, state that they hear the BC tone in the ear which is masked. If occlusion of the defective ear results in perception of the tone in the closed ear, it can be inferred that the patient has some type of medio-tympanic involvement in the ear in question. However, if the AC loss is significantly greater than the maximal BC loss that can be measured with the audiometer, occlusion may not result in perception of the sound by BC. In such instances the examiner must rely on the AC measurements and on the ear history and physical examination when he makes the diagnosis.

4. The occlusion test can be substituted for the BC threshold sensitivity measurements in patients with medio-tympanic impairments, if desired.

If an impaired ear presents a Bing-positive reaction, it can be assumed with a high degree of certainty that the patient has the same hearing levels for both AC and BC. However, if the patient reacts with a Bing-negative response, it is necessary to obtain the BC threshold.

5. If a patient's AC and BC thresholds are approximately equal in a given ear but the tympanic membrane appears abnormal (is retracted or scarred or contains calcium plaques), the occlusion test will inform the examiner whether or not the tympanic structures possess normal mobility.

6. The Bing test can be used to learn if or when a patient with an acute otitis media has recovered complete function after medication, myringotomy, or paracentesis. Restoration of middle ear function after middle ear surgical procedures also can be evaluated by means of this test.

Csovanyos (19) reports a positive Bing test after mobilization of a case of otosclerosis; Csovanyos also found that ". . . the Bing test, when done on patients with Ménière's disease, indicates the presence of a conductive lesion. As soon as the intralabyrinthine pressure subsides, the Bing test becomes positive. This is an objective sign of improvement of Ménière's Disease." The term "conductive," as used above, implies a mechanical conductive lesion within the inner ear.

It is not unusual for patients to maintain that the BC sound is "softer" when the ear is occluded with a finger because they expect sounds to be softer when the ear is plugged. If the examiner wishes to obtain audiometric BC measurements while the canal is occluded, it is advisable to use some type of insert earplug. A finger, either the examiner's or the patient's, generates undesirable masking noises. A Vaseline-impregnated small ball of cotton, placed in the opening into the meatus and then covered with an air tight film or seal of Vaseline in the concha, provides dependable occlusion and avoids excessive air pressure in the canal.

Many European otologists value the occlusion test to the extent that they often test the patient's bone sensitivity twice: first with open ear canals (relative BC), and then with occluded canals (absolute BC). If the relative and absolute values coincide, the patient has tympanic or mixed pathologies; if the absolute measurements show significantly better BC sensitivity than the relative measurements, the patient has normal middle-ear function.

Sullivan, Gottleib, and Hodges (20) added the differences between the relative and absolute measurements at 250, 500, and 1000 c/s on normal ears and called the sum the "occlusion index." They reported a mean occlusion index of 60 dB with a standard deviation of 19 dB on a group of 28 normal subjects.

It is not unusual to read in some of the older textbooks on otology, as well as in a few of the more recent ones, that increased BC sensitivity

TABLE 6.1

Frequency	(22)	(23)	(23)	(20)	(21)	Means
c/s			dB			
125	19	27	26	13	17	20.4
250	21	23	24	20	23	22.2
500	23	18	20	23	20	20.8
1000	12	14	17	18	11	14.4
2000	2	1	3	9	X	3.75
4000	X	0	1	3	X	1.33
8000	X	0	1	1	5	1.75

The numbers in parentheses in the boxheads refer to the reference list at the end of the chapter, giving the sources in which the respective studies are discussed. The numbers in the last six columns show the decreases in intensity in dB required to reach the BC thresholds after the ears were occluded, for each of the frequencies in the first column.

resulting from occlusion of the canal is an artifact, resulting from attenuation of room masking noise while the meatus is closed. This viewpoint possessed a certain amount of validity when most hearing tests were performed with tuning forks in ordinary treatment rooms and the examiner used his own auditory sensitivity for comparison and evaluation of the sensitivity of the patient. However, considerable research under more ideal and objective test conditions has established once and for all the fact that BC sensitivity in normal middle ears is increased while the ear is occluded. Siegenthaler, Cohen, and Rhodes (21) reviewed the differences between relative and absolute BC in the normal ear as reported in four studies, including their own. A condensed version of the summary appears in Table 6.1.

Unfortunately, earphones used to present masking noises, which fit snugly against the auricle, also increase the BC sensitivity for frequencies below 2000 c/s because of their occlusion effect in ears with medio-tympanic pathologies. This is particularly undesirable because the effectiveness of a given intensity level masking noise while making BC measurements differs when applied to an ear with tympanic (Bing-negative) and an ear with medio-tympanic (Bing-positive) pathology. A masking procedure which increases the BC sensitivity in the ear in which the BC sound is to be masked partially defeats its own purpose. The Rainville BC test is subject to the same aberration. Naunton (9) discusses the importance of the occlusion effect in clinical bone-conduction audiometry at considerable length and points out, "The magnitude of the occlusion effect is shown to be unrelated to the degree of air-conduction threshold loss."

Watson and Gales (24) avoided this masking noise dilemma by producing the noise with an earphone or small loud-speaker in one end of an enclosure having a minimal volume of 2000 cc. When the enclosure was coupled tightly to the auricle by placing the auricle in a padded hole at the opposite end of a box or large diameter tube, the occlusion effect was avoided.

A word of caution must be emphasized about one aspect of the Bing test. As is universally known, patients with unilateral tympanic pathologies generally refer BC sound to the involved ear (Weber test). BC measurements on this ear usually show normal BC sensitivity. Occlusion of the opposite ear, which increases the BC sensitivity of the normal ear approximately 20 dB at low frequency levels, rarely shifts the lateralization from an ear with tympanic pathology (and normal BC) to the occluded normal ear (with increased BC). This puzzling paradox is called a "false-Bing" phenomenon by Fournier (25). As is the case with all hearing measurements, the test results must be evaluated in relation to the patient's ear history and physical examination, as well as with the outcome of the other tests.

Békésy Audiometry.

Description of the Instrument. It is not surprising that several different types of more or less "automatic" audiometers have been constructed in the present age of automation. Such instruments usually are designed so that the desired frequency and intensity parameters are produced mechanically according to a programmed sequence. In the more sophisticated instruments, the listener's responses determine the intensity levels at which the tones are presented; also, the most consistent threshold response is printed out by means of some type of indicating mechanism, such as a teletype tape punch, an automated typewriter, or an IBM card-punch recorder, to facilitate the processing of masses of data.

Only one type of automatic device for measuring auditory threshold sensitivity—the Békésy audiometer (26)—will be discussed in the present chapter. An accumulation of considerable data and testing experience with this instrument since its introduction in 1947 has demonstrated that the Békésy audiometer testing technique reveals more clinically significant information about the auditory characteristics of pathological ears than any other single type of auditory threshold sensitivity test devised to date.

The instrument, as first described, measured auditory sensitivity over a continuously variable frequency range from 100 to 10,000 c/s in 15 min.— approximately 2 min. per octave. The variable audio-frequency oscillator dial is driven by an electric motor, which also is coupled to a mechanism which pulls a co-ordinated audiogram blank under a recording stylus. The instrument's gain control, driven by an instantly reversible motor, covered an intensity range of 140 dB at an intensity rate of change of 140 dB per min.—2.33 dB per second. The patient's response key controls the action of the instantly reversible motor in such a way that pressing the key decreases the intensity and releasing the key increases the intensity of the test tone. (The reverse key action was built into the original instrument.) Synchronized with the intensity-changing mechanism is a stylus which records on the audiogram blank the variations in the intensity output of the gain control as the measurement proceeds. The recording stylus moves at a right angle (y-axis, intensity ordinate) to the direction in which the audiogram blank is moved (x-axis, frequency abscissa).

The test is started with the test tone adjusted to the desired initial frequency and the intensity-control mechanism is set at its minimal intensity output position. The patient is instructed to press the signal key whenever and as long as the test tone can be heard and to release it as soon as the tone becomes inaudible. When the instrument is turned on, the action of the instantly reversible motor increases the intensity of the test tone until the patient hears it and presses the signal key, whereupon the intensity decreases as long as the key is pressed. When the tone becomes inaudible and the key is released, the intensity increases until the sound is heard and the key is pressed again, and so on throughout the test.

The responses recorded on the audiogram draw a continuous series of up and down (peak and valley) sloping straight lines, commonly called a "tracing." The lengths (or heights) of the lines indicate the intensity ranges between audibility and inaudibility as the intensity of the test tone is varied by the patient's reactions with the signal key. The angle of the slope of the lines which comprise the tracing is a function of the attenuation rate in dB per second and the velocity with which the audiogram blank is pulled at the right angle to the movement of the recording stylus.

Perhaps the most valuable feature of the instrument is inherent in the psychophysics of the tone-presentation procedure. Although several investigators are of the opinion that the Békésy audiometer test technique is that of the method of adjustment, the methodology and test results bear several striking resemblances to the method of limits. The listener responds as soon as he hears the tone on an increasing intensity presentation and makes a response when the tone becomes inaudible on a decreasing intensity presentation. Audibility occurs at an intensity level a few dB higher than inaudibility—the overlapping or criss-crossing which is characteristic of the method of limits. The threshold lies approximately midway between the "just audible" and "just inaudible" intensities of the stimulus and the recorded tracing.

In addition to measuring threshold sensitivity over a desired frequency range, two other aspects of the Békésy tracing possess significant diagnostic implications: (1) the variability or intensity range between the audible and inaudible points of the tracing and (2) drifts in threshold sensitivity for discrete uninterrupted tones during a given testing time interval.

The Amplitude of the Tracing. Although it has been suggested that the intensity range between the audible and inaudible points indicated by the tracing constitutes a measure of the difference limen for intensity (DLI), it may be more appropriate to regard this intensity variation as the range in dB of the zone of threshold uncertainty. This intensity range hereafter will be referred to as the *excursion* of the tracing.

The excursion is subject to considerable individual variation, even in persons with normal hearing. Lundborg (27) obtained continuously variable frequency sensitivity measurements on 50 listeners with normal hearing with an instrument equipped with a 2-dB step attenuator having an intensity rate of change of 2.33 dB per sec. He reported that the normal excursion varied between 6 and 12 dB, with the majority between 6 and 9 dB. "Exceptionally, patients with normal hearing may be observed who record a minimum or maximum difference limen, with extreme limits at 5 dB and 20 dB." Corso (28) analyzed the excursion widths of 10 normal university students over a continuously variable frequency range from 250 to 8000 c/s. With an attenuation rate of change of 2 dB per sec., the following mean excursions occurred: 8.77, 7.21, and 10.53 dB over testing times of 1, 2, and 4 min. per octave, respectively.

Most of the systematic research to date on the excursion has been confined to discrete frequency measurements. Table 6.2 summarizes the results of four such studies on a total of 77 normal individuals.

The standard deviation is a measure of subject variability and may be interpreted as follows: at 250 c/s, the top E is 8.2 dB with an SD of 2.6 dB. This means that 68.26% (a little more than two thirds of a normal distribution) of the excursions fall within a dB range of 5.6 to 10.8 dB (8.2 − 2.6 and 8.2 + 2.6). The 68.26% figure is derived from the following statistical consideration: if under a normal distribution curve perpendiculars are erected from the base line at the mean and at points one standard deviation either side of the mean, the part of the area under the curve included within these perpendiculars will be 68.26% of the total area under the curve.

The attenuation rates used in the four studies varied from 2 to 2.5 dB per second. The order of presentation of the different frequencies was randomized and short practice sessions were given before making the measurements in three of the studies. Inspection of the data in Table 6.2 indicates that the excursion decreases slightly in intensity range from low to high frequency levels. The weighted means show that the excursion is about 1.5 dB greater at 250 and 500 c/s than it is at 4000 c/s.

The excursion of the Békésy tracing also varies in magnitude with the

TABLE 6.2

Mean values and standard deviations of the excursions (in dB) at the indicated discrete frequency levels

Study	No. of Subjects in Study	Frequency (c/s)										
		250		500		1000		2000		4000		8000
		E*	SD†	E	SD	E	SD	E	SD	E	SD	E
						dB						
(29)	30	8.2	2.6	7.4	2.4	7.0	2.8	6.6	2.1	6.7	1.8	
(30)	21	6.8	3.7			5.5	2.9			5.2	3.9	
(31)	16	9.4	4.3	9.7	3.9	8.5	4.0	9.2	4.2	8.4	3.5	
(32)	10	8.5		7.9		6.6		6.1		5.5		5.5
Weighted mean		8.1		8.1		6.9		7.3		6.5		5.5

The numbers in parentheses in the first column refer to the reference list at the end of the chapter, giving the sources in which the respective studies are discussed.

* The numbers in the columns headed "E" show the magnitudes of the excursions for the given frequencies.

† The numbers in the columns marked "SD" show the standard deviations for the associated excursions.

attenuation rate in dB per second. Von Békésy (26) pointed out that increasing the attenuation rate from 1.5 to 3.66 dB per sec. resulted in an increase in the excursion amplitude. Epstein (33), obtaining measurements on seven normal, relatively sophisticated listeners, found "... ranges of from 4–9 dB, 5–17 dB, 8–15 dB, and 10–30 dB for attenuation rates of 1, 2, 3 and 6 dB per second respectively." Small and Minifie (32), testing 10 normal university students at discrete frequency levels with attenuation rates of 2.5 and 5.0 dB per sec., obtained the mean excursion values in Table 6.3.

As the attenuation rate increases, not only does the width or magnitude of the excursion become greater but the threshold sensitivity (mid-point between the excursion extremes) falls at a lower intensity level. Corso and Wilson (34), testing 10 university students over a continuously variable frequency range (300 to 7000 c/s), found the sensitivity was approximately 5 dB more acute when the attenuation rate was 5.0 dB per sec. than when it was 1.5 dB per sec. Stream and McConnell (35) made measurements on 42 normal subjects at 250, 1000, and 4000 c/s with attenuation rates of 2.5 and 4.5 dB per sec. They found that "... in all cases the faster rate of attenuation yielded a slightly better threshold. ..."

It is mandatory that the attenuation rate with which Békésy audiometer measurements are obtained be known and recorded for two reasons. (1)

TABLE 6.3

Mean excursion values (in 10 university students)

Discrete Frequency Level	Mean Excursion Values		Difference
	5.0	2.5	
c/s	dB/sec		dB
250	12.3	8.5	3.8
500	10.5	7.9	2.6
1000	9.6	6.6	3.0
2000	8.1	6.1	2.0
4000	7.4	5.5	1.9
8000	8.1	5.5	2.6

Threshold sensitivity varies slightly but systematically with changes in attenuation rate. Threshold responses occur at lower intensity levels at the more rapid attenuation rates. (2) The magnitude or width of the excursions varies with attenuation rate, becoming larger as the rate is increased. The significance of the size of the excursion will be discussed later.

Very little difference in sensitivity of normal ears results between measurements made with pulsed and sustained tones. Corso and Wilson (34), testing 10 normal university students over a continuously variable frequency range (300 to 7000 c/s), reported, "For frequencies below 2000 c/s, tone-pulsing appears to increase the threshold values, but these differences are not statistically significant as indicated in the analyses for 1000 [c/s] and 300 [c/s]. Above 2000 [c/s], tone-pulsing appears to lower significantly the mean threshold value, with the largest differences occurring in the 3000–4000 [c/s] region." (There was slightly less than 3-dB difference at 3000, 4000, and 6000 c/s.) Palva (31) reported that in the case of discrete frequencies: "The size of the tracings is similar regardless of whether interrupted or continuous tones are used."

Not unexpectedly, but fortunately, threshold sensitivity measurements obtained on the Békésy audiometer agree very closely with those made on the commonly used discrete frequency clinical audiometer. Corso and Wilson (34) stated that "... there is considerable agreement between the mean threshold values obtained on a Bekesy-type audiometer and those obtained by a conventional discrete-frequency audiometer" at an attenuation rate of 1.5 dB per sec. Burns and Hinchcliffe (36) reported that "... the measurement of the threshold of hearing either by the Bekesy technique or by pure-tone manual audiometry gives essentially similar results." Twenty normal subjects between the ages of 20 and 58 years of age were used. The attenuation rate of the Békésy audiometer was 2 dB per sec.

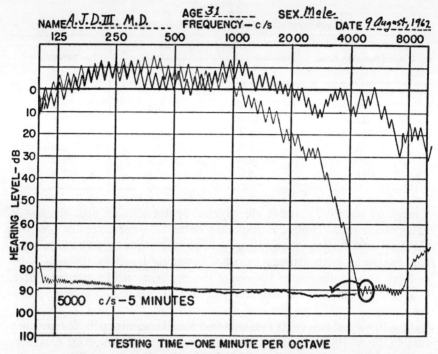

FIG. 6.2. Continuous variable frequency Békésy audiogram

Figure 6.2 shows a Békésy audiogram obtained on a patient with a normal right ear but with a high-frequency loss in the left ear. The etiology of the impairment is unknown. The testing time was 1 min. per octave and the attenuation rate was 2.5 dB per sec. with a "stepless" gain control. Visual inspection of the tracing shows an excursion of approximately 5 dB over the frequency range through which the sensitivity of both ears was normal. Obviously, the excursion is smaller above 4000 c/s in the left ear, being about 3 dB wide at the 5000-c/s level, included within the heavy "O" on the audiogram. The narrower, almost horizontal tracing to the *left* of the "O" shows the patient's responses to a discrete 5000-c/s tone over a 5-min. testing interval. It is readily apparent that the threshold range is smaller for the discrete tone than for the same frequency when it is encountered within a continuously variable frequency continuum.

In addition to providing a graphic record of the results of all the conventional clinical pure-tone measurements, the Békésy audiometer can be used for recording the results of a test for the detection of unilateral malingering (37, 38) and has been used in a feedback loop to record variations in the sound pressures required to elicit cochlear potentials in experimental animals (39, 40). The instrument also has been found to be of significant value in the detection of threshold recruitment and of temporary threshold drift. As a matter of fact, the potential of the technique is limited only by the ingenuity of the clinician or investigator. Hirsh (41) presents a concise review of some of the clinical and research applications of the instrument.

Recruitment Tests. The recruitment phenomenon remains an intriguing and controversial subject. Considerable clinical research awaits completion before the maximal significance and value of the various tests can be assessed and utilized. The early papers by Pohlman and Kranz (42) and by Fowler (43–47) serve as introductions to the phenomenon. Reviews by Luscher and Zwislocki (48), Harris (49), Bangs and Mullins (50), Hirsh, Palva, and Goodman (51), Hedgecock (52), Harris, Haines, and Myers (53), Ewertson, Filling, Terkildsen, and Thomsen (54), Eisenberg (55), and the comprehensive monograph by de Bruine-Altes (56) summarize much of the pertinent literature. Over a dozen so-called recruitment tests have been devised.

For the sake of brevity and the avoidance of excessive misinformation, only the most commonly used tests and generally accepted ideas about the subject are mentioned in this chapter. The following conclusions about recruitment appear to have considerable support at the present time (1964): (1) recruitment (R) is characterized by an abnormally rapid increase in loudness as intensity is raised above the threshold sensitivity of certain pathologic ears; (2) R is rarely (if ever) experienced by patients with exclusively middle ear pathology; (3) R is symptomatic of lesions involving the organ of Corti (see Yantis (57)); (4) R is not associated with lesions involving the VIIIth cranial nerve and higher acoustic centers (see Dix, Hallpike, and Hood (58) and Eby and Williams (59)); (5) R usually is present in pathologies associated with acoustic insult, oto-toxicities, and Ménière's disease at certain stages; (6) patients with R experience disproportionate difficulty in perceiving speech; (7) R tests are supra-threshold measures; and (8) the loudness-balance tests are the procedures of choice in the detection and measurement of the phenomenon.

The Alternate Binaural Loudness-Balance Test. This test is applicable to patients with somewhat better hearing in one ear than the other. Ideally, the equipment should consist of a pure-tone oscillator; a masking noise with a built-in attenuator; two attenuators, each capable of at least a 100-dB intensity range, in 1- or 2-dB steps; appropriate earphones; and a device for switching the test tone without audible transient clicks from one ear to the other as often as desired. The switching should be designed so that the masking noise is presented to the better ear while the test tone is in the worse ear to avoid shadow curve errors. Tone presentations of approximately 1 sec. in duration and silent intervals of comparable length are suitable for the balance measurements.

After the threshold sensitivity measurements in each ear have been obtained (with the 1- or 2-db step attenuators), the tone is presented at a 5-dB sensation level (SL) in the "constant" ear—usually the worse ear. Then, while the tone is switched from one ear to the other, the patient adjusts the "variable" attenuator to the better ear until he judges the constant and the variable tones to be equally loud. A minimum of three loudness balances should be obtained and averaged for each SL in the constant ear. The patient must not be permitted to see or know the values at which he sets the variable attenuator while making his loudness-balance judgments. After completing a set of balances at a given SL in the constant ear, and after a rest of several seconds, the task is resumed at the additional desired intensity levels.

It is advisable to repeat the measurements with the role of the ears reversed, i.e., with the better ear the constant and the worse ear the variable. If both sets of data do not agree, the accuracy of the recruitment measures is questionable.

The above laboratory approach can be approximated with the conventional clinical audiometer—at the expense of a decrease in the accuracy of the measurements. Assume a patient with normal hearing in the right ear and a loss of 40 dB in the left at, e.g., 2000 c/s. Present this frequency in the "constant" left ear at the 10-dB SL (50-dB hearing level) for about a second, turn the tone off, quickly turn the ear selector switch to the right ear, adjust the attenuator to the 25-dB hearing level, and then turn on the 2000-c/s tone. If the tone is heard as softer in the right ear, again present the tone at the same 10-dB SL in the left ear and then switch to, e.g., the 30-dB hearing level in the right ear. Repeat this maneuver, varying the intensity of the variable tone in the right ear until the patient judges the loudness to be identical in each ear (to the nearest 5-dB step in the right ear). Continue in like manner at the desired sensitivity and frequency levels. Masking must be used when indicated.

Figure 6.3 shows a "ladder-gram" of a set of balance measurements. The top solid line, sloping downward from left to right, connects the threshold values of the 2000-c/s tone in the two ears. The top broken line, connecting the 30-dB (right ear) and 50-dB (left ear) hearing levels, indicates that a 2000-c/s tone at the 10-dB SL in the left ear is equal in loudness to the same tone at the 30-dB hearing level in the normal right ear. The bottom horizontal line superimposed on the 80-dB hearing level line indicates that a 2000-c/s tone at the 40-dB SL in the left ear is equal in loudness to the same tone at the 80-dB hearing level in the normal right ear. When a tone at a given intensity level is perceived with the same loudness in a hard-of-hearing ear as in the opposite normal (or near normal) ear, recruitment is said to be "complete." Whenever a tone at a given intensity is heard as

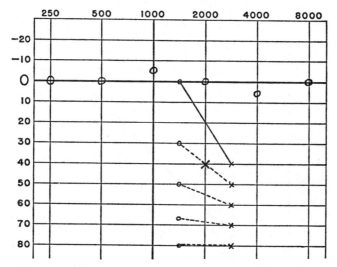

FIG. 6.3. Alternate ear loudness level balance ladder-gram

louder in the defective ear than in the normal ear, the patient is said to experience "hyper-recruitment" or "over-recruitment."

Figure 6.4 shows an additional method of presenting equal-loudness level data. The straight diagonal line A at the 45° angle or slope plots the equal-loudness levels of persons with bilaterally normal ears. This curve indicates that tones of given intensities in one ear are equally loud in the opposite ear at the same corresponding intensity levels. Curve B shows the plot of the data comprising the "ladder-gram" of Figure 6.3. Curves having the type of slope presented by B are called asymptotic, and patients with similar "growth of loudness" curves are said to have asymptotic recruitment. Line C, being parallel to line A, shows the same rate of growth of loudness as does the normal ear, and therefore no recruitment.

Monaural Bi-Frequency Equal Loudness Level Test. This method of measuring recruitment is applicable to patients who have significantly better threshold sensitivity over part of the audiometric frequency range than for the remainder of the range. Figure 6.5 shows both equal-loudness level balances and Békésy audiometer threshold measurements at 2000 and 4000 c/s in the patient's right ear. (The patient had approximately identical sensitivity in each ear. When this is the case, the use of masking is not indicated.) This approach necessitates the use of two different audio-frequency generators, or a single generator, the frequency of which can be altered quickly in octave steps. The two different frequencies are alternated in one ear only.

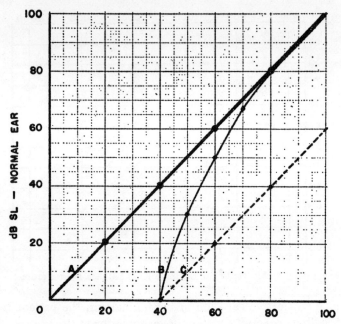

Fig. 6.4. Rate of growth of loudness curves. A = Alternate ear equal loudness level balances in two normal ears. B = 40-dB shift in one ear from masking or cochlear pathology. C = 40-dB shift in one ear from tympanic pathology.

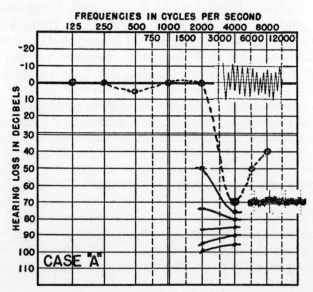

Fig. 6.5 Monaural bi-frequency equal loudness level contours and Békésy thresholds at 2000 and 4000 c/s.

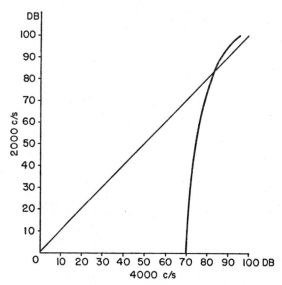

FIG. 6.6 Asymptotic recruitment of case "A"

After the threshold sensitivity for the two frequencies in the ear under test was obtained, the intensity of the 4000-c/s tone—the "constant" tone—was set at the 5-dB SL. Then, while the two frequencies were presented alternately in the right ear, the patient varied the intensity of the 2000-c/s tone—the variable tone—until both tones were perceived with equal loudness. The data of Figure 6.5 indicate that a 4000-c/s tone at the patient's 5-dB SL was equal in loudness to a 2000-c/s tone at his 50-dB SL. At high intensity levels the patient experienced over-recruitment (Fig. 6.6).

The measurements shown on Figure 6.5 were obtained on a 52-year-old man who had worked in a noisy machine shop for 30 years. He was constantly aware of a high-frequency tinnitus, especially at night while the environment was quiet.

Figures 6.7 and 6.8 present measurements comparable to those in Figures 6.5 and 6.6, respectively, but on a different patient and at 1000 and 2000 c/s. This patient also had essentially identical threshold sensitivity in each ear. No history of noise exposure could be elicited. No specific diagnosis of a certain type of cochlear or neural deafness could be made—other than medio-tympanic involvement.

The approximately straight growth of the loudness curve in Figure 6.8 differs significantly from the asymptotic curve of Figure 6.6. The abrupt rise of the asymptotic curve before it parallels the diagonal line indicates that the loudness of the 4000-c/s tone increases more rapidly just above the threshold than at higher loudness levels; and the approximately straight growth of loudness curve of Figure 6.8 indicates that the loudness of the

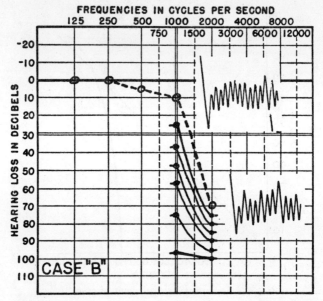

Fig. 6.7. Monaural bi-frequency equal loudness level contours and Békésy thresholds at 1000 and 2000 c/s.

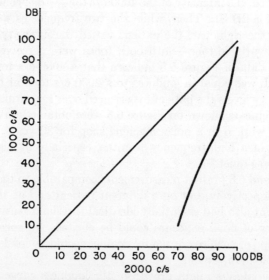

Fig. 6.8. Straight-line recruitment of case "B"

2000-c/s tone increases at about the same rate per dB increase of the intensity above the threshold. Four different types of slopes of growth of loudness curves have been described by Harris, Haines, and Myers (53).

The ordinary clinical pure-tone audiometer also can be used in obtaining monaural bi-frequency loudness level balances in somewhat the same way as it is used in obtaining the alternate-ear single-frequency balances. To make the bi-frequency balances, the ear-selector switch is left in position for the desired ear and the frequency-selector switch alternates between the desired frequency levels. The gain-control settings are manipulated as in the alternate-ear presentations, with one control designated as the constant and the other as the variable.

Unfortunately, the loudness-balance tests are of little value in persons with unilateral flat losses and those with flat and equal bilateral losses.

The Békésy Audiometer Threshold Recruitment Test. The response the listener makes to the Békésy audiometer stimulus is related to the rate at which the intensity of the test tone increases and decreases in loudness above and below his threshold sensitivity. It has been learned that patients with asymptotic recruitment exhibit exceptionally small excursions in their Békésy audiograms and that patients with delayed or straight-line recruitment show significantly wider excursions in their responses. In Figure 6.5, the Békésy audiometer excursions at 2000 c/s have an intensity range of about 8 dB, and at 4000 c/s the range is about 2 dB. This patient had an asymptotic growth of loudness curve (Fig. 6.6). In Figure 6.7, the excursions at 1000 c/s have a range of about 7 dB and at 2000 c/s a range of about 8 dB. This patient had an approximately straight-line growth of loudness (Fig. 6.8).

The differences in the Békésy excursions of the original measurements shown in Figures 6.5 and 6.7 have induced some investigators to conclude that the Békésy threshold test is not a reliable indicator of the presence or absence of recruitment. The author of this chapter prefers to interpret the data shown in Figures 6.5, 6.6, 6.7, and 6.8 as indicative of two different manifestations of the recruitment phenomenon, each having different etiological and anatomic localization implications.

A more stable and accurate evaluation of threshold recruitment is obtained by performing the Békésy test at discrete frequency levels, as in Figure 6.2 at 5000 c/s. Threshold recruitment can be quantified by means of a timing device and an electro-mechanical counter, as used by Bangs (29). Recruitment is not an all-or-none symptom.

Many investigators feel that an excursion range as small as 3 to 5 dB is symptomatic of threshold recruitment. Because of the rather wide ranges in individual variation in the intensity range of the Békésy excursion in normal ears, estimation of the presence or absence of recruitment on the basis of the absolute value of the excursion range is open to criticism. It seems preferable to compare the excursions in the impaired ear with the excursions in the opposite better ear, or to compare the excursions at frequency levels which differ significantly in sensitivity.

The three common etiologies associated with recruitment—noise insult, oto-toxins, and Ménière's disease—usually show both asymptotic recruitment on the loudness-balance tests and threshold recruitment on the Békésy audiometer test.

The Short-Increment Sensitivity Index (SISI) Test. Jerger, Shedd and Harford (60) have described a test which differentiates between patients with certain cochlear disorders and patients with normal hearing, middle ear lesions or VIIIth nerve disorders. The patient is presented with the desired continuous discrete frequency at the 20-db SL. Every 5 seconds the intensity is increased 1 dB for $\frac{2}{10}$ second. Whenever the patient hears the intensity increase, he pushes a signal key. Twenty increases are presented in a series. The test is scored in terms of the percentage of the number of intensity increases that are perceived. Patients who score from 60 to 100 % at frequencies above 1000 c/s usually have cochlear disorders. Patients with lower scores usually have middle-ear lesions or VIIIth nerve disorders.

The Uncomfortable Loudness Level Recruitment Test. This is a subjective test which requires a minimum of time and equipment. Bangs and Mullins (50) found this procedure an exceedingly useful clinical aid. The test is administered by instructing the patient to increase the loudness of the test tone with the audiometer's volume control until the sound becomes uncomfortably loud. If the patient can tolerate the tone only a few dB above his threshold, recruitment is present. It is also advisable to repeat this maneuver in the better ear as a control. If the patient can tolerate the tone at a significantly higher SL in the good ear than in the involved ear, the examiner can be a little more certain of the accuracy of the patient's subjective reports.

Several additional recruitment tests are described in the references in the bibliography. As stated earlier, additional research is needed to clarify many pertinent questions about the recruitment phenomenon.

Pathological Temporary Threshold Drift

In 1952, Reger and Kos (61) reported the noteworthy results of Békésy audiometer threshold sensitivity measurements on a patient with an acoustic neurinoma. The patient's sensitivity for discrete frequencies at 1000, 2000, and 4000 c/s decreased or deteriorated with dramatic rapidity. This finding has been confirmed subsequently by Thompson and Hoel (62), Jerger, Carhart, and Lassman (63), Yantis (64), Sørensen (65), Pestalozza and Cioce (66), and Harbert and Young (67).

Figure 6.9 reproduces the original measurements made on a patient with a bilateral acoustic neurinoma. The left ear had no vestibular response and no reaction to sound at 110-dB hearing levels, permitting the measurements on the right ear without the necessity for masking. The data show a decrease in the threshold sensitivity of 40 dB in less than 3 min. at 500 c/s

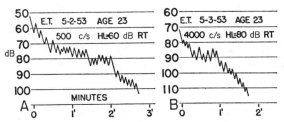

FIG. 6.9. Pathological temporary threshold drift of a patient with an acoustic neurinoma.

and a decrease of 30 dB in less than 2 min. at 4000 c/s. This rapid decrease in auditory sensitivity has been called threshold fatigue, tone decay, abnormal auditory adaptation, abnormal perstimulatory adaptation, temporary threshold shift, and temporary threshold drift. Temporary threshold drift (TTD) is preferred by this writer. TTD has been reported in patients with acoustic neurinomas, cerebellopontine angle tumors, one patient with a pinealoma, and two patients with multiple (or disseminated) sclerosis (68).

A very high percentage of patients with acoustic neurinomas have the TTD response. Brand and Rosenberg (69) have reported the smallest percentage to date of TTD in 10 patients with neurinomas or cerebellopontine angle tumors. Four did not show an abnormal reaction on the Békésy audiometer threshold test. Sørensen (65) reports that, "In all patients with tone decay, the threshold of hearing returns to the prestimulatory level within half a minute after the interruption of the tone."

This abnormally rapid TTD does not become obvious during conventional clinical pure-tone audiometry. Apparently, the manually interrupted tone, with alternating sound pulses and silent intervals of relatively brief durations, does not produce sufficient stress to decrease the threshold sensitivity in ears which are vulnerable to uninterrupted tones. Pathological ears, which are susceptible to significant shifts from threshold intensities, recover their pre-stimulation sensitivity very rapidly while the tone is off. Also, the "on" effect associated with steep wave-front pulse stimuli is not present in uninterrupted tones.

As is to be expected, discrete frequency interrupted-tone tests by means of the Békésy audiometer do not show TTD in ears which are susceptible to marked threshold shifts to uninterrupted tones. Jerger (70) feels that there is a unique relationship between interrupted and uninterrupted tracings in relation to the site of lesions within the auditory system and categorizes four different basic types of relationship. In each of the four types, the threshold sensitivity of the steady tone either coincides with that of the interrupted (pulsed) tone or shows less sensitivity than the pulsed stimulus. Harbert and Young (67) have reported that a patient with an acoustical neurinoma showed "extreme adaptation" for pulsed tones and did not perceive the steady tone when tested with the Békésy instrument.

Jerger and Herer (71) have found greater hearing losses for interrupted than for continuous tones in three patients with non-organic hearing impairments. This finding has been confirmed by Resnick and Burke (72) and Peterson (73).

Carhart (74) has described a method for measuring "abnormal auditory adaptation" which can be performed with any clinical audiometer. After obtaining the patient's threshold sensitivity, the observer increases the intensity of the test tone to 5 dB above the threshold level. The patient is requested to signal whenever and as long as he can hear the steady tone. If he can hear it for 1 min. at the 5- or 10-dB SL, it is assumed that the stability of the sensitivity is within normal limits, and the test is terminated. If the patient hears the tone for less than 1 min., immediately the intensity is increased an additional 5 dB, and so on until the tone is heard over the complete 1-min. interval. Some patients show marked "tone decay" before the tone is heard for 1 min. In extreme cases, the tone may not be heard at the 100-dB hearing level for the specified time.

Additional case reports and research on abnormal temporary threshold drift and recovery following termination of exposure to the test tone may prove to have greater diagnostic potential than suspected at the present time.

MIDDLE-EAR IMPEDANCE

Measurement of middle-ear impedance permits quantification of the relationship between sound pressure and the resultant motion of the eardrum and attached ossicles. Impedance measures give an indication of the physical condition of the middle ear. At low frequencies the normal drum behaves like an elastic membrane enclosing a volume of air. Its displacements are proportional to the incident sound pressure. If the impedance at the eardrum is known, the amount of sound energy transferred to it can be calculated. At frequency levels near the resonant frequency of the middle-ear system—about 1500 c/s—the drum reflects very little of the sound energy that impinges upon it. This natural frequency of vibration of the middle ear depends upon the ossicular masses, the volume of the tympanic cavity, and the elastic properties of the various ligaments that hold the ossicles in place.

Pathological physical changes in the ossicles and their supports reflect different values of impedance from those found in the normal ear. Stapes ankylosis and/or interruption of the ossicles produce opposite effects: ankylosis results in an increase of the impedance above normal, and ossicular interruption decreases the impedance below normal.

By means of impedance measurements it is possible to differentiate between tympanic and medio-tympanic pathologies. It is suggested that incipient otosclerosis may be detected before confirmation can be established by other techniques. Impedance measurements are uniquely adapted to detection of ossicular discontinuity—a finding difficult to obtain with any other procedure at the present time except surgical exploration. The test is of considerable value in detecting a disarticulated prosthesis following certain types of surgery on the middle ear.

Since the contracting middle-ear muscles alter the impedance of the drum, certain test procedures which elicit reflex contraction of these muscles may be employed as localization aids. The intra-tympanic muscles of normal ears contract bilaterally (a consensual reaction) whenever tones are perceived at approximately the 80-dB hearing level in either ear.

If a patient with a severe unilateral loss is suspected of malingering or psychogenic disorders, a change in impedance in the normal ear when a 90-dB hearing level tone is presented to the "defective" ear confirms relatively normal sensitivity in the ear in question. The middle-ear muscle reflex is not elicited in patients with tympanic pathologies. If the middle-ear muscles of a patient with a significant hearing impairment contract when exposed to a 90- or 100-dB hearing level tone, the reaction is thought to be due to recruitment of loudness. Impedance measurements are objective since they require no overt response from the patient.

Middle-ear impedance is measured by means of an impedance bridge. The procedure is both a science and an art, since considerable skill in the operation of the instrumentation is required in order to obtain valid measurements.

Details of the instrumentation, measurement technique, and clinical uses of middle-ear impedance have been described by Zwislocki (75), Feldman (76), and Thomsen (77).

DIPLACUSIS, PITCH DISCRIMINATION, AND TONE QUALITY

Diplacusis is the perception of a given frequency as two different pitches in the two ears. Patients with unilateral impairments due to labyrinthine hydrops usually perceive a given frequency as higher in pitch in the involved ear than in the normal ear. Some patients with unilateral impairments, usually resulting from accidental noise exposure to one ear, also experience diplacusis. Shambaugh (78) presents a historical background and evaluation of the diplacusis phenomenon.

Pitch discrimination usually is measured in a single ear in terms of the smallest difference in frequency between pairs of pulsed tones that can be perceived as differing in pitch. Butler and Albrite (79) reported, "The performance of the perceptively deafened group was significantly inferior to that of the conductive group at 3000 and 4000 c/s." Harris, Haines, and Myers (80) found that some patients with recruitment have normal pitch discrimination, whereas others with recruitment exhibit markedly reduced pitch-discrimination ability.

Some patients with cochlear and/or neural pathologies experience unusual tone quality perceptions while listening to pure-tone stimuli. Pure steady tones have been described as sounding like the noise made by "frying bacon"; like the noise made by dragging a tree limb filled with leaves on the ground; and as a "chirping" noise. Many pure tones appear to have a "grating" or "rasping" sound and may be unpleasant or irritating. Investigators presenting high intensity level pure tones for the measurement of recruitment, diplacusis, pitch discrimination, or other sensory function should first learn if the pure tone in the pathological ear approximates the quality of the same tone in the normal ear. If not, the accuracy of the measurement can be questioned.

LOCALIZATION IMPLICATIONS OF THE PURE-TONE HEARING TESTS

Patients with tympanic pathologies usually give the following reactions to the various hearing tests: (1) relatively flat AC losses not exceeding the 60-dB hearing level; (2) approximately normal BC sensitivity; and (3) negative Bing or occlusion test (no change in the loudness when the external canal is occluded).

Patients with medio-tympanic (cochlear or neural) pathologies exhibit the following reactions: (1) usually, but not always greater impairments for high frequency than for low frequency sounds; (2) approximately equal hearing impairments for both AC and BC sound; (3) positive Bing or occlusion test (increase in loudness at low frequency levels for BC sound when the external canal is occluded); (4) loudness recruitment (in patients with cochlear pathologies); and (5) rapid temporary threshold drift (in patients with neural pathologies, particularly of the VIIIth nerve).

Detailed analysis of audiometric curves is discussed by Carhart (81, 82). It cannot be over-emphasized that the history and the physical examination of the ears, nose, and throat are nearly always more essential in formulating the diagnosis than are the results of the hearing tests. However, there are instances in which the results of the hearing tests must be considered, in relation to the history and physical examination, before a defensible rational diagnosis can be made.

EQUIPMENT CALIBRATION

Accurate maintenance of audiological equipment involves the use of artificial ears for calibration of AC receivers and the use of artificial mastoids for calibration of BC vibrators. Such equipment is expensive and must be handled with care. Calibration of audiometers demands a background in electro-acoustics and electronics and should be attempted only by experts in these areas.

The clinician can check the calibration of his equipment by testing the AC and BC sensitivity of several young adults who present negative ear histories and physical examinations under ideal test conditions. Tests conducted in excessive room noise will shift the threshold sensitivity more for frequencies below 1000 c/s than for higher frequencies. The BC measurements will be shifted more than the AC measurements since the earphone-cushion assembly will attenuate room noise by several dB and the BC sensitivity measurements are obtained with open ear canals. The examiner should keep a permanent and dated serial record of his own auditory sensitivity and repeat the measurements from time to time. Then if at any time he has reason to doubt the calibration of his audiometer, he can repeat the measurements on himself and compare them with the earlier results.

If the audiometer output has not decreased by more than approximately 20 dB, a correction factor can be applied to subsequent measurements if the owner of the equipment wishes to do so. However, if the output of the audiometer decreases by more than 20 dB, it is advisable to have it calibrated by a professional who has access to adequate frequency wave-form and intensity standards—including frequency counters, distortion analyzers, artificial ears, and artificial mastoids.

REFERENCES

1. Reger, S. N., and Kos, C. M.: Anatomic localization implications of the functional hearing tests; revision of terminology. Arch. Otolaryng., 67: 394, 1958.
2. Carhart, R., and Jerger, J. F.: Preferred method for clinical determination of pure-tone thresholds. J. Speech & Hearing Disorders, 24: 330, 1959.
3. Glorig, A., and House, H. P.: A new concept in auditory screening. Arch. Otolaryng., 66: 228, 1957.
4. Hanley, C. N., and Gaddie, B. G.: The use of single frequency audiometry in the screening of school children. J. Speech & Hearing Disorders, 27: 358, 1962.
5. Liden, G., Nilsson, G., and Anderson, H.: Narrow-band masking with white noise. Acta oto-laryng., 50: 116, 1959.
6. Rittmanic, P. A.: Pure-tone masking by narrow-noise bands in normal and impaired ears. J. Auditory Res., 2: 287, 1962.
7. Zwislocki, J.: Acoustic attenuation between the ears. J. Acoust. Soc. America, 25: 752, 1953.
8. von Békésy, G.: Vibration of the head in a sound field and its role in hearing by bone conduction. J. Acoust. Soc. America, 20: 749, 1948.
9. Naunton, R. F.: Clinical bone-conduction audiometry. The use of a frontally applied bone-conduction receiver and the importance of the occlusion effect in clinical bone-conduction audiometry. Arch. Otolaryng., 66: 281, 1957.
10. Studebaker, G. A.: Placement of vibrator in bone conduction testing. J. Speech & Hearing Res., 5: 321, 1962.

11. Rainville, M. J.: New method of masking for the determination of bone conduction curves. Translations of the Beltone Institute for Hearing Research, No. 11, 1959.

12. Lightfoot, C.: The M-R test of bone-conduction testing. Laryngoscope, *70:* 1552, 1960.

13. Jerger, J. F., and Tillman, T.: A new method for the clinical determination of sensorineural acuity level (S.A.L.). Arch. Otolaryng., *71:* 948, 1960.

14. Keys, J. W., and Milburn, B.: The sensorineural acuity level (S.A.L.) technique. Arch. Otolaryng., *73:* 710, 1961.

15. Palva, T., and Palva, A.: Masking in audiometry. III. Reflections upon the present position. Acta oto-laryng., *54:* 521, 1962.

16. Goldstein, D. P., Hayes, C. S., and Peterson, J. L.: A comparison of bone-conduction thresholds by conventional and Rainville methods. J. Speech & Hearing Res., *5:* 244, 1962.

17. Bing, A.: Ein Neurer Stimmgabelversuch. Wien. Med. Blatter, *41:* 4, 1891.

18. *Dorland's Illustrated Medical Dictionary,* Ed. 23, edited by L. B. Arey *et al.,* p. 1376. W. B. Saunders Company, Philadelphia, 1957.

19. Csovanyos, L.: The Bing test in the diagnosis of deafness. Laryngoscope, *71:* 1548, 1961.

20. Sullivan, J. A., Gottleib, C. C., and Hodges, W. E.: Shift of bone conduction threshold on occlusion of the external ear canal. Laryngoscope, *57:* 690, 1947.

21. Siegenthaler, B. M., Cohen, A., and Rhodes, D.: Additional data on bone-conduction shift when the external auditory meatuses are occluded. Arch. Otolaryng., *66:* 223, 1957.

22. Pohlman, A. G., and Kranz, F. W.: The influence of partial and complete occlusion of the external auditory canals on air and bone transmitted sound. Ann. Otol. Rhin. & Laryng., *35:* 113, 1926.

23. Kelley, N. H., and Reger, S. N.: The effect of binaural occlusion of the external auditory meati on the sensitivity of the normal ear for bone conducted sound. J. Exper. Psychol., *21:* 211, 1937.

24. Watson, N., and Gales, R.: Effects of occlusion enclosures and masking devices on bone conduction threshold. J. Acoust. Soc. America, *14:* 207, 1943.

25. Fournier, J. E.: The "false-Bing" phenomenon—some remarks on the theory of bone conduction. Laryngoscope, *64:* 29, 1954.

26. von Békésy, G.: A new audiometer. Acta oto-laryng., *35:* 411, 1947.

27. Lundborg, T.: Diagnostic problems concerning acoustic tumors; Study of 300 verified cases and Békésy and audiogram in differential diagnosis. Acta oto-laryng., Suppl. 99, p. 1, 1952.

28. Corso, J. F.: Evaluation of operating conditions on a Békésy-type audiometer. Arch. Otolaryng., *61:* 649, 1955.

29. Bangs, T. E.: Testing for auditory sensitivity at threshold using a Békésy audiometer. Laryngoscope, *72:* 387, 1962.

30. Siegenthaler, B.: Reaction time, difference limen, and amplitude of excursion on the normal Békésy audiogram. J. Auditory Res., *1:* 285, 1961.

31. Palva, T.: Self-recording threshold audiometry and recruitment. Arch. Otolaryng., *65:* 591, 1957.

32. Small, A. M., and Minifie, F. D.: Intensive differential sensitivity at masked threshold. J. Speech & Hearing Res., *4:* 164, 1961.

33. Epstein, A.: Variables involved in automatic audiometry. Ann. Otol. Rhin. & Laryng., *69:* 137, 1960.

34. Corso, J. F., and Wilson, J. F.: Additional variables on the Békésy-type audiometer. Arch. Otolaryng., *66:* 719, 1957.
35. Stream, R., and McConnell, F.: A comparison of two methods of administration in Békésy-type audiometry. J. Auditory Res., *1:* 263, 1961.
36. Burns, W., and Hinchcliffe, R.: Comparison of the auditory threshold as measured by individual pure tone and by Békésy audiometry. J. Acoust. Soc. America, *29:* 1274, 1957.
37. Reger, S. N., Reneau, J. P., and Watson, J. E.: Quantitative evaluation of the Stenger test. Internat. Audiology, *2:* 144, 1963.
38. Watson, J. E., and Voots, R. J.: A report on the use of the Békésy audiometer in the performance of the Stenger test. J. Speech & Hearing Disorders *29:* 36, 1964.
39. Reger, S. N., Voots, R. J., and Watson, J. E.: Use of the Békésy audiometer in the measurement of cochlear microphonics. Laryngoscope, in press.
40. Voots, R. J., Reger, S. N., and Watson, J. E.: Use of the Békésy audiometer technique in animal research. J. Auditory Res., *4:* 55, 1964.
41. Hirsh, I. J.: Békésy's audiometer. J. Acoust. Soc. America, *34:* 1333, 1962.
42. Pohlman, A. G., and Kranz, F. W.: Binaural minimum audition in a subject with ranges of deficient acuity. Proc. Soc. Exper. Biol. & Med., *21:* 335, 1924.
43. Fowler, E. P.: Marked deafened areas in normal ears. Arch. Otolaryng., *8:* 151, 1928.
44. Fowler, E. P.: A method for the early detection of otosclerosis; a study of sounds well above threshold. Arch. Otolaryng., *24:* 731, 1936.
45. Fowler, E. P.: Measuring the sensation of loudness. Arch. Otolaryng., *26:* 514, 1937.
46. Fowler, E. P.: The use of threshold and louder sounds in clinical diagnosis and the prescribing of hearing aids. New methods for accurately determining the threshold for bone conduction and for measuring tinnitus and its effects on obstructive and neural deafness. Laryngoscope, *48:* 572, 1938.
47. Fowler, E. P.: The recruitment of loudness phenomenon. Laryngoscope, *60:* 680, 1950.
48. Luscher, E., and Zwislocki, J.: Comparison of the various methods employed in the determination of the recruitment phenomenon. J. Laryng., *65:* 187–195, 1951.
49. Harris, J. D.: A brief critical review of loudness recruitment. Psychol. Bull., *50:* 190, 1953.
50. Bangs, J. L., and Mullins, C. J.: Recruitment testing in hearing and its implications. Arch. Otolaryng., *58:* 582, 1953.
51. Hirsh, I. J., Palva, T., and Goodman, A.: Difference limen and recruitment. Arch. Otolaryng., *60:* 525, 1954.
52. Hedgecock, L. D.: The measurement of auditory recruitment. Arch. Otolaryng., *62:* 515, 1955.
53. Harris, J. D., Haines, H. L., and Myers, C. K.: Loudness perception for pure tones and for speech. Arch. Otolaryng., *55:* 107, 1952.
54. Ewertsen, H. W., Filling, S., Terkildsen, K., and Thomsen, K. A.: Comparative recruitment testing. An evaluation of some new and older methods. Acta otolaryng., Suppl. 140, p. 116, 1957.
55. Eisenberg, R. B.: Loudness, recruitment and differential diagnosis. Arch. Otolaryng., *68:* 199, 1958.
56. de Bruine-Altes, J. C., and Huizing, H. C.: The monaural masking method for recruitment testing in symmetrical deafness. Acta oto-laryng., *37:* 385, 1949.

57. Yantis, P. A.: Locus of the lesion in recruiting ears. Arch. Otolaryng., *62:* 625, 1955.
58. Dix, M. R., Hallpike, C. S., and Hood, J. D.: Observations upon the loudness recruitment phenomenon, with especial reference to the differential diagnosis of disorders of the internal ear and VIIIth nerve. J. Laryng. & Otol., *62:* 671, 1948.
59. Eby, L. G., and Williams, H. L.: Recruitment of loudness in the differential diagnosis of end-organ and nerve fiber deafness. Laryngoscope, *61:* 400, 1951.
60. Jerger, J., Shedd, J., and Harford, E.: On the detection of extremely small changes in sound intensity. Arch. Otolaryng., *69:* 200, 1959.
61. Reger, S. N., and Kos, C. M.: Clinical measurements and implications of recruitment. Ann. Otol. Rhin. & Laryng., *61:* 154, 1952.
62. Thompson, G., and Hoel, R.: 1957. Cited by Yantis (53).
63. Jerger, J., Carhart, R., and Lassman, J.: Clinical observations on excessive threshold adaptation. Arch. Otolaryng., *68:* 617, 1958.
64. Yantis, P. A.: Clinical application of the temporary threshold shift. Arch. Otolaryng., *70:* 779, 1959.
65. Sørensen, H.: Clinical application of continuous threshold recording. Acta otolaryng., *54:* 403, 1962.
66. Pestalozza, G., and Cioce, C.: Measuring auditory adaptation: the value of different clinical tests. Laryngoscope, *72:* 240, 1962.
67. Harbert, F., and Young, J. M.: Threshold auditory adaptation. J. Auditory Res., *2:* 229, 1962.
68. Reger, S. N.: Pathologic temporary threshold shift. Internat. Audiology, *1:* 274, 1962.
69. Brand, S., and Rosenberg, P. E.: Problems in auditory evaluation for neurosurgical diagnosis. J. Speech & Hearing Disorders, *28:* 355, 1963.
70. Jerger, J.: Békésy audiometry in analysis of auditory disorders. J. Speech & Hearing Res., *3:* 275, 1960.
71. Jerger, J. F., and Herer, G.: An unexpected dividend in Békésy audiometry. J. Speech & Hearing Disorders *26:* 390, 1961.
72. Resnick, D. M., and Burke, K. S.: Békésy audiometry in nonorganic auditory problems. Arch. Otolaryng., *76:* 38, 1962.
73. Peterson, J. L.: Nonorganic hearing loss in children and Békésy audiometry. J. Speech & Hearing Disorders, *28:* 153, 1963.
74. Carhart, R.: Clinical determination of abnormal auditory adaptation. Arch. Otolaryng., *65:* 32, 1957.
75. Zwislocki, J.: Acoustic measurement of the middle ear function. Ann. Otol. Rhin. & Laryng., *70:* 599, 1961.
76. Feldman, A. S.: Impedance measurements at the eardrum as an aid to diagnosis. J. Speech & Hearing Res., *6:* 315, 1963.
77. Thomsen, K. A.: Employment of impedance measurements in otologic and otoneurologic diagnostics. Acta oto-laryng., *45:* 159, 1955.
78. Shambaugh, G. E., Jr.: Diplacusis: a localizing symptom of disease of the organ of Corti. Arch. Otolaryng., *31:* 160, 1940.
79. Butler, R. A., and Albrite, J. P.: The pitch-discriminative function of the pathological ear. Arch. Otolaryng., *63:* 411, 1956.
80. Harris, J. D., Haines, H. L., and Myers, C. K.: Recruitment, pitch tests, and speech-tone hearing discrepancies. Arch. Otolaryng., *62:* 66, 1955.
81. Carhart, R.: Audiometry in diagnosis. Laryngoscope, *68:* 253, 1958.
82. Carhart, R.: Atypical audiometric configurations associated with otosclerosis. Ann. Otol. Rhin. & Laryng., *71:* 744, 1962.

7

Speech Audiometry

J. Donald Harris, Ph.D.

THE NEED FOR SPEECH AUDIOMETRY

The need for speech audiometry arises because speech is by far the most important class of sounds we wish to hear. Pure-tone audiometry often gives an erroneous or even misleading notion as to how an individual can handle speech communication. Fortunately, it is not difficult to arrange for accurate tests of speech reception, and they can be as quick and accurate as tests with pure tones.

Speech as a Representative Acoustic Signal

Evolution has brought the human ear and voice so in accord that the human voice in its intensity range, its frequency range, and its temporal aspects very nearly exhausts the capacities of the human ear. If the usual speaking voice were much louder it would seem uncomfortable; if it were lower in frequency, the timbre would sound dull; if it were more rapid, it would mask itself. What minor mismatches exist can be thought of as built-in safety factors on the part of the ear. Thus, speech can serve not only as a test for communicability, but also as an extremely handy representative signal with which to examine an ear. For these reasons speech can be used to examine speech communication, while, at the same time, first-order information is provided on the ear's reception for many other classes of sound within the dynamic ranges of speech, such as sounds of nature, traffic, music, etc.

The Relation between Audiometric Loss for Speech and for Pure Tones

Historically, pure tones preceded speech as objectively controlled stimuli with which to assess hearing. What was needed as an interim measure was some way to assess hearing for speech from a knowledge of hearing for pure tones.

When an ear exhibits audiometric loss at one or more pure-tone frequencies, a formula can be used to relate this loss to a predicted loss for actual speech. The predicted loss will depend on the pure tones at which audiometric loss occurs, and also upon the particular sample of speech considered. No really final formula has been advanced, but there is a wide area of general agreement between the two evaluating procedures.

For the widely-used spondee lists of two-syllable equal-stressed words, and for colloquial speech, the 50% correct speech thresholds can be assessed most conveniently by Fletcher's formula (1) as modified by Quiggle and his group (2).

In the Fletcher formula, speech loss = 5 dB plus average hearing loss for pure tones at 500, 1000, and 2000 cycles per second (c/s). The slightly better formula of Quiggle and associates (2) gives greater relative weight to 1000 c/s and none to 2000 c/s.

$$\text{Speech loss} = 6.9 + 0.22\ HL_{500} + 0.35\ HL_{1000} + 0.21\ HL_{1500}$$

In case the audiometric data are not available at 1500, then 2000 c/s may be substituted as follows:

$$\text{Speech loss} = 6.9 + 0.22\ HL_{500} + 0.47\ HL_{1000} + 0.09\ HL_{2000}$$

The data at 2000 c/s, however, do not improve the prediction made by a formula using only 500 and 1000 c/s.

$$\text{Speech loss} = 7.1 + 0.23\ HL_{500} + 0.54\ HL_{1000}$$

It has been concluded by Graham (3) that since the multiple regression equation does not materially improve prediction for spondees, a simple average of the loss at the two best of the frequencies 500, 1000, and 2000 c/s should be used, as Fletcher proposed in 1950. Any formula can work only for large numbers, not for an individual ear. Individual ears may be miscategorized by more than ± 10 dB in about 5% of cases, even with the best formula.

For other types of speech material, notably the widely used phonetically balanced monosyllable lists, the formula (4) definitely must include 2000 c/s as follows:

$$\text{Speech loss} = 3 + 0.35\ HL_{500} + 0.23\ HL_{1000} + 0.41\ HL_{2000}$$

Furthermore, for speech in noise or for distorted voices the formula must include 3000 c/s (5–7). Since much of daily speech is noisy or distorted in many ways, the best estimate for speech loss in everyday life can be had by averaging the loss at 1000, 2000, and 3000 c/s.

It must be noted that these formulas are not always applicable when cochlear or central disorders exist or when there are unusual language backgrounds. They apply only to the intensity of speech needed to furnish 50 % correct judgments. Predicted hearing for speech will occasionally differ rather widely from actual hearing for any of these reasons. It is largely because of such discrepancies that actual speech audiometry is being recommended more and more widely, not only to assess threshold, but also supra-threshold, discrimination loss (8).

In summary, pure-tone audiometry is in many situations no real substitute for the assessment of social handicap using actual speech material, and a vigorous search for the best materials and equipment should be made.

RAPPORT WITH PATIENT

In addition to the usual audiometric precautions concerning rapport, more than usual care must be taken with speech materials. In understanding speech, patients often present language problems which have no real relation to the actual status of their hearing mechanism. The audiometrist must assure himself that the patient knows exactly what is expected of him, and must give him adequate practice prior to the test proper. He must observe the patient's reaction time in order to pace the test properly. Only experience with all types of personality and all types and degrees of hearing defect will enable the audiometrist to meet these special situations as they arise.

SPEECH MATERIALS

A very wide variety of speech materials exists in the literature for research and other special purposes. Clinical speech audiometry in this country, however, depends almost exclusively on word lists originally prepared at the Harvard Psycho-Acoustic Laboratory. These are the so-called spondee and phonetically balanced (PB) lists, of equally stressed spondees and of monosyllables respectively, whose phonemic makeup roughly matches that of American colloquial speech (9).

Somewhat altered lists of spondees for the speech reception threshold (SRT) and of PB words for discrimination loss are available from several sources (10-12). It is also possible to use conversation (13) as material for SRT.

There are now standardized lists of sentences sampling American colloquial speech (14), and standardized lists of individual phoneme intelligibility (15). Conversion factors relating thresholds on these tests to the zero hearing level on speech audiometers (which are calibrated in terms of spondee lists) will presumably be available shortly.

The audiometrist's report of any speech test should include mention of the material used for testing. Differences of more than a few dB have been noted in some cases from one type of speech material to another.

THE CLASSICAL SPOKEN- AND WHISPERED-VOICE TESTS

The spoken voice may be summarily dismissed as of little if any real value unless the examiner has some means of measuring the volume of his vocal output. The usual testing alley contains a drop of only about 15 dB as the tester moves from the 15-ft. distance up to within 6 in. of the ear. This means that experienced testers, in order to measure losses of more than 15 dB, must and do superimpose a voice intensity change on the reduced intensity with distance. It has been calculated (16) that one experienced tester, in his spoken voice test, uses a sound of which the log intensity varies linearly with the final voice score. Thus, the intensity for a 20/20 voice score could be heard at 43 ft. by a normal listener, while the intensity yielding a 1/15 voice could be heard over ⅖ of a mile! Evidently only experienced testers can so regulate their voices.

After much practice, and with the aid of a sound-level meter to help regulate and standardize voice intensity, an otologist can derive some information from the freely spoken-shouted voice (17, 18). (See the section later in this chapter on "Instruments for Monitoring Live Voice" for a list of handy sound-level meters.) However, precision of speech testing by this procedure cannot be very reliable, and in any case the shouted voice is a somewhat distorted signal.

The whispered voice is rather more successful in assessing mild to moderate speech losses. With care, it can be a serviceable quick screen. In one sample of 5248 ears (19) the whispered voice test screened out all but 92 ears which had an average loss of 15 dB through the speech range 250 to 4000 c/s. The 92 ears, or 1.75%, represents the selection error. A standard error of about 3 ft. expresses the precision of which this test is capable in well supervised hands. This means that a score of, for example, 10/15 will mean something between 7/15 and 13/15 on two out of three patients.

Table 7.1 gives a fair idea of the conversions among some of the classical categories of hearing tests.

ELECTRONIC SPEECH AUDIOMETRY

General

The spoken-shouted voice test as administered with a sound level meter can be materially improved when the speaker uses a normal conversational level throughout, and amplification is provided electronically. He may either talk into a microphone, monitoring his level with a volume indicator (VU meter), or record his speech on disk or tape. The extra precision ac-

TABLE 7.1

Conversion table for scores of speech intelligibility (38)

General Classification	Percentage Hearing Loss for Speech[a]	Average Audiogram Loss at 500, 1000, and 2000 c/s	Loss Below Normal Level of Speech[b]	Spoken Voice-Distance Fraction[c]	Whispered Voice-Distance Fraction
		dB			
Normal or near normal	0	0	0	15/15	Not reliable
	1–19	7	6	15/15	able
	10–19	17	16	14/15	15/15
Somewhat hard of hearing	20–29	30	26	10/15	7/15
	30–39	42	36	6/15	3/15
Needs hearing aid for effective social intercommunication	40–49	52	46	4/5	0.5/15
	50–59	65	56	3/15	No reliable data
	60–69	77	64	1/15	
	70–79	No reliable	74	0.75/15	
	80–89	data	80	0.5/15	
	90–99			0/15	
	100				

Each column independently calculated.

[a] Calculated from audiogram by American Medical Association method of computing percentage loss.

[b] Data from phonograph voice test and monitored voice test: both tests give similar results.

[c] Data adapted from Fowler (39).

[d] No scores can be obtained representing loss of less than 20 dB in the usual testing situation with a noise level of 20 to 30 dB as found in the usual testing alley.

quired, and the re-testing advantages, are obvious when such devices are used.

Two speech tests have been standardized to date: (1) *speech reception threshold (SRT) test*, or the intensity in dB with respect to a normal group at which 50 % of spondee words can be understood; and (2) *discrimination loss test*, or the percentage of phonetically balanced (PB) words understood at an intensity 40 dB over the individual's SRT.

Equipment

The American Standards Association has set forth specifications for speech audiometers (20). Since then a good tradition of acceptable speech audiometry has grown up in the manufacturing industry and among audiologists. With standard speech audiometers commercially available, it is no longer appropriate to provide suggestions as to how a home-made instrument can be patched together from hi-fi equipment and calibrated on the spot. It is imperative that a commercial speech audiometer which meets A.S.A. specifications be acquired by anyone considering performing speech audiometry.

Care. It cannot be emphasized too strongly that the tester should be thoroughly familiar with his equipment. All directions from the manufacturer pertaining to use and maintenance should be scrupulously followed. It is certainly not implied that the audiometrist be an electronics engineer, but he must know the mechanics of the speech audiometer so that he can perform quickly the operations required. He must also be so familiar with the instrument that he will know when it is not operating correctly or is not in calibration. He must be able to analyze the instrument to locate the general site of any defect in order to know whether he should repair it himself, as with a broken phone cord; call in a local repairman, as with tube checks; or send the whole unit back to the factory for repair or periodic overhaul.

Calibration. Determining whether a speech audiometer is within the A.S.A. specification limits as to distortion, gain, attenuation, frequency response, etc., is beyond the capacity of the usual local electronic repairman. man. Very expensive distortion meters, wow meters, microphones, filters, sound level meters, and an echo-free room are required to perform a complete physical calibration. This should be done at the factory during an annual preventive maintenance check. However, the audiometrist can determine whether his instrument is calibrated properly as to gain simply by collecting average thresholds on a half dozen normal-hearing young ears. Using his own ear as a relatively stable transfer standard, the audiometrist can regularly check the zero hearing level setting for unusual variation. (This can be done daily.)

Choice of Recorded or Monitored Live-Voice Test

Although a well run clinic will have both live-voice and recorded tests available, for the most part a recorded-voice test is preferable for several reasons. It has a handy 1000-c/s tone on the disk or tape for exact calibration, it is insensitive to the peculiarities of the tester's own speech, it furnishes excellent inter-clinic comparisons, it provides for item analysis, and it has several other minor advantages.

On the other hand, every audiologist will encounter a large number of patients who cannot follow a rather fast-paced test in general American dialect. Here the monitored *live voice* has certain advantages. With children, disturbed patients, the aged, the unintelligent, or the patient from another language background it offers the necessary flexibility. Often a child, or even an adult, will respond well only to a near relative, such as a mother or sibling, who can quickly be trained to assist. For such cases the monitored live voice definitely should be available. Its disadvantages are that it is not so objective and is certainly more expensive to calibrate since it demands an echo-free space between a calibrating loudspeaker and the audiometer's microphone.

Thus, the choice to be made is not whether the monitored live voice or the recorded voice should be installed in a clinic. All sources of speech should be available to the tester. The choice depends upon whether a patient can handle the standardized program recorded on a disk or tape. An informed guess may serve, or an actual preliminary sample test may be necessary.

Over-all Instructions for Monitored Live-Voice Audiometry

All commercial speech audiometers are furnished with complete instructions for the care of the monitored live-voice test equipment. These instructions should be studied and followed carefully.

Instructions as to how to administer the usual standardized SRT and discrimination loss tests are summarized below, and the step-by-step technique outlined later in this chapter, under "Directions for Speech Testing."

The audiometrist talks into a microphone 6 to 12 in. from the mouth and speaks *across* the diaphragm rather than *into* it. If the audiometrist's room has a relatively high noise level, it may be necessary to reduce this distance to a few inches. The audiometrist then trains himself to speak spondee words at a level to read "0" in the VU meter* on the instrument panel. However, for the same VU reading, two voices may vary several dB in intelligibility. It is necessary, therefore, for the audiometrist to examine approximately six ears with known normal hearing and adjust the auxiliary gain control provided so that for his particular voice a VU reading of "0" and a hearing level dial setting of "0" actually result in 50% intelligibility for the normal group. This should be done for earphone listening and for loudspeaker listening in the patient's adjoining room.

If the system is suspected of being out of calibration, it is necessary to repeat the whole procedure with another normal group. If the original settings cannot be approximated within a few dB, the instrument is probably faulty and should be checked for a broken connection, a bad microphone (often dropped), a burned-out attenuator, etc., and/or returned to the factory for correction and physical recalibration.

Once these settings are achieved, the accuracy of the test depends upon the accuracy of the audiometrist in approximating VU "0" on the peaks of the spondees.

---

* A VU meter is used to monitor the *input* from a microphone prior to amplification. In this context it is used to keep the tester's voice constant with respect to volume or intensity.

When being tested for SRT, the patient is asked to repeat the test words. The audiometrist simply presents the speech material into the microphone and notes the responses of the patient over the intercom system between the rooms. As the test progresses, the intensity settings are governed by what the audiometrist knows or observes about the patient's hearing. If the ear is suspected to be nearly normal, speech could well be started at 30 dB over normal "0."

Ten words are given and the percentage correct noted; then the intensity is reduced until less than 50% correct response is reached. The dB value which should yield 50% can easily be found by interpolating, thus: 20 dB yields 80%, 10 dB yields 20%, and therefore a setting (hearing level) of 15 dB should yield 50%. Again, 45 dB yields 60%, 40 dB yields 20%, and therefore a setting of about 43 dB should yield 50%. In order not to give a spurious impression of extreme reliability, all hearing levels should be rounded off to the nearest even number of decibels.

The discrimination loss is found by first finding an SRT for spondees, presenting PB speech to the patient at an intensity at least 40 dB over the SRT. One list of 50 PB words should suffice to determine the percentage of correct response. This figure subtracted from 100 gives discrimination loss.

(In addition to the instructions later in this chapter, the reader is referred to Newby's book *Audiology* (12), which provides voluminous procedures which have not been improved upon.)

General Instructions for Recorded-Speech Audiometry

For many situations it is possible to record speech on disk or tape and present it through the audiometer circuit to an earphone or speaker (10, 11, 21). The disadvantage of the variance associated with the individual voice is thus avoided. Disks of spondees and of PB lists with answer sheets and complete instructions are now available.* In addition, many other countries have followed the lead in recording similar spondee and monosyllabic words in their native language.

Both disks and tapes have a 1000-c/s tone pre-recorded at the same VU intensity as the original voice. There is a meter on the speech audiometer with a reference point to which the needle must rise when this tone is on. A monitoring switch on the phonograph or tape recorder is used to adjust this setting. At this point, the hearing-loss dial setting of "0" will yield about 50% intelligibility for normal ears. If it does not, the recording unit and/or the audiometer must be checked for operational trouble.

When the instructions are followed as to gain and settings, the speech

---

* Disks: Technisonic Studios, 1201 South Brentwood Boulevard, Richmond Heights, 17, Missouri. Tapes: Allison Laboratories, 11301 East Ocean Avenue, La Habra, California.

signal can be fed to the patient's earphone at any sequence of intensities required, exactly as described in the section on the monitored live-voice test, and SRT and discrimination loss can then be derived.

A great advantage of recorded-speech audiometry is the high reliability of the results on the same ear from day to day and from clinic to clinic. This considerably facilitates and makes more precise any continuous, long-term assessments of hearing changes which are the result of age, therapy, industrial noise trauma, etc. In addition, it is easier for the audiometrist to administer and is to be preferred when feasible.

Advantages of Electronic Speech Audiometry

Precision.

Better Financial-Legal Status. Hearing loss for speech, measured in dB, yields a quantitative index which may be entered on disability rating tables and graphs. Especially when financial and legal considerations apply, it is highly desirable to be as objective and reliable as possible, within a clinic and from one clinic to another.

A good speech test which is accurate within ± 2 dB is infinitely better than a *predicted* speech score derived from a pure-tone audiogram. According to Quiggle and his associates (2), the error of prediction from pure-tone hearing level to speech hearing loss will be between 5 and 10 dB in one case out of three.

Earlier Detection of Slight Losses Otherwise Overlooked. It is usually considered that a pure-tone loss of 15 dB is within normal limits, and group screening audiometry is often performed at that level. An occasional dip to 15 dB at one or even two frequencies is usually well compensated at other frequencies. However, if a speech audiogram is administered to screen at 15 dB, any "fail" on the test is a matter for concern. Such an ear is immediately labeled as on the verge of being "somewhat hard of hearing" (see Table 7.1), and appropriate action may be taken. Such ears would almost never be labeled correctly with the earlier crude speech testing methods.

Better Documentation of Initial or Slight Gains after Therapy. In cases when recovery of a hearing loss can be expected to be gradual, an accurate test of the course of recovery is indispensable to be sure that the proper regimen is being followed.

Better Assessment of Differences among Hearing Aids. Only an accurate test of speech reception, preferably of distorted speech, will serve to pick out the better of two similar hearing aids (22). Without such tests, hearing aid selection depends almost entirely upon the subjective impressions of the patient.

Complete Shape of Intelligibility Function Is Provided. By providing a graph showing how intelligibility improves as the voice intensity increases, speech audiometry can render important assistance to the diagnostician since certain types of defects cannot handle high intensities without "garbling." A distorted or "overloaded" intelligibility curve is pathognomic of perceptive, often central, loss. At the same time, the intelligibility curve indicates how much the patient could profit from a hearing aid. To fit certain ears of the "overload" type with an aid is almost deliberately to lead those patients to an even more frustrating experience. This frequently happens on a try-it-and-see basis without complete speech audiometry.

Use of the Social Adequacy Index Is Made Possible. The social adequacy index (8, 23) is very handy for predicting a patient's true capacity to handle ordinary speech when only his speech threshold (the 50% correct point on his intelligibility curve) and his maximal speech-handling capacity (the maximal percentage correct on that curve) are known. This index has proved of widespread service but obviously cannot be calculated without careful speech audiometry.

A slight drawback to the use of the social adequacy index is that the PB recordings are not standardized enough to measure a person's discrimination with the same precision with which his threshold level is measured.

Present and Future Research and Clinical Uses

Familiarity with the equipment will allow the audiometrist to provide oto-audiological data over and above simply providing two points on the intelligibility curve. The following are some of the extra tests which are available on a two-channel audiometer with either tape, disk, or microphone input.

Speech Testing by Monaural Phone with Contralateral Masking Noise. The purpose of this test is to assess speech reception in an ear defective by air conduction to the extent of 40 dB or more (mean loss at 500, 1000, and 2000 c/s) with respect to the better ear. SRT and discrimination score (DS) are computed as usual, except that a masking noise of the order of 40 dB is inserted in the better ear.

Alternate Binaural Speech-Loudness Balancing for Recruitment. The purpose of this test is to ascertain whether loudness recruitment for pure tones is in fact parallelled by loudness recruitment for speech. The experimental operations are exactly those for pure-tone work except that consecutive discourse is used as the signal. The question is whether an enhancement of loudness for speech in a particular ear actually yields enhanced intelligibility. This information bears on whether an ear would benefit from a hearing aid.

Lombard Test for Malingering. The purpose of this modification of the Lombard test is to quantify the intensity rise in the patient's voice when masking noises of higher and higher intensities are fed to the ear. By asking the patient to speak in his usual conversational voice into the microphone input of a live-voice speech audiometer, it is possible to maniuplate the attenuator dial so that the VU meter peaks at "0." While he continues to talk, masking noise is inserted in slowly increasing levels until the attenuation must be increased a significant amount to keep the VU peak at "0." Research by this technique should yield information on the level of masking, in relation to the threshold, at which the voice reflex begins for a normal or for abnormal populations.

Delayed Speech Feedback (Side-tone). With almost any tape recorder-reproducer, it is possible to pick up, amplify, and lead to the ears a speech signal from the second of two heads over which the tape passes. Delay will thus be inserted between the speaker's direct perception of his own voice and his perception of his voice through the earphones. The time of the delay is that taken by the tape to move to the second head (approximately $\frac{2}{10}$ sec.). Since most talkers experience a noticeable distortion in their speech when this time delay is of the order of that found with the usual $7\frac{1}{2}$ IPS tape recorder, it is possible to make a shrewd guess as to whether the subject actually hears the speech in the earphones, by observing the presence or absence of a speech distortion. This test can be used in some cases to detect malingering; and it is a handy research tool with which to explore the parameters affecting the feedback certainly present in all speech production.

Monaural and Binaural Hearing-Aid Evaluation. When the audiometer is furnished with a loudspeaker, almost any speech input can be used to determine the gain in intelligibility yielded by a hearing aid. The purpose of the monaural-binaural evaluation comparison is to determine whether in fact a binaural aid is indicated. There are some data to show that the slope of the intelligibility function is steeper in the binaural situation than in the monaural (24). In these cases, two aids would be considered better than one. This test would, then, have both practical and theoretical use.

Speech Reception by Bone Conduction. The purpose of this test would be to assess the possible usefulness of a bone-conduction hearing aid. Although such aids are prescribed less often than previously, this may not remain true. The technique of assessing SRT by BC would be identical with that for AC.

Insulation of Ear-Protective Devices for Speech. Inasmuch as the insulation of ear-protective devices is not necessarily linear with frequency, so that it might be difficult from pure-tone information to predict the insulation for actual speech, it is perfectly feasible to take SRT measurements in a free-field loudspeaker situation with or without ear-protective devices when the signal is actual speech.

The tests in this list can in certain cases yield vital information to the diagnostician or therapist. The choice of which tests or modifications to use is ordinarily not decided by the audiometrist but by his medical supervisor. However, these tests can be so standardized that the audiometrist will extract the same information from the patient as if the supervisor had himself performed the operations.

Other Possible Uses. Many uses and extensions of speech audiometry are at present being investigated. Multiple-voice tests using stereophonic equipment may relate to social adequacy in groups. A variety of masking distortion tests are being proposed (5, 25–28). When standardized, these tests among others may become the clinical tools of the speech audiometrist in the not-too-distant future.

Three of the most powerful audiological tools now in common use, recruitment (29), electrodermal (EDR) audiometry (30), and bone conduction testing, have been found to be as reliable and meaningful with speech materials as with pure tones.

On a research level, considerable thought is being given to the probability that a fairly elementary test such as that with the spondees or PBs does not really indicate what some individuals can and cannot hear of speech. Guberina (31) uses phonemes and monosyllables but presents any one sound through only one of three octave band-pass filters: namely, that one which gives maximal intelligibility for that sound. In this approach Guberina specifies the frequency content of individual sounds and relates these to the audiogram, in a more precise way than we have discussed above. In repeating some of Guberina's work and especially considering a series of about 15 persons with very depressed tonal hearing at 750 c/s who yet had quite passable communication ability, Maspétiol and associates (32) concluded that some individuals develop extreme ability to "fill in" missing frequency regions by a "phonemic supplementation."

Huizing and co-workers (33, 34) also use three band-pass filters (below 900, 900 to 1800, and above 1800 c/s) to gain a better insight into the speech-discriminative functions of impaired ears. Amplification and ear training are indicated in the frequency region where the most good could be expected.

The use of speech material distorted in other ways besides frequency filtering is being extensively used by Bocca and associates (25, 26) to explore the speech defects in those cases (old age, tumor) in which the audiogram and SRT may be essentially normal. Their patients showed profound defects for distorted speech, as by speed-up, interruption, long sentences, alterations of rhythm and accent, and elimination of meaning. This line of attack is also being pursued by Tato and Quirós (28), who suggest an even wider range of distortions, partly from the literature and partly from a systematic outline of all the things which could be varied in in speech.

It is an old observation that for normal ears binaural speech will meld perfectly if the signal is split into high- and low-tone components and led separately to the two ears. Matzker (35) uses this principle to determine subcortical lesions (where melding must occur); Groen and Hellema (24) suggested that in cases of peripheral deafness, but not of central deafness, the binaural intelligibility curve will be several dB steeper than the monaural.

In summary, it is seen that there are many practical and theoretical reasons for using speech audiometry with standardized electronic equipment wherever possible, in preference to earlier speech-testing methods.

INSTRUMENTS FOR MONITORING LIVE VOICES

Very inexpensive hand-held sound survey meters which can perform the simple function suggested by Fowler (17) are manufactured by:

H. H. Scott Company, 111 Powder Mill Road, Maynard, Massachusetts;

Mine Safety Appliances Company, Pittsburgh 8, Pennsylvania;

General Radio Company, West Concord, Massachusetts; and

Korfund Company, 35A4 Cantiague Road, Westbury, Long Island, New York.

Other more elaborate units which might be used if they are available, or the purchase of which might be justified on additional grounds, are manufactured by:

General Radio Company, West Concord, Massachusetts;

Boeing Airplane Company, Renton, Washington (Speech Interference Meter);

Bruel and Kjaer Company, 3036 West 106th Street, Cleveland 15, Ohio;

Allison Laboratories, 11301 East Ocean Avenue, La Habra, California;

Industrial Acoustics Company, 341 Jackson Avenue, New York 54, New York;

Rudmose R.A. No. 100 Sound Analyzer Tracor, Austin, Texas;

Doe Instruments, Ltd., London, England (handled by Korfund Company above); and

Western Electric Company.

STANDARD SPEECH AUDIOMETERS COMMERCIALLY AVAILABLE

Speech Audiometers.

Grason-Stadler Model 162, and

Panacoustic Model SA-101 A.

Pure-Tone Wide-Range Audiometers with Speech Audiometry Accessories.

Allison Model 21B,C (recorded- and live-voice equipment standard);

Otarion Models 900, 1000 (recorded- and live-voice equipment standard);

Beltone Models 14A, 15A (recorded- and live-voice equipment available);

ADC Model SC-1 (live-voice equipment available: unit may be adapted for recorded speech); and

Maico Models H-1, H-1B, MA-8.

A subcommittee of the Committee on Conservation of Hearing, American Academy of Ophthalmology and Otolaryngology has to date listed only the Grason-Stadler Model 162 of the above models (36). It is expected that other models will be tested and listed subsequently.

THE SOCIAL ADEQUACY INDEX (SAI) (8, 23)

A patient's articulation curve shows how his intelligibility score in per cent climbs as speech is made progressively louder. Such a curve gives a complete picture of that patient's ability to understand speech at all intensity levels. But a complete curve is time consuming and costly; some way to sample the total possible information must be found. The SAI does this by collecting intelligibility scores at only three intensity levels and averaging these scores.

Figure 7.1 illustrates the general thought behind the SAI and some of the actual procedure. Threshold for faint speech (SRT) is most quickly measured by the spondees or by connected discourse (13); percentage of intelligibility for the PB lists is then found at an intensity at least 35 dB above SRT. Figure 7.1 will show that at this intensity one is measuring an ear's ability to handle loud speech. Let us take the case of the ear in Figure 7.1 with an SRT for connected discourse of 44 dB and a discrimination loss of 0 %. No "faint" speech will come through, only 58 % of "average," and only 40 % of "loud" speech, for an average, or SAI, of 33.

Figure 7.2 eliminates these calculations altogether: one simply locates the intersecting cell of SRT and discrimination loss and reads SAI directly. It is worth noting here that an SAI of 33 has been suggested as a threshold of handicap (37).

DIRECTIONS FOR SPEECH TESTING

Speech Reception Threshold (SRT) Test

Purpose of Test. To determine the decibel level at which the content of speech can be understood at the 50 % correct level, with respect to standards established on normal ears.

Equipment Needed. A speech audiometer which meets the specifications for such equipment as established by the American Standards Asso-

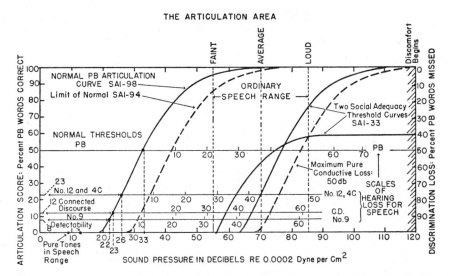

FIG. 7.1. The phonetically balanced (PB) articulation curve and the thresholds
for the various speech tests are based on receiver listening on the apparatus employed in Laboratory No. 2 of the Central Institute for the Deaf, 1944 to 1948. The
articulation curves apply to the PB word lists of the Psycho-Acoustic Laboratory as
recorded at the Technisonic Studio (Central Institute for the Deaf) spoken by Rush
Hughes. Slightly different shapes of curves and different values for thresholds may
be found with other apparatus and other recordings.

The section of the normal PB articulation curve from 5 to 55% correct is straight
with a slope of 50/13 (3.85% per dB). The slight "tail" to the left at the bottom
leaves the base line at 19 dB. The curve crosses the 50% correct line at 33 dB, and the
upper half is adequately defined by the following representative points: 36 dB, 60%;
40 dB, 73%; 46 dB, 86%; 56 dB, 96%; and 70 dB, 100%.

SAI refers to the Social Adequacy Index tabulated in Figure 7.2. It is the average
percentage of PB words that would be correctly understood by the listener at the
three speech levels indicated by the *dashed lines.*

ciation. The input may be either a microphone into which the experimenter
may speak, or a stored program (tape or disk). The speech material in
general use is a list of 36 two-syllable words listed in references 9 to 13.

Instructions to Patient. "You will hear a list of words through your
earphones (or speaker in the case of free field testing). These will consist
of two-syllable words such as baseball, armchair, etc., with the accent on
both syllables. First I will make the words loud enough for you the hear
them easily, then the loudness will gradually get weaker. You must repeat
into the microphone every word just as you hear it. If you are not sure,
guess. The words will finally become so weak that no one could hear them
all, so do not worry if toward the end of the test you can not repeat some
words. Do you have any questions?"

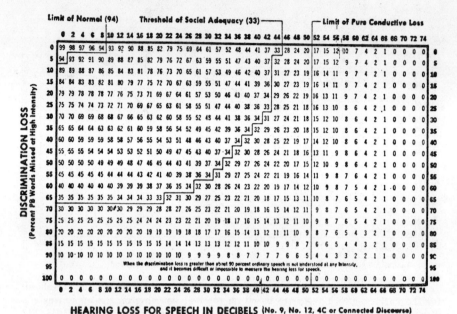

HEARING LOSS FOR SPEECH IN DECIBELS (No. 9, No. 12, 4C or Connected Discourse)

FIG. 7.2. Social Adequacy Index (SAI). Table to derive SAI from speech reception threshold and discrimination loss. PB words = phonetically balanced words.

Technique. The audiometrist must make sure that he understands the equipment thoroughly and has had training and practice under direction for many weeks before he attempts this test entirely by himself. In this preliminary training he will become familiar with the controls of the equipment so as to be sure, for example, that the tester's microphone, or the phonograph table, or the tape recorder, as the case may be, is connected correctly to the amplifier and earphone or speaker. In case the tester uses a microphone he must have practiced on the carrier phrase "You will say" which precedes every test word until the VU meter is peaking correctly on the "0" reading.

Live-Voice Administration. Speak a few test words slowly, preceding each by a carrier phrase with the attenuator set such that the patient could be expected to hear the test items clearly. This should be at an intensity level perhaps 30 to 40 dB above a reasonable estimate of the patient's hearing. If the patient responds promptly and correctly, decrease the loudness by 10 dB and repeat a few more test items. Continue decreasing intensity in 10-dB steps until the patient first shows signs of faltering. At that first point decrease the loudness in 5-dB steps, and then in 2- or even 1-dB steps until the tester is satisfied that a level is reached at which the patient's responses are approximately 50% correct.

Repeat for the other ear. In case a hearing aid is being used, a loudspeaker in a sound-treated room is to be used. In case there is a difference of approximately 40 dB between the two ears, a masking noise should be led to the better ear just as in pure-tone audiometry.

Recorded-Speech Administration. In case the program is stored on disk or tape, simply be sure the proper connections are made and follow the directions carefully as provided by the manufacturer of the recorded material and by the audiometer manufacturer. Together with the recorded speech material is stored a 1000-c/s tone with which the gain of the amplifier can be adjusted so that the tone yields "0" on the VU meter. Because the carrier phrase is recorded at the same level as the tone, and both at a level 10 dB louder than the test words themselves, it is necessary to subtract 10 dB from the attenuator dial reading to arrive at the correct SRT for the ear.

Expected Results. A correctly derived SRT will predict the speech level at which a subject is just able to follow the train of thought of colloquial consecutive cold-running speech. The term "cold" is used for non-emotional speech delivery.

Speech Discrimination Test

Purpose. To determine the percentage of speech intelligibility when loudness conditions are optimized for the ear.

Equipment Needed. As with the SRT, except that phonetically balanced (PB) word lists are used. These may be obtained from the same source as the spondee lists.

Instructions to Patient. "You are going to hear a list of 50 one-syllable words with which everybody is familiar. You are to repeat each word into the microphone as best you can. If you are not sure, guess."

Technique. This test is always performed subsequent to a determination of SRT. Set the attenuator dial to a level 40 dB above the patient's SRT, and present the entire list of 50 PB words. The reported score is the percentage of words correctly repeated (number correct × 2). Either with a stored program or with a live-voice administration the gain is set with respect to the SRT.

Some patients will be able to write the words rather than repeat them into the patient's microphone. This is preferable where possible. Note that spelling should in no way count.

Expected Results. A correct derived discrimination score (DS) will indicate the percentage of isolated words which an ear can hear under the most favorable loudness conditions. Conversely, subtracting the DS from 100 will yield the discrimination loss, which is useful in some circumstances.

REFERENCES

1. Fletcher, H.: *Speech and Hearing.* D. Van Nostrand Company, Inc., New York, 1929.

2. Quiggle, R. R., Glorig, A., Delk, J. H., and Summerfield, A.: Predicting hearing loss for speech from pure tone audiograms. Laryngoscope, 67: 1, 1957.
3. Graham, J. T.: Evaluation of methods for predicting speech reception threshold. A. M. A. Arch. Otolaryng., 72: 347, 1960.
4. Harris, J. D., Haines, H. L., and Myers, C. K.: A new formula for using the audiogram to predict speech hearing loss. A. M. A. Arch. Otolaryng., 63: 158, 1956. (See Errata, p. 477.)
5. Harris, J. D., Haines, H. L., and Myers, C. K.: The importance of hearing at 3kc for understanding speeded speech. Laryngoscope, 70: 131, 1690.
6. Harris, J. D., Haines, H. L., and Myers, C. K.: The relation of auditory acuity to normal and to distorted speech. Arch. Otolaryng., in press.
7. Kryter, K. D., Williams, C., and Green, D. M.: Auditory acuity and the perception of speech. J. Acoust. Soc. America, 34: 1217, 1962.
8. Walsh, T. E., and Silverman, S. R.: Diagnosis and evaluation of fenestration. Laryngoscope, 56: 536, 1946.
9. Egan, J. P.: Articulation testing methods. Laryngoscope, 58: 955, 1948.
10. Hirsh, I. J., Davis, H., Silverman, S. R., Reynolds, E. G., Eldert, E., and Benson, R. W.: Development of materials for speech audiometry. J. Speech & Hearing Disorders, 17: 321, 1952.
11. Hudgins, C. V., Hawkins, J. E., Karlin, J. E., and Stevens, S. S.: The development of recorded auditory tests for measuring hearing loss for speech. Laryngoscope, 57: 57, 1947.
12. Newby, H. A.: Audiology. Appleton-Century-Crofts, Inc., New York, 1958.
13. Fasconer, G. A., and Davis, H.: The intelligibility of connected discourse as a test for the 'Threshold of Speech.' Laryngoscope, 57: 581, 1947. (Discs available at cost from Central Institute for the Deaf, 818 S. Euclid, St. Louis, Mo.)
14. Silverman, S. R., and Hirsh, I. J.: Problems related to the use of speech in clinical audiometry. Ann. Otol. Rhin. & Laryng., 64: 1234, 1955.
15. Fairbanks, G.: Test of phonemic differentiation: the rhythm test. J. Acoust. Soc. America, 30: 595, 1958.
16. Harris, J. D.: Free voice and the pure tone audiometer for routine testing of auditory acuity. Arch. Otolaryng., 44: 453, 1946.
17. Fowler, E. P., Jr.: The discovery and evaluation of otic cripples. Arch. Otolaryng. 45: 550, 1947.
18. Harris, J. D.: Some suggestions for speech reception testing. Arch. Otolaryng., 50: 388, 1949.
19. Shilling, C. W., Harris, J. D., and Everly, I. A.: Hearing tests: an evaluation. Navy M. Bull., 44: 100, 1945.
20. American Standards Association: Standard Z24.13-1953, Specifications for Speech, Audiometers, 1953.
21. Manual of Instruction for Auditory Test No. 9: Threshold of Hearing for Words, 1C No. 73, NDRC Research on Sound Control, Psycho-Acoustic Laboratory, Harvard University, May 20, 1944.
22. Harris, J. D., Haines, H. L., Kelsey, P. A., and Clack, T. D.: Speech intelligibility and the electroacoustic characteristic of low fidelity circuity. J. Auditory Res., 2: 357, 1960.
23. Davis, H.: The articulation area and the social adequacy index for hearing. Laryngoscope, 58: 761, 1948.
24. Groen, J. J., and Hellema, A. C. M.: Binaural speech audiometry. Acta oto-laryng., 52: 397, 1960.

25. Bocca, E., Calearo, C., and Cassinari, V.: Cortical deafness. Rev. laryng., *78:* 777, 1957.
26. Bocca, E.: Clinical aspects of cortical deafness. Laryngoscope, *68:* 301, 1958.
27. Harris, J. D.: Combinations of distortion in speech: the 25% safety factor by multiple-cueing. A. M. A. Arch. Orolaryng., *72:* 227, 1960.
28. Tato, J. M., and Quirós, J. B.: Die Sensibilisierte Sprachaudiometrie. A. M. A. Arch. Otolaryng., *51:* 593, 1960.
29. Harris, J. D., Haines, H. L., and Myers, C. K.: Loudness perception for pure tones and for speech. A. M. A. Arch. Otolaryng., *55:* 107, 1952.
30. Ruhm, H. B., and Carhart, R.: Ojective speech audiometry: a new method based on electrodermal response. J. Speech & Hearing Res., *1:* 169, 1958.
31. Guberina, P.: L'audiometrie verbo-tonal. Rev. laryng., *77:* 20, 1956.
32. Maspétiol, R., Robert, P., and Semette, D.: Le phénomène de suppléance phonémique auditive. Acta oto-laryng., *49:* 325, 1958.
33. Huizing, H. D., and Taselaar, M.: Triplet testing and training—an approach to band discrimination and its monaural or binaural summation. Laryngoscope, *68:* 535, 1958.
34. Huizing, H. C., Kruisinga, R. J. H., and Taselaar, M.: Triplet audiometry: an analysis of band discrimination in speech reception. A. M. A. Arch. Otolaryng., *51:* 256, 1960.
35. Matzker, J.: *Ein Binauraler Hörsynthese-Test zum Nachweis zerebraler Hörstörungen.* Georg Thieme Verlag, Stuttgart, 1958.
36. Listing of audiometers. Tr. Am. Acad. Ophth., *64:* 761, 1960.
37. Silverman, S. R., Thurlow, W. R., Walsh, T. E., and Davis, H.: Improvement in the social adequacy of hearing following the fenestration operation. Laryngoscope, *58:* 607, 1948.
38. Harris, J. D.: Interpretations of measurements of auditory threshold. In *Encyclopedia of Vocational Guidance,* Vol. 1, p. 443. Philosophical Library, New York, 1947.
39. Fowler, E. P., Sr.: Hearing standards for acceptance, disability rating and discharge in the military services and in industry. Laryngoscope, *51:* 937, 1941.

8

Screening Tests

Aram Glorig, M.D.

Screening is a mass survey technique which seeks to identify those persons whose hearing is outside normal limits and requires further evaluation. It is possible in survey work to use any of a wide variety of audiometric measuring procedures, including threshold tests. Most of the standard threshold tests, however, were devised for diagnostic rather than survey purposes, and are not economical of either time or money.

In screening it is not necessary to make a complete audiometric evaluation or to concentrate on factors of hearing such as sensitivity, pitch recognition, discrimination, and tolerance. It is necessary only to obtain the answer to one question: Does this person hear the tone when it is presented at a pre-determined dB level (re audiometric zero)? If he does hear it, he may be presumed to have hearing within "normal" limits. If he does not, then he must be referred for a complete audiometric evaluation.

Considerable work has been done to develop techniques and measuring instruments which permit such an assessment. Although there are several variations within these categories, the tests and instruments fall into three general groups: Individual pure-tone sweep-check screening devices, group screening, (manual or automatic), and limited frequency screening (monitoring audiometry).

INDIVIDUAL PURE-TONE SWEEP-CHECK TEST

This test requires an audiometer with air-conduction earphones, properly calibrated to meet the screening criteria of the American Standards Association. The person being tested is seated so that he cannot see the operation of the audiometer and is instructed to raise his hand (or finger) when he hears a tone through the earphone. The intensity dial of the audiometer is set at a pre-determined level, preferably 5 dB (15 dB on the Proposed International Standard). The test frequencies of 1000, 2000, 3000 and/or

170

4000, and 6000 c/s are then presented in this order. If the person being tested fails to respond to the tone at 1000 and/or 2000 c/s or if he fails to hear the tone at *any two of the three frequencies* of 1000, 4000, and 6000 c/s, he should be referred for a threshold audiogram.

The sweep-check test is preferred by many audiometrists because it presents great reliability in case finding. Using this method, a good audiometrist can screen a cooperative person in approximately 2 min. This, of course, does not compare favorably with the numbers who can be screened by group methods in the same amount of time, but it still represents the most reliable and most practical screening method available today.

GROUP SCREENING TESTS

The primary advantage of a group test is that many persons can be tested at one time by a single audiometrist. However, accuracy may be sacrificed in favor of time and economy. The common group tests recommended for use today are: the Massachusetts test, the pulse-tone group tests (Regar-Newby or Glorig), and the Johnston group pure-tone screening test.

The Massachusetts Test

This test requires a pure-tone audiometer with multiple earphones which are matched in their frequency response at the three test frequencies of 500, 4000, and 6000 c/s. Because of the utilization of multiple earphones, the audiometer must be carefully re-calibrated according to a specific time and procedural schedule, and the necessary corrections made.

In testing, a sequence of tonal bursts is given with six "yes" or "no" options at each frequency. Those being tested circle "yes" or "no" on a special form depending upon whether or not they heard a tone at the time they were to listen. The forms are scored by counting the "no" responses, and if the number of "no" responses at any frequency differs by more than two from the number presented, it constitutes a failure. With 40 earphones in use, as many as 150 persons can be tested and graded in 1 hour. Investigators have found that the Massachusetts test provides accurate screening from grade 3 up. Because of the type of cooperation required of the listener, it is not recommended below this level.

Pulse-Tone Group Tests

In these tests a set number of pulses, or spurts of tone, are presented automatically. Those being tested indicate by writing on a test blank the number of pulses heard each time they see the signal to listen. Two excellent procedures of this type have been developed by Reger and Newby and by Glorig. Each employs an automatic audiometer and the test is so identified.

Reger-Newby Group Screening Audiometer. An automatic audiometer produces varying numbers of tonal spurts at each frequency. The spurts are counted and recorded on a form by the subjects. The attention of the group is caught by a flashing light on the instrument at the time the pulse tones are to start. Once the starting point has been dialed, the instrument continues automatically until the completion of the test. Forty persons can be screened simultaneously with this method. It is acceptable for grade 3 and above.

Glorig Automatic Group Screening Audiometer. This device automatically screens up to 40 persons in 3 min. by means of a pulse-count technique. The attention of the group is captured by a panel of lights. A varied number of pulse tones at each frequency is then presented, first to one ear and then to the other. The subject records the number of beats heard at each frequency, thereby providing results for both ears at the same time. This technique is excellent for a large group. Using this method 100 persons per hour have been screened and re-checked. Inasmuch as the test administers itself, a specially trained testing administrator is not required. It is accurate for all groups down to the level of the 3rd grade.

Johnston Group Pure-Tone Screening Test

This test eliminates the need for a written response, making it practical for the lower grades. A pure-tone audiometer is modified to accommodate 10 earphones, and the sweep technique is used. The subjects are seated in a semi-circle around a table and are instructed to keep their eyes closed. They are told to raise their hands when they hear a tone. They are warned, however, that not all of them will hear the tone because a few of the earphones will be disconnected each time, so they are to ignore others being tested. By checking the raised hands against the earphones carrying the signal, the tester can tell immediately who fails to hear the tone.

In addition to the tests described, other methods recently developed include: (1) familiar sounds screening test for pre-school children (University of Denver); (2) a group speech audiometric test (Stanford); and (3) the binaural group hearing test (Palo Alto).

LIMITED-FREQUENCY SCREENING

This is a special screening technique (devised by Glorig) in which only one frequency, 4000 c/s, is used. The technique is based on the finding that in many audiograms the largest degree of hearing loss occurs at 4000 c/s. The screening test level is pre-set 20 dB above audiometric zero (A. S. A., 1951), and it is extremely simple to administer. The time required for each subject is 20 sec., including recording time. No special training is required to administer the test, and valid results can be obtained even when the test environment does not meet stringent noise-level requirements. This test is of particular value in industry and the military.

PROCEDURES

The Testing Program

Any screening program must be pre-planned and must include the following examinations and procedures.

Screening

A screening program must include the following examinations: (1) routine hearing examinations at birth; (2) routine hearing checks at all physical examinations (birth to 3 years); (3) screening tests of the pre-school group (3 to 5 years); (4) sweep-check screening tests of the school population (5 to 18 years); and (5) pre-placement and monitoring audiograms in industry and the military.

Inasmuch as a screening test is only the first step in a hearing conservation program, adequate follow-up must be provided and must include threshold audiometric tests for anyone failing a screening test; audiological evaluation, medical referral and follow-up treatment for those failing the threshold test; and educational and vocational referral following medical treatment.

Birth to 3 Years—Screening Examinations. This is the critical period for hearing impairment diagnosis, yet there is no organized program for the detection of hearing problems in this age group. Modern techniques of applying hearing aids to children within the 1st year of life require that new standards be established to implement the detection and reporting of hearing problems in infancy. Such early detection will also provide the means for a program of preventive medicine which will fully cover the child population at the optimum time. The attending physician or pediatrician should incorporate routine checks of hearing into each physical examination. The following procedures are recommended.

Birth. The attending physician must check for the following reactions:
Step 1. Moro's reaction.
  Technique: Clap hands sharply within 3 ft. of the infant's ear.
  Response: Total bodily startle response is to be expected. (First reaction should be carefully observed because repetition leads to extinction of response.)
Step 2. Eye-blink reflex.
  Technique: In quiet environment snap fingers within 1 ft. of the child's ear.

Response: Blinking of the eyes can be expected. (This technique probably cannot be repeated successfully.)

Screening the hearing of newborn infants has not yet become a common practice, but a number of reports have been made on experimental neonate screening programs in this country and abroad. These investigations suggest strongly that it will be feasible to implement mass screening programs in the near future. Although the methods and procedures have not been agreed upon, a survey of the possible approaches to such a program points to the direction that will be taken.

The detection of hearing problems at birth will be the primary step in a comprehensive hearing conservation program. Until school age is reached, there is no other time when the child population is so easily available as in the newborn nursery. Mass screening techniques at birth may give us answers to many questions that have confounded us: What is the true incidence of congenital deafness? Can early training and habilitation of the hearing-impaired child improve his chances for integrating into the hearing world? Will the auditory behavior of the newborn infant give any clues to later performance or to the existence of central involvements? These questions are being asked by many investigators, and their answers may be at hand.

Successful screening of newborn infants is dependent on two factors: the selection of effective acoustic stimuli that reliably evoke auditory responses in infants, and the establishment of criteria for the infants' auditory responses that can be agreed upon by observers. Both of these factors have been reported on in a variety of ways.

The kinds of acoustic stimuli that have been employed in screening neonates vary widely. Fröding (1) used a metal gong of 126- to 133-dB SPL; Suzuki and Sato (2) employed recorded animal sounds through loudspeakers to obtain free-field startle responses; Richman, Grossman, and Lustman (3) used a cowbell of 113-dB intensity; Hardy and his associates (4) reported using a 60-dB clacker, in a modification of the techniques of Ewing and Ewing (5); Wedenberg (6, 7) designed a special audiometer producing pure tones in half-octave steps, 500 to 4000 c/s, with build-up time of less than 2 msec., with output measured at 50 cm. from the loudspeaker, 70- to 115-dB SPL; Downs and Sterritt (8) report a narrow band of filtered white noise, 2500 to 3500 c/s, with a 1-msec. rise, measured at 90-dB SPL 6 inches from the loudspeaker. The last two reports indicate that it is possible to screen newborn infants with measurable acoustic stimuli that will differentiate between losses that are greater in the high frequencies than in the low frequencies. It is evident that if any acoustic stimulus is to be standardized, it must be measurable and reproducible with great precision. Pure tones or filtered bands of noise will be most likely to meet these criteria.

The response categories that have been described by these investigators show remarkable unanimity. The auro-palpebral reflex (termed APR by Wedenberg) is the easiest response to observe and the most consistent. The complete or partial Moro reaction is also described by all workers, and is sometimes referred to as a "startle" response. Other responses that have been reported are the waking or arousal response; cessation of activity and vocalization; and, less common, orienting of eyes and head to source, movement of eyeballs, and change of expression. It seems fairly certain that if any standardization of response categories can be made, it will rest on the APR and the Moro reaction. These two lend themselves to more reliable inter-observer agreement.

Based on the evidence currently available, an ideal neonate screening program would incorporate the following methods:

1. The use of an acoustic stimulus which differentiates in some way between the various frequency ranges that are important for identifying hearing losses. The frequencies above 1000 c/s and up to 4000 c/s would be most definitive.

2. A stimulus intensity range of from 90- to 100-dB SPL, measurable at a reasonable distance from the source. Six to 18 inches would be practical in the usual nursery situation.

3. A rapid onset of the stimulus of from 1 to 2 msec. Acoustic treatment should ensure that no signals other than the specified one would be represented.

4. A definition of response categories that would allow any observer to duplicate the observations of other observers.

5. A longitudinal follow-up program that will demonstrate the validity of the observed responses and correlate them with conditions found in later life. Such a follow-up program requires definitive testing procedures, which appear to be at hand. For example, the recording of evoked responses to auditory stimuli through analog computers appears to offer the definitive evaluations required of an early testing program.

Neonate screening programs incorporating these methods will in time answer some of the most searching questions in the field of hearing and deafness.

Six-Week Check. The attending physician must check for the Moro reaction and eye-blink reflex (steps 1 and 2 above).

Three-Month Check. Attending physician must repeat steps 1 and 2 above and

Step 3. Test for orienting response.

Technique: Present repeated sound 3 ft. to one side of the child's ear, and behind his line of vision.

Response: A delayed, clumsy head turning in the general direction of the sound may be expected within 20 sec. (The sound source may be a small rubber squeeze toy which emits a "whooshing" sound but does not have a loud squeal or whistle. A small clacker or rattle may also be used. (In orienting test, if child responds to clacker but not to squeeze toy, or small high-pitched bell, a high frequency loss may be suspected.))

Step 4. Check for speech awareness.

Technique: Expose child to normal conversation in quiet environment.

Response: At this age, a momentary cessation of activity may be observed in response to conversation in quiet environment.

Six-Month Check. The attending physician should repeat steps 3 and 4 above and

Step 5. Test for speech awareness.

Technique: Say the child's name in normal conversational tone behind line of vision in a quiet environment. (Conversation should be eliminated for at least 60 sec. prior to this test.)

Response: Head turning in direction of the speaker may be expected.

Six Months to 1 Year. The attending physician should repeat step 5 above and counsel the parents to observe the child's response to sound. Particular attention should be paid to responses to speech and environmental sounds out of the line of vision. Failure to respond consistently to these sounds should be reported by the parent to the physician at once. In addition, failure of child to "babble," and, by 1 year, to imitate "babbling" sounds, should also be reported. At 1 year, physician should repeat step 5.

One to 3 Years. Attending physician should repeat step 5 above routinely.

If at any of the above stages the child does not produce a satisfactory response to these screening techniques, or if the parent has any reason to believe that the child is not hearing properly, the physician should refer the child to an audiological evaluation center for an examination.

Three to 5 Years. The pre-school group is attracting more attention recently, primarily because it is now established that this age group *can* be tested and that appropriate techniques are available. The major problem rests in assembling these youngsters for testing. The physician should continue his check of his patient's hearing, particularly with reference to general development of speech, adequacy of vocabulary, and distinctness of articulation throughout this age range. He should also check hearing after any disease or illness, using orienting response and speech awareness tests.

In addition to the physician's assessments, screening tests of pre-school children, individually and in groups, are becoming a common practice wherever appropriate facilities for testing children are available. The recommended procedures for sweep-check screening this age group follow.

Sweep-Check Screening Test.

Method: Individual pure-tone sweep-check test.

Equipment: Pure-tone air-conduction audiometer.

Level: 5 dB re audiometric zero (15 dB proposed International Standard).

Frequency: 1000, 2000, 3000 and/or 4000, and 6000 c/s.

Environment: Sound-treated room. If not possible, select quietest room.

Technique: a. Assemble children in a group and explain the entire testing procedure.

b. Conduct a "dress rehearsal" with the audiometer, allowing the children to hear the tones (greatly amplified). Demonstrate "finger lift" response.

c. In the testing room, assemble children in groups of four, with one being tested and three observing. Repeat the instructions to each child.

d. Sweep-check test each child.

e. Re-screen failures.

f. Refer children failing test for threshold test.

Supplementary Techniques. Several special techniques have been developed which are specifically designed for this age group, and which may be used for a screening program. These should be used only with the advice and supervision of a qualified audiologist. They include play audiometry, filtered familiar sounds with picture recognition, and puppet-show and peep-show techniques.

Five to 18 Years. The public school system has assumed the major responsibility for testing this age group. The major need is to bring the varied programs into alignment so that all communities adhere to the same standards and meet the same criteria. The recommended procedures for public school screening follow:

Frequency of Testing. Testing shall be conducted *annually* in grades Kindergarten, 1, 3, 5, and 7. Testing shall be conducted annually for all transfers into the school system, including the high-school-level student. Testing shall be conducted annually for all students with a history of hearing impairment until the testing reveals a return to "normal" range as the result of medical care, or until, following treatment, the audiograms show no decline for 3 successive years.

Sweep-Check Screening Test.

Method:	Individual pure-tone sweep check test.
Equipment:	Pure-tone air-conduction audiometer.
Level:	5 dB (15 dB proposed International Standard).
Frequencies:	1000, 2000, 3000 and/or 4000, and 6000 c/s.
Environment:	Sound-treated room, or the quietest room in the building.
Technique:	a. Assemble entire class in classroom. Give instructions to entire group, including a demonstration of the audiometer. Demonstrate position of earphones; allow group to hear tone.
	b. Screen one student at a time, cautioning class to be very quiet during testing.
	c. Sweep-check each student.
	d. At the completion of testing the group, re-screen anyone who fails to respond to the tone at the level of 5 dB at 1000 and/or 2000 c/s or who fails to respond to the tone at the level of 5 dB at two out of the three frequencies of 3000, 4000, and 6000 c/s.

Industrial and Military Programs. These programs are administered by the medical departments of the companies or the military services. A discussion of the principles and some of the special considerations of these groups is presented in Chapter 12.

THE HEARING-CONSERVATION PROGRAM

Screening may be viewed as an independent technique, but it should always be reviewed in the context of a hearing-conservation program. Most screening tests are presently administered as part of state or local hearing-conservation programs, although industrial and military screening surveys are often independent operations. Unfortunately, these programs are characterized by a high degree of individuality in their methods and procedures.

In the preceding discussion of some of the screening methods, it was emphasized that screening is but the initial step in a process which includes complete medical and educational follow-up. What is now needed is to bring all screening programs into alignment so that there is some continuity and agreement from state to state. Inasmuch as screening tests provide the only opportunity many people will have for an assessment of their hearing, the techniques and criteria used to detect hearing problems must be standardized so that uniform procedures will be used in all communities.

The soundest way to achieve these standardized procedures is to establish a *national* hearing-conservation program, the goals of which would be: (1) The acceptance of screening-test procedures which discover, within human ability, *all* persons having a hearing loss; (2) The establishment of follow-up programs which assure medical evaluation and care for every person with a hearing loss; and (3) The assurance of educational and vocational programs which provide complete services for all types of hearing rehabilitation needs.

Organization

The steering committee for a national hearing-conservation program would establish a national set of standards. (Fortunately, several excellent professional committees are already in existence which could assume this function.) Once these national standards had been agreed upon, all communities would use the same procedures in detecting hearing loss, adopt the same criteria for failure of hearing tests, administer the tests in the same manner, organize programs for medical referral and follow-up, and provide for educational and vocational rehabilitation. Individual hearing-conservation programs, therefore, would remain state and local efforts but would conform to these national standards.

The responsibility for the program would rest with the medical profession, since hearing impairment is a medical problem. The most logical supervisors for such state programs are the state departments of health. Many programs are now under the aegis of other organizations, such as departments of education. This type of non-medical supervision is not recommended because these departments lack authority to ensure proper medical referral and follow-up. Further, under such programs no provision is made for testing any but the school child.

Under the direction of competent medical authority, evaluation of hearing would begin at birth and continue *routinely* throughout the lifetime of the individual. It would be responsibility of the medical authority to:

1. Supervise the entire program.
2. Adopt the national standards as official operating procedure.
3. Establish a procedure whereby all physicians would make an official report to the state department of health of all cases of suspected hearing loss.
4. Establish audiological evaluation centers wherever need exists, utilizing the services of existing facilities such as hospital clinics, university clinics, etc., wherever possible.
5. Work in conjunction with other interested agencies to provide for educational follow-up and/or vocational rehabilitation.

TABLE 8.1
Hearing conservation chart*

Ages and Screening Tests	By Whom	Location	Criteria for Failure	Referral to	Criteria for Rehabilitation	Rehabilitation
0-3 months 1. Moro's reflex to sudden sound 65 dB or more Sound source: handclap at 3 ft.; wooden clacker (calibrated) 2. Eye-blink reflex to sudden sound 30 dB or more Sound source: finger snap at 2 ft.; small frog clacker; bell and baby rattle (calibrated) (Note: Reflexes extinguish on repeated presentation of stimuli.)	Attending physician or pediatrician	Quiet delivery room or nursery soon after birth & pediatrician's office at 6-week & 3-month check	Lack of specific responses to the sound stimuli	Completely equipped oto-audiological evaluation center with complete examination and testing facilities for all age groups	Ave. level of 30 dB or more; following completion of medical treatment refer to audiology center for rehabilitation [E]	Level of 30-60 dB ave.: continued observation and retesting; parents counseled to institute home program of structured auditory stimulation Level of 60 dB and over: continued testing; diagnostic testing with amplification and assessment of potential with hearing aids
3-12 months 1. Repeat Moro's reflex and eye-blink test as above. 2. Orienting response (localizing) to soft noises 30 dB or more Sound source: soft squeeze toys and bells at 4 ft. for high pitches; clackers for low 3. Observe cessation of activity and/or orientation to conversational voice ("attending")	Pediatrician, or attending physician at each examination; trained personnel of well-baby clinics	Quiet environment in doctor's office or at well-baby clinic	1. Lack of specified responses to the sound stimuli 2. Failure to orient until sound exceeds 65 dB 3. Failure to localize on the appropriate side	Same as above	Same as above	Level of 30 dB ave. or greater: diagnostic training with hearing aids and fitting of appropriate hearing aid; structured home program of auditory stimulation with emphasis on bombardment with verbal and sound stimuli
12 months-3 years 1. Repeat (2) and (3) above 2. Observe definite attentive localization of all meaningful soft sounds of 30 dB	Same as above	Same as above	Same as above	Same as above	Same as above	Same as above
3-6 years 1. Individual pure-tone sweep-check test	Pediatrician, or attending physician at each examination; trained personnel of testing clinics; public health personnel; specially trained volunteers	Doctor's office, well-baby clinic, area testing clinic, pre-schools, camps, etc.; always in sound-treated room	No response to signal at HL of 5 dB at 1000 c/s and/or 2000 c/s or no response at HL of 5 dB at 2 of 3 frequencies of 3000, 4000, & 6000 c/s	Same as above	Ave. level 15 dB or more in speech range following completion of medical treatment	15-25 dB ave.: consideration of possible hearing aid use. If no hearing aid recommended, L/R and A/T and speech rehab. where indicated 25-65 dB ave.: hearing aid fitting and auditory training with aid; speech rehab. and L/R where indicated 65-100 dB ave.: hearing aid fitting and auditory training with aid; speech rehab. and L/R where indicated; consideration of placement in special classes, or in oral school for deaf with more severe losses.

180

	5-18 years					
1. Individual pure-tone sweep-check test	Trained lay personnel; audiometrists; school nurses; school therapists; Public Health personnel	Sound-treated room, or quietest classroom in building	Same as above	Same as above	Same as above	Same as above
18 years and over						
1. Individual pure-tone sweep-check test	Industrial, medical, & military audiometrists; trained lay personnel; Public Health personnel, hearing society or other agency audiometrist	Sound-treated rooms in facility—plant, factory, military camp, doctor's office, college entrance physical examination rooms	Dependent upon age & medical history of patient	Same as above	Ave. level 30 dB or more following completion of medical treatment	20-30 dB ave.: consideration of hearing aid, depending on individual needs; L/R and A/T where indicated 30-65 dB ave.: hearing aid fitting; HAO, A/T, and L/R where indicated 65-100 dB ave.: hearing aid fitting; HAO, A/T, and L/R where indicated; and speech insurance

* From Gloria, Downs, and Overfield, 1962, unpublished.
† For greater detail, the film "Auditory Screening for Infants" is highly recommended. Obtainable from Division of Maternal & Child Health, Maryland State Dept. of Health, 301 W. Preston St., Baltimore 1, Md.

181

This medical supervision does not mean that the staff would be entirely medical; in fact, this would not be practical. The responsibility for the administration of the program would rest with qualified audiologists whose training and experience meet certification requirements of the American Speech and Hearing Association.

It would be the audiologist's responsibility to:

1. Make certain that the national standards were met in actual practice.
2. Administer a referral and follow-up system based on physicians' reports (see 3. above).
3. Develop and administer pre-school screening programs.
4. Administer (in co-operation with the department of education) the screening of school-age children.
5. Act as liaison with industry and the military services to assist them with their hearing programs.
6. Select, train, and supervise volunteer workers to carry out pre-school screening programs.
7. Select, train, and supervise personnel for threshold testing programs.
8. Act as liaison with other agencies whose services are required to complete the total program.

A structure such as the one roughly described would permit full opportunity for inter-departmental planning and co-operation. It is assumed that all interested agencies would have specific responsibilities in the total program, and each would make a maximal contribution because of this increased co-operation.

An explanation of the 5-dB screening level set forth in this chapter may be in order, inasmuch as it deviates by 10 dB from the customary 15-dB screening level now in use.

The first screening instrument used in this country, the Western Electric 4 C speech audiometer, utilized a 9-dB criterion for screening. This technique missed some high-frequency losses, but it compared well with a 15-dB pure-tone screening criterion. This is understandable when one considers that the 9-dB criterion was based on a laboratory standard of average normal threshold, whereas the pure-tone reference has been based on the present United States audiometric standard now known to be 10 to 20 dB higher than a laboratory standard. Therefore, the Western Electric audiometer, despite the drawback of frequency range, screened at a lower level relative to true threshold than a 15-dB pure-tone screen.

Further, when European screening programs have been reported using a 15- or 20-dB criterion, this level is equivalent to 5 or 10 dB on American audiometers.

From both medical and educational viewpoints, a 5-dB level of screening is also desirable. Children are frequently found with significant ear pathology whose air-conduction thresholds are as low at 0 to 5 dB. Often such children show −15 or −20 thresholds by bone conduction, indicating a significant air-bone gap. The traditional 15-dB screening level misses these children entirely.

In addition, it has been felt that a hearing loss of 15 to 25 dB in children constitutes an impairment which requires special attention or training of some kind. When it is considered that a 15-dB screening level may permit children with a 15-dB threshold level to be overlooked, it is evident that this is an unrealistic criterion.

In order to screen successfully at a level of 5 dB in the usual school environment, the lower frequencies cannot be used because of the noise. The choice of frequencies therefore becomes 1000 c/s and up, in order to eliminate the many false positives which would be found if 250 and 500 c/s were used. Fortunately, experience indicates that the higher frequencies will detect most significant hearing losses, particularly when several are used in combination.

The new screening level of 5 dB will be less disturbing to workers when the new proposed audiometric standards have been adopted. As soon as the change is made to the new sound pressure standard, screening will again be done at 15 dB on the hearing level dial, using the criterion that is being suggested. Accordingly, it will be most opportune to incorporate the screening level change now.

REFERENCES

1. Fröding, C. A.: Acoustic investigation of newborn infants. Acta oto-laryng., *52:* 31, 1960.
2. Suzuki, T., and Sat, I.: Free field startle response audiometry. Ann. Otol. Rhin. & Laryng., *70:* 997, 1961.
3. Richmond, J. B., Grossman, H. J., and Lustman, S. L.: Hearing test for newborn infants. Pediatrics, *11:* 634, 1953.
4. Hardy, W. G., Hardy, J. B., Brinker, C. H., Frazier, T. M., and Dougherty, A.: Auditory screening of infants. Ann. Otol. Rhin. & Laryng., *71:* 759, 1962.
5. Ewing, A. W. G., and Ewing, I. R. G.: *Educational Guidance and the Deaf Child*, edited by A. W. G. Ewing. Manchester University Press, Manchester, England, 1957.
6. Wedenberg, E.: Determination of the hearing acuity in the newborn. Nord. med., infants. Pediatrics, *50:* 1022, 1956.
7. Wedenberg, E.: Objective auditory tests on non-cooperative children. Acta oto-laryng., Suppl. 175, 1963.
8. Downs, M., and Sterritt, G.: Toward a method of screening newborn infants—a preliminary investigation. J. Auditory Res., *4:* 69, 1964.

SUGGESTED ADDITIONAL READINGS

1. American Public Health Association and the American School Health Association, School Health Section: Report of the Committee for Hearing Conservation, J. School Health, *29:* 71, 1959.

2. Barr, B.: Pure tone audiometry for pre-school children; clinical study with particular reference to children with severely impaired hearing. Acta oto-laryng., Suppl. 121, p. 1, 1955.

3. Carhart, R., and Jerger, J. J.: Preferred method for clinical determination of pure-tone thresholds. J. Speech & Hearing Disorders, *24:* 330, 1959.

4. DiCarlo, L. M., and Gardner, E. F.: The efficiency of the Massachusetts pure tone screening test as adapted for a university testing program. J. Speech & Hearing Disorders, *18:* 175, 1953.

5. DiCarlo, L. M., and Gardner, E. F.: The efficiency of three group pure tone screening tests for public school children. Exceptional Child, *24:* 351, 1958.

6. Downs, M.: The familiar sounds test and other techniques for screening hearing. J. School Health, *26:* 77, 1956.

7. Glorig, A., and House, H. P.: A new concept in auditory screening. A. M. A. Arch. Otolaryng., *66:* 228, 1957.

8. Johnston, P. W.: An efficient group screening test. J. Speech & Hearing Disorders, *17:* 8, 1952.

9. Leshin, G. A.: Pre-school hearing conservation on a statewide basis. J. Speech & Hearing Disorders, *25:* 346, 1960.

10. Lierle, D. M.: Report of the Committee on Conservation of Hearing. Tr. Am. Acad. Ophth., March–April, 1959.

11. Newby, H. A.: Evaluating the efficiency of group screening tests of hearing. J. Speech & Hearing Disorders, *13:* 236, 1948.

12. Newby, H. A.: Group of pure tone testing in the public schools. J. Speech & Hearing Disorders, *12:* 357, 1947.

13. Newhart, H., and Reger, S. N.: Manual for a school hearing conservation program. American Academy of Ophthalmology and Otolaryngology, 1956.

14. Siegenthaler, B. M., and Sommers, R. K.: Abbreviated sweep check procedures for school hearing testing. J. Speech & Hearing Disorders, *24:* 249, 1959.

9

Audiometry and Diagnosis

Kinsey M. Simonton, M.D.

AUDIOMETRY

Definition. Audiometry is the testing of hearing. The definition will be used in this chapter in its broadest sense, to include all methods available in and applicable to the office of the otologist to determine the hearing ability of his patient.

Purpose. The purpose of audiometry is to aid in the diagnosis of the causative conditions and estimation of the degree of hearing loss, so that the otologist may advise the patient and his family of the prognosis for future hearing and of treatment or rehabilitation measures available for the individual patient.

NON-AUDIOMETRY EVALUATION

Evaluation of the patient's hearing problem begins with his entry into the physician's office. Observation of his manner, his voice, and his hearing for conversation at the first meeting may provide a rough index of the nature and degree of his hearing disability. The patient who watches a speaker closely may be proficient at speech reading. The voice is often soft in conductive disability and flat and toneless with sensori-neural losses. When a louder than normal voice is required for communication in a small, quiet office, significant hearing handicap is probable.

The clinical history is the first step in audiologic diagnosis. Techniques of taking the history vary. A wise rule is to allow the patient to tell his own story. Pertinent information may then be obtained by questioning. The following outline presents points of particular importance:

Time and age of onset of loss of hearing
Illness, accident or other unusual circumstances at onset

Concurrent symptoms, vestibular disturbance, pain or fullness in the
    ear, headache, neurological disturbance, infection of the ear or
    respiratory tract, tinnitus
Personal history
    Acute infectious diseases
    Aural infections
    Respiratory infections
    Noise exposure
    Drugs
        Dihydrostreptomycin
        Neomycin
        Kanamycin
        Quinine
    Trauma to head
Family history
    Loss of hearing in parents or siblings, age at onset, and suspected
    cause
    German measles during first trimester of mother's pregnancy
    Conditions in which disability is apparent: groups, noise
    Patient's reaction to his disability

The physical examination may reveal the cause of impaired sound conduction. A clue to lesions of the VIIIth cranial nerve may be found in the
function of other cranial nerves, although physical examination of the ear
usually does not show abnormality in sensori-neural lesions.

AUDIOMETRIC EXAMINATION

This type of examination includes all methods of testing hearing in
which sound is used to elicit a response from the patient. Nine tests or
methods of testing hearing will be considered.

Voice Test. Commonly used and easily applied, the voice test, whether
spoken or whispered, is inaccurate because of poor control of the intensity
of the signal. Some information as to whether the predominant loss is for
high or low tones can be obtained by use of words made up predominantly
of sibilant sounds (sister) or vowel sounds (football). The spoken voice of
a familiar person is said to be the best test for young children (1).

Watch Test. A useful screening test for persons with normal hearing,
but one which is unduly selective for patients in the presbycusis age group,
is the watch test. Rough calibration can be achieved by determining the
distance at which the watch is heard by normal ears. The watch tick is
principally made up of high frequency sounds (higher than 3000 c/s).

Noisemakers. Whistles, bells, snappers, and various noisemaking toys
are useful for testing young children. Responses are reflex (eye blink) in

the young child, or learned (turn or look toward sound). These tests may allow an estimate but not a close measure of the degree of loss. Ingenuity is required to avoid response from visual stimuli.

Handclap. Similar to other noisemakers, the handclap has the additional disadvantage of creating an air movement which may evoke a response by skin sensation.

Tuning Forks. The use of tuning forks is rapidly becoming a lost art. This is unfortunate since the tuning forks are, next to the electric audiometer, the otologist's most useful test instrument. Quantitative tests can be done by use of calibrated forks or by comparison of the end point for the patient's ear with the examiner's ear. The threshold for the examiner's ear should be known. Quantitative tests with forks are time-consuming and lack accuracy. Judgment of the end point of audibility (threshold) of a gradually decaying sound is difficult. Qualitative tests with tuning forks are informative practical tests recommended for every otologist for preliminary evaluation of his patient's problem and as a check on the patient's response to other tests. The most useful qualitative tests are those of Weber, of Rinné, and of Schwabach.

Weber's Test. This test is used to classify unilateral hearing losses. The stem of a vibrating tuning fork is held at the midline of the skull and the tone is best heard in the affected ear in conductive lesions, and in the non-affected ear in sensori-neural lesions.

Rinné's Test. The tone of the tuning fork is alternately presented by air conduction 1 cm. from the concha and by bone conduction with the stem of the fork pressed firmly against the skull behind and above the ear. In a normal (positive Rinné) response, air conduction is heard approximately twice as long as is bone conduction. In an abnormal (negative Rinné) response, bone conduction is heard longer than air conduction. Responses may be of any degree, as decreased positive or equal. Abnormal response indicates decreased sound conduction in the external or middle ear. The Rinné test is recommended as a check on accuracy of bone-conduction audiometry in patients considered for operation to improve hearing. The 256, 512, and 1024 forks are most useful. Forks of lower frequency may be felt as a vibration, while those of higher frequency are heard by air conduction when bone conduction is being tested.

Schwabach's Test. Measurement of the time during which a tuning fork is heard by air conduction and by bone conduction provides a quantitative test of both conductive and sensori-neural function. The test is done with calibrated forks or by comparison with examiner's ear. Shortened hearing for bone conduction indicates the presence of a sensori-neural lesion. Lengthened hearing by bone conduction indicates a conductive lesion.

Masking of the normal ear is often useful when testing patients with unilateral hearing loss by the methods mentioned. The Bárány noisemaker or a stream of compressed air flowing across the concha is effective.

The Electric Audiometer. The electric audiometer is an instrument designed to deliver a sound of controlled intensity. Electric audiometry is superior to the previously described tests since repeated presentation of sounds of controlled intensity allows more accurate judgment of threshold by the patient and since the threshold intensity can be read from the dials of the instrument for recording. These features allow the test to be repeated in order to follow the progress of the patient's hearing and allow comparisons between tests done by different audiometrists at different times. The electric audiometer is the essential instrument in current audiometric techniques.

The following audiometric tests desirable for otological diagnosis are recommended for the otologist's office practice: (1) threshold tests for pure tones delivered by air conduction and bone conduction and threshold tests for speech, (2) tests for speech discrimination delivered at intensities above threshold, (3) tests to demonstrate disturbed cochlear function, loudness-balance tests for recruitment of loudness, short-increment sensitivity index (SISI) tests, tests of adaptation and fatigue, and tests for diplacusis binauralis dysharmonica, and (4) tests for functional hearing loss—The Lombard, Stenger, and Doerfler-Stewart tests.

More sophisticated tests are useful in neuro-otological diagnosis and should be available to the otologist through audiology clinics, although they may not be practical for the office of the individual otologist. These are Békésy audiometry, psychogalvanic skin-resistance tests, distorted speech (by filters or reduced intensity), and delayed feedback tests. A completely objective method of determining thresholds for pure tones by use of evoked cortical potentials averaged by computer has recently been described. This test will be useful for testing young children, mentally retarded children, and persons suspected of psychogenic hearing loss (2).

EQUIPMENT

Many audiometers are available on the market. Different models are designed to meet specific needs. The choice of audiometer should be dictated by the use to which it is to be put. Audiometers for office use fall into three general classes.

Auditory Screeners

These are simple battery-powered instruments which provide one or two frequencies at two levels of intensity. Their purpose is to determine quickly those persons whose hearing is normal and who do not require further study. This simple test may satisfy the needs of the general practitioner, pediatrician, or internist and may be used as a preliminary screening test in the office of the otologist. Single-frequency screening at 4000 c/s is reported to demonstrate 98.5 % of losses in speech frequencies (3). Study of a smaller selected group of patients with hearing deficiency failed to confirm this thesis and demonstrated that auditory screening is not dependable when done by people who are inexperienced in testing of hearing (4).

Portable Audiometers

These light-weight instruments provide pure-tone tests at frequencies from about 250 to 8000 c/s at intensities from −10 to 100 dB in 5-dB* steps. Determination of the threshold audiogram is thus possible. Bone-conduction and speech circuits are available on some models. Instruments so equipped are suitable for limited diagnostic audiometry and may suffice in the office which does only a small amount of otological diagnosis.

Clinical or Diagnostic Audiometers

These instruments are larger and incorporate more features than the portable models. They are designed to provide most of the audiometric tests commonly used in otological diagnosis.

Essential Features.

Air Conduction. Air-conduction testing should be available at frequencies from 125 to 10,000 c/s in octave and half-octave intervals and at intensities from −10 to 100 dB in steps no greater than 5 dB.

Bone Conduction. Bone-conduction testing should be available at frequencies from 250 to 4000 c/s and at intensities from −10 to 60 dB in 5-dB steps.

Speech Circuit. A speech circuit equipped for use with phonograph records, tape, or live voice and incorporating a voltmeter for use in monitoring the input intensity in live-voice tests should be available.

Masking Circuit. A masking circuit which delivers saw-tooth or white noise at controlled intensities up to 100 dB should be included. White noise is preferred.

Tone Interrupter. A tone interrupter which should be free of clicks or extraneous noise and which should provide a build-up from zero to full intensity within 0.1 sec., but not less than 0.02 sec., should be available.

Double Earphones. The instrument should have double earphones with balanced output and adequate insulation against ambient noise provided by a pad of sponge rubber or similar material.

Desirable Features.

Pulsed Tones. Pulsed tones may aid the patient in determination of his threshold.

---

* All dB in this chapter are re the 1951 ASA audiometric zero.

Reversing Switch. A reversing switch to transfer the signal from one ear-phone to the other is helpful.

Double-Attenuator Circuit. Such a circuit adds to the convenience of the binaural loudness-balance test.

Short-Increment Sensitivity Index (SISI). The short-increment sensi-tivity index is also desirable.

The calibration of the clinical audiometer should be checked daily by the operator. This is done by determining his own threshold. Bone-conduc-tion calibration can be compared with air conduction by comparison of air-conduction and bone-conduction thresholds on patients known to have pure sensori-neural loss (5). In addition, the instrument should be returned to the manufacturer at yearly intervals for calibration and servicing. (See Chapter 6.)

Accessory instruments which are useful in the office in which the major practice is otology or in audiology clinics are equipment for psychogalvanic skin-resistance tests and delayed-feedback-tape equipment for speech tests. Both instruments are used in the study of psychogenic or functional loss of hearing. The former is used in audiometry on young children. A free-field amplifier is useful for evaluation of hearing aids and for determining the speech-reception threshold with a hearing aid.

The Békésy Audiometer. The Békésy audiometer is a self-recording automatic audiometer. The signal intensity changes at a constant rate. The direction of change is controlled by the subject by pressing and releasing a key. Intensity is increased until it is barely perceived, then decreased until the tone is no longer heard. The resultant tracing is a saw-toothed curve which crosses the threshold. The signal may be a fixed frequency or a gradually changing frequency and is presented as either a continuous or periodically interrupted tone.

Békésy audiometry is useful for threshold determinations and also offers information of value in differential diagnosis. Jerger (6) classifies the Békésy audiometer tracings into four types based on the relationship of tracings made with continuous and interrupted tones.

Type I (Conductive Loss). This type is characterized by inter-weaving or super-position of tracings of continuous and interrupted tones.

Type II (Ménière's Disease, Stimulation Deafness). The continuous-tone tracing drops below the interrupted-tone tracing at high frequencies (1000 c/s), but the gap seldom exceeds 20 dB. The amplitude of the tracing is small in high tones.

Type III (Retrocochlear Lesions, Acoustic Neuroma). The continuous-tone tracing drops away from the interrupted-tone tracing very rapidly and at low frequencies. In fixed-frequency tracings the interrupted-tone tracing is horizontal while the continuous-tone tracing drops rapidly and may not stabilize. The amplitude of the excursions is constant. This demonstrates abnormal adaptation.

Type IV (Retrocochlear Lesions). This type resembles Type II except that the separation of the tracings for interrupted and continuous tones occurs through both low and high frequencies.

Distorted speech signals are achieved by passing the signal through a low-pass filter or by presenting the signal at reduced intensity. These signals are useful in demonstrating lesions of the auditory areas of the cerebral cortex.

The audiometrist, whether he be otologist, audiologist, or technician, should be thoroughly familiar with the equipment in use and should be experienced in testing hearing. Above all, he should constantly question the results obtained in testing the patient; he should look for inconsistencies in the results obtained and should be willing to repeat the test or do other tests if the accuracy of the result is doubted. Audiometric technicians may be trained in the office, but better results will be obtained from attending a course in audiometry at a recognized school.

The technique of audiometry should follow a definite pattern from patient to patient and from test to test. Variations of test methods will produce results which are inconsistent and will not allow comparison between repeated tests on a given patient or between tests on different patients.

SPEECH TESTS

Speech tests are tests of hearing which use the spoken voice as the signal. They are of two types: threshold and above threshold. Speech tests should be presented in a language with which the patient is familiar.

The source of the signal is important in speech tests. Commonly used sources are phonograph recordings, tape recordings, and live voice. Phonograph records wear with repeated use and should be replaced when deterioration of the speech signal is evident. The number of playings that a disk recording will stand without significant deterioration varies with the type of disk, the record player used, and the general care of the disks. A trained listener or a panel of instructed listeners can judge the adequacy of speech recordings for clinical testing. (Recorded tests are available from Technisonic Studios, 1201 Brentwood Boulevard, St. Louis 17, Missouri.)

Tape recordings have a longer useful life than disks. It is customary in some laboratories to transcribe the standard speech tests from new disks to tape for routine clinical use.

Live voice must be monitored by a voltmeter (VU meter). The intensity delivered at the earphone of the audiometer varies directly with the input intensity at the microphone. The speaker attempts to have the swing of the VU meter needle center at the "0" reading when spondaic words are being used. The VU meter will vary depending on the phonetic content of phonetically balanced (PB) words. Results of the live-voice test vary owing to differences of inflection with repeated reading of the word lists.

The speech-reception threshold (SRT) is a test of threshold using a speech signal. The speech material used is the Harvard Spondaic Word List, which contains two-syllable words having equal emphasis on the first and second syllables. The speech reception threshold is the intensity level at which half of the spondaic words are repeated correctly. The speech reception threshold compares closely with the average of the thresholds for pure tones at 500, 1000, and 2000 c/s and is thus a convenient check on the accuracy of the pure-tone threshold.

The speech-discrimination test is an above-threshold test to determine the ability to interpret speech signals. Interpretation of speech signals involves both hearing and mental processes. The results obtained by the discrimination test reflect the efficiency of the sound-conducting mechanism, the state of the cochlea and of nerve transmission, as well as the mental acuity of the patient. The results are unfavorably influenced by unfamiliarity with the language being used for the test. Material used is a series of lists of mono-syllabic words, each list prepared to contain relatively similar amounts of each phonetic component. The words in the lists are referred to as phonetically balanced (PB) words. Two sets of recorded words are available, the Rush Hughes recording of Harvard Phonetically Balanced Word Lists and Auditory Test W-22. The former is more difficult and usually results in lower scores.

Discrimination tests are given at two or more intensities. The first intensity may be the level of most comfortable loudness (MCL), which is the level judged by the patient to be most comfortable to his ear, or an arbitrary intensity level 30 dB higher than the SRT. The second test is given at an arbitrary level 15 dB more intense than the first if this is not unpleasantly loud to the ear being tested. Further tests may be given at higher intensities if indicated. Each test consists of 50 words. The percentage of words repeated correctly is recorded as the score. Results are commonly recorded on a graph with the intensity as the ordinate and the percentage of words heard correctly as the abscissa. The speech-reception threshold is recorded on the zero abscissa. The test is administered with sufficient time interval between words to allow accurate responses.

The tester should establish norms for the discrimination tests in his own environment and with his own equipment. Live-voice tests give a higher score, and tapes may give a lower score than tests by phonograph recordings.

Additional Tests

The test for threshold of discomfort (TD) also may be administered with the use of a speech signal. The threshold of discomfort is the intensity which elicits a painful sensation in the ear. Since the threshold of discomfort is usually 110 to 120 dB, this test cannot be administered to normal ears on the standard audiometer. (See also Chapter 7.)

The SISI (short-increment sensitivity index) test is a measure of ability to detect small changes in intensity (difference limen). A pure tone is presented continuously at an intensity 20 dB above threshold. At intervals of 5 sec. the intensity is increased 1 dB for a period of 200 msec. Twenty pips are presented and the score is recorded as the percentage recognized by the subject. Subjects with end-organ lesions, such as Ménière's disease or acoustic trauma, identify a high percentage of the pips. Subjects with conductive or retrocochlear lesions identify few or none. Subjects with presbyacusis show a wide range of response. As administered by Jerger and his associates (7), the sequence of presentation of the pips is varied to reduce error. This variability is not available in the SISI test incorporated in commercial audiometers.

TESTS FOR FUNCTIONAL LOSS OF HEARING

Tests for functional loss of hearing, malingering, or hysteria are tests of the ingenuity of the examiner as well as of the hearing of the patient.

The history presented by the patient may raise suspicion of functional loss of hearing, particularly in medico-legal cases in which claims for compensation are based on hearing defects.

Test results which suggest functional hearing loss are lack of consistency on repeated testing with pure tones or speech on the same or different days, inconsistency in the judgment of threshold in a single test, and wide difference in threshold determined by pure tone and by speech.

The Lombard Test. This test is based on the principle that a speaker unconsciously regulates the intensity of his own speech according to the environment. In noisy surroundings, a speaker automatically raises his voice to compensate for the masking effect of the noise. The Lombard test is administered by having the patient read aloud while a masking noise is presented and gradually increased or decreased in intensity. If the patient's voice demonstrates fluctuations of intensity as the masking is raised and lowered, it may be assumed that the masking is being heard. Results of the test are considered negative when changes in the level of masking do not cause fluctuations in the loudness of the patient's speech. The limitations of this test are obvious. The results must be recognized as giving only gross evidence of hearing acuity.

The Stenger Test. If a masking noise or tone presented to a supposedly defective ear at an intensity no greater than the admitted threshold causes a shift in threshold in the unmasked ear, the other ear can be assumed to hear the masking tone.

The Doerfler-Stewart Test. The normal or organically defective ear can interpret speech in an environment of masking noise 10 to 20 dB louder than the level of the speech. The patient with functional loss often ceases to repeat speech when the masking level is much fainter than would be expected to disturb an organic loss.

The Delayed-Feedback Test. The voice of the patient being tested is recorded on tape and fed back to his ear approximately 0.1 sec. later. When heard, this produces disturbance in rhythm and flow of speech. This is an effective test but one which requires special equipment.

The Psychogalvanic Skin-Resistance Test. This test is a conditioned-reflex test judged by reduced resistance of the skin to transmission of a galvanic current owing to sweating when under stress. Two electrodes connected to a galvanometer are placed on the skin of the subject, who is then conditioned by simultaneous presentation of an audible sound stimulus and a mildly painful electric shock. Each presentation of the stimulus is accompanied by a swing of the galvanometer. After conditioning, the occurrence of a response when the tone is presented without the shock indicates that the tone is heard. This test requires special equipment, time for conditioning, and skill in interpretation. It is not practical for most office situations.

ESTABLISHMENT OF TYPES OF HEARING LOSS

Data gathered by audiometric methods must be interpreted in order to establish the anatomico-physiological type of hearing loss. The type of hearing loss is of great value in determining the cause of the loss and in planning the management of the patient.

Cases of hearing loss are divided into three broad anatomico-physiological classes on the basis of audiometric data. These are conductive loss and sensori-neural loss (nerve type and end-organ or sensory type).

Conductive Loss

Causes. Lesions in the external and middle ear, including the oval window, stapedial footplate, and round window, which interfere with transmission of air-borne vibrations to the cochlea cause conductive loss of hearing.

History. The patient will have relatively good hearing in noisy environment (paracusis willisiana). The conductive lesion equally attentuates the environmental (masking) noise and the signal. Sounds of intensity equal to the environmental noise are usually loud enough to reach the cochlea and be heard. The patient understands well when the voice signal is of adequate intensity. He prefers increased loudness on radio or television.

Pertinent Tests and Results.

1. Tuning Forks. Rinné's test, negative results; Weber's test, tone referred to defective ear; Schwabach's test, increased hearing by bone conduction.

2. Pure-Tone Audiometry. Air-conduction threshold is greater than bone-conduction threshold. The difference between the air and bone thresholds is called the air-bone gap and is a measure of the degree of conductive impairment. The bone-conducted stimulus is transmitted to the cochlea by vibration of the skull and is not influenced greatly by the state of the conductive apparatus. An exception is the Carhart notch in otosclerosis (8). The bone-conduction threshold often decreases 5 to 10 dB in the frequency zone of 500 to 2000 c/s after surgical treatment of otosclerosis.

3. Speech Audiometry. The speech-reception threshold approximates the pure-tone air-conduction threshold. Speech-discrimination scores are poor at low intensity but approach 100 % when delivered at intensities above the threshold. The normal sensori-neural system is capable of perceiving and interpreting stimuli which reach it.

4. Accessory Tests. SISI, score low; Békésy audiometer curve, Jerger, type I.

Sensori-Neural Loss, Nerve Type

Causes. Lesions of cells or fibers of the auditory nerve system at any point from the spiral ganglion to the cerebral cortex are causative factors.

History. The patient has poor hearing for speech in a noisy environment, and his ability to interpret speech is reduced. Increase in loudness may not improve ability to understand.

Pertinent Tests and Results.

1. Tuning Forks. Rinné's test, positive results; Weber's test, tone referred to better ear; Schwabach's test, hearing by bone conduction decreased.

2. Pure-Tone Audiometry. Thresholds for air conduction and bone conduction approximate one another. Threshold values are greater for high tones than for low tones. Recruitment of loudness may be absent or present in slight degree near the threshold. Diplacusis is absent. The pain threshold is at normal intensities.

3. Speech Audiometry. The speech-reception threshold approximates the pure-tone air-conduction threshold. Speech-discrimination scores improve as intensities are increased above the most comfortable level, but they do not reach normal levels. The scores also vary significantly with the shape of the pure-tone threshold curve. The best scores are achieved by the person whose pure-tone threshold is approximately equal for intensities from 500 through 3000 c/s. Poorer scores are achieved by the person whose threshold gradually increases by 10 or more dB per octave from 500 to 3000 c/s. Abrupt changes in pure-tone thresholds limit speech discrimination in a variable manner depending on the frequency at which the increase in threshold occurs. An abrupt increase in threshold for tones above 1000 c/s results in slight impairment of discrimination demonstrable in the test with the phonetically balanced words and noticed by the patient when listening conditions are unfavorable (noise of conversation when in groups, long distance from speaker). Discrimination disability is progressively increased when the abrupt drop takes place at lower frequencies. The disability is moderate when the threshold drop includes 2000 c/s and is severe when 1000 c/s is included.

"Phonemic regression" is the term applied when discrimination of speech is distinctly lower than anticipated from the pure-tone threshold curve. The phenomenon is seen in persons of advanced age or those with degenerative brain disease. The factors mentioned above explain the difficulties encountered in efforts to devise a method of computing percentage loss of hearing from the pure-tone threshold curve.

4. Accessory Tests. SISI, score variable, usually low for low frequencies, high for high frequencies. Békésy audiometer curves, type I or type II of Jerger.

Acoustic neurinoma is differentiated from other lesions of the neural system by the presence of abnormal auditory adaptation (Carhart test; Békésy Audiometer curve, type III of Jerger) and by discrimination scores significantly lower than those expected from the pure-tone curve.

Sensori-Neural Loss, End-Organ Type

The term end-organ deafness is misleading, since the audiometric picture associated with the term is characteristic of the early stages of endolymphatic hydrops but is not found in late stages of hydrops or in other lesions of the cochlear end organ, such as stimulation loss, noise-induced hearing loss or presbycusis. Pathological changes in the cochlea in these conditions have not been fully defined, but a clue to the audiometric differences is found in the studies of cochlear pathology which are available.

The reports of Hallpike and his associates (9, 10), Lindsay (11), and others suggest that in endolymphatic hydrops the initial pathological change is distention of the cochlear duct and that initially Corti's organ is not destroyed and the spiral ganglion remains intact.

Reudi (12) studied the effects of acoustic trauma on the guinea pig cochlea. He found the initial change in the outer hair cells, followed by loss of the inner hair cells. After degeneration of Corti's organ, spiral ganglion cells are lost.

Schuknecht's (13) studies of presbycusis on the cat and on the human ear showed two types of damage—epithelial atrophy and neural atrophy—co-existing in the same cochlea. These changes closely parallel the changes described by Crowe, Guild, and Polvogt (14) in human ears with high-tone deafness. Schuknecht believes that changes in the two areas develop simultaneously.

Loss of spiral ganglion cells may explain the absence of distortion of hearing in lesions of the cochlea other than endolymphatic hydrops.

At the present time audiometric studies provide no clear-cut differentiation between cochlear lesions other than hydrops and lesions of the neural system. More sophisticated tests may provide this differentiation in the future.

The term "end-organ" loss is too broad to fit the pathology, and I therefore suggest that the term "sensory" loss be substituted.

Sensori-Neural Loss, Sensory Type

Causes. Endolymphatic hydrops is a causative factor. Classically, any pathology which produces changes in the function of the hair cell and basilar membrane may be included. Examples are noise-induced hearing loss and streptomycin-type deafness.

History. The patient's loss of hearing is of variable degree; his hearing for speech in noisy environment is extremely poor, and he experiences distortion of pitch in music and poor tolerance of loud sounds (low threshold of pain). Associated vestibular dysfunction is often present.

Pertinent Tests and Results.

1. Tuning Forks. Rinné's test, positive; Weber's test, tone referred to better ear; Schwabach's test, hearing by bone conduction decreased.

2. Pure-Tone Audiometry. In patients with this type of loss of hearing, thresholds of air conduction and bone conduction approximate one another. Air-conduction thresholds typically are higher for low than for high frequencies. The recruitment of loudness is of high degree as indicated by the loudness-balance test. Diplacusis binauralis dysharmonica is present. Also the patient's pain threshold is at less than normal intensities. The SISI score is high. Békésy audiogram is Jerger's type II (15).

3. Speech Audiometry. The speech-reception threshold approximates the pure-tone air-conduction threshold. Speech-discrimination scores decrease as intensities are increased above the most comfortable loudness level owing to distortion of loudness and pitch.

Loss of hearing may be the result of a combination of any two or more of the anatomico-physiological types. The findings reflect the combination of causes.

DIAGNOSIS

The diagnosis of the causative conditions of loss of hearing is based on the patient's history and on the physical and audiometric findings. Classification of the type of loss of hearing on an anatomico-physiological basis by audiological methods limits the area to be considered in determination of the cause.

Conductive Loss.

1. Occlusion of the external auditory canal
    Causes
    Inflammation
      Acute
      Chronic
    Exostosis
    Stenosis
      Congenital
      Acquired
        Traumatic
        Inflammatory
    (Diagnosis is usually obvious from history and physical examination. Inflammatory stenosis is unusual; it results from chronic otitis externa.)
    Audiometry: conductive loss up to 50 dB.
2. Otitis media
    Serous
      History: loss of hearing and fullness in the ear without pain.
      Examination: tympanic membrane retracted, normal luster but altered color: blue, amber, or brown. Moves sluggishly.
      Audiometry: conductive loss 15 to 40 dB. May show slight elevation of bone-conduction threshold from splinting of round and oval windows.
    Suppurative, acute
      History: recent onset of pain, fullness and hearing loss. Associated upper respiratory disease.
      Examination: tympanic membrane intact: bulging, inflamed or with opaque, white appearance. Membrane perforated; drainage in canal.
      Audiometry: conductive deficit up to 40 dB.
    Suppurative, chronic
      History: long-standing discharge.

Examination: tympanic membrane perforated. Discharge, polypi.

Audiometry: conductive loss up to 60 dB depending on degree of damage to middle ear.

Suppurative, adhesive

History: hearing loss dated to prior inflammation.

Examination: tympanic membrane normal or scarred.

Audiometry: conductive loss up to 50 dB.

3. Perforations

History: prior infection or trauma.

Examination: tympanic membrane perforated.

Audiometry: conductive loss up to 30 dB. If no other pathology, patch over perforation will improve hearing.

4. Tympanosclerosis

History: prior inflammation.

Examination: waxy or chalky deposits in tympanic membrane with or without perforation.

Audiometry: normal hearing (lesion in tympanic membrane only) up to 50 dB conductive loss (lesion fixes ossicles).

5. Ossicular chain broken

History and examination: chronic otitis media. Perforation.

Audiometry: conductive loss of 50 to 60 dB.

6. Congenital fixation of ossicles

History: hearing loss since childhood.

Examination: tympanic membrane normal.

Audiometry: conductive loss 40 to 60 dB.

Pathology: usually head of malleus fused to epitympanum.

7. Otosclerosis

History: insidious onset at age 20 to 50. Rarely younger or older. Positive family history.

Examination: tympanic membrane normal.

Audiometry: conductive loss up to 60 dB, usually greater for low tones. Bone-conduction threshold elevated 5 to 10 dB for speech frequencies.

8. Middle ear tumor (usually glomus jugulare)

History: loss of hearing, pulsating tinnitus.

Examination: reddish mass in middle ear, may appear as polyp in canal.

Audiometry: degree of loss depends on size of tumor.

Sensori-Neural Loss, Nerve Type. Sensori-neural loss, nerve type, results from many causes. The etiology is not always certain and is often of academic interest only. Diagnosis is usually made by the history and

occasionally by associated evidence of neurological disease. The following
outline presents some of the common etiologies of sensori-neural loss:

1. Congenital
    Heredity
    Developmental abnormality
    Infection of mother
        German measles in first trimester of pregnancy
        Syphilis
    Rh incompatibility between mother and child
2. Acquired
    Advanced age
    Acute infectious diseases
        Meningitis
        Encephalitis
        Viral diseases
        Mumps
        Acute exanthemas
        Syphilis
    Drugs
        Dihydrostreptomycin
        Kanamycin
        Neomycin
        Quinine
    Labyrinthitis
        Viral
        Suppurative
    Vascular occlusion, posterior-inferior cerebellar artery or its
        successive branches leading to the cochlea
    Tumors, intracranial
        Acoustic nerve
        Cerebellopontine angle
        Other
    Degenerative disease of brain
    Trauma, fracture of the base of the skull, severe concussion of
        brain
    Stimulation, exposure to high-intensity noise
    Concussion of cochlea due to explosions
    Operation for otosclerosis (occurs in a small percentage of cases)

The differential diagnosis between tumors of the VIIIth nerve and
cerebellopontine angle and Ménière's disease is of considerable significance.
Recent developments in surgery for acoustic neuroma place a premium on
early diagnosis. Disturbed hearing is often the earliest sign of acoustic

neuroma. This diagnosis should be considered in every case of sensori-neural hearing loss.

Cerebellopontine angle lesions

    History: initial symptom, hearing loss, tinnitus, or vestibular dysfunction, usually instability but may be severe vertigo. Cranial nerves V, VI, or VII may be involved. Symptoms usually progressive. Intracranial hypertension and cerebellar signs occur late.

    Examination: disturbance of cranial nerves V through VIII. Reduced vestibular function, spontaneous nystagmus. Increased cerebro-spinal fluid protein. Radiography to show enlargement of internal acoustic meatus or decalcification at petrous apex. Contrast radiography to show filling defect of internal meatus. Planography.

    Audiometry: sensori-neural loss of any degree. Speech-reception threshold corresponds to pure-tone threshold. Discrimination loss greater than pure-tone loss. Recruitment usually absent (may be present in early case). SISI score, low. Abnormal adaptation on Carhart or Békésy (Jerger, type III or IV).

Endolymphatic hydrops (Ménière's disease)

    History: hearing loss, tinnitus and episodic rotatory vertigo. Any one may be initial symptom. Variable hearing improving during remissions. Bilateral in 4 to 10%. Fullness in affected ear.

    Examination: in attack: nystagmus, vasomotor lability, labyrinth suppression. In remission: may have residual loss of vestibular and cochlear function.

    Audiometry, early stage: hearing fluctuates. Sensori-neural, low tones predominate. Speech reception threshold corresponds to pure-tone threshold. Distortion, i.e., recruitment of loudness, diplacusis, marked discrimination loss which increases with increased intensity. High SISI score. Late state: high-tone loss predominates. Fluctuation absent. Distortion less prominent.

Central lesions. Jerger (15) reports that in lesions of the brain stem discrimination loss in the ear opposite the lesion is found associated with normal pure-tone threshold. He has also found that the ear opposite a lesion of the cerebral cortex will give normal response to pure-tone tests but will fail when the task is made more difficult, as by a low-pass filter or by the use of faint speech signals.

MANAGEMENT OF THE PATIENT

The management of the patient is guided largely by the audiometric diagnosis. Loss of hearing due to conductive lesions is often amenable to therapy. Occlusion of the external auditory meatus, with the exception of congenital atresia, and some cases of traumatic atresia are corrected by simple means, and treatment should always be the choice. Traumatic atresias should have the benefit of surgical treatment if nerve function is good. Operation is often indicated in cases of bilateral congenital atresia, but it is seldom indicated in unilateral cases in which the hearing of the opposite ear is good.

In cases of acute otitis media, serous, mucoid, or suppurative, treatment is again the method of choice. Myringotomy with removal of the fluid, treatment of infection in the ear, and correction of disease of the naso-pharynx or nose which contribute to dysfunction of the Eustachian tube are indicated.

Perforation of the tympanic membrane may be treated by closure of the perforation by tissue graft or, if small, by the caustic and paper-patch technique. The physician must be sure that no infection or squamous epithelium is covered by the graft and that the ossicular chain is intact. The latter point is determined by use of the acoustic probe or by the air-conduction test before and after application of a paper patch over the perforation. Gain in hearing by touching the malleus with the probe or by covering the perforation indicates a functioning ossicular chain. The probe may be attached to the bone-conduction unit of the audiometer or to a cardboard paddle which vibrates with the sound of the voice.

Elimination of the disease is the primary consideration in cases of chronic suppuration of the middle ear and mastoid, including cholesteatosis. Reconstructive procedures for restoration of hearing will fail uniformly if suppuration or cholesteatoma matrix is covered by a graft or flap.

Audiometric data are an important factor in decision for operation to correct hearing deficit from otosclerosis or destructive lesions of the middle ear. Tests should include Weber's test with forks, pure-tone air and bone audiometry, and speech-discrimination tests.

The surgeon should be assured that the nerve function is adequate to support hearing and that the conductive element of the hearing loss is great enough that its correction will allow satisfactory improvement of hearing. Amplification with a hearing aid compensates for conductive loss of hearing, and this means of rehabilitation should be offered to all patients because the benefit of surgical therapy is never certain.

Sensori-neural hearing loss of the nerve type is rarely amenable to medi-cal or surgical therapy.* Rehabilitation by hearing aid, speech reading, and auditory training is indicated. The benefits to be gained from amplifica-

---

* Exceptions are occasional cases of sensori-neural loss which begin abruptly and progress rapidly. Improved hearing has been noted following therapy with corti-costeroids or with vasodilators. Therapy has been empiric. Neither the causative lesion nor the diagnostic criteria have been determined (16).

tion can be estimated from audiometric data. The pure-tone air-conduction threshold is useful for this purpose but is best supported by the speech-discrimination curve. In general, results from amplification are better when the air-conduction threshold is approximately equal through the speech frequencies of 500 to 2000 c/s than when the threshold curve is highly irregular or drops sharply at 500 or 1000 c/s. Amplification usually is not needed when the air-conduction threshold is 30 dB or less; it gives satisfactory results with thresholds between 30 and 65 dB; worthwhile benefit is obtained if the threshold lies between 65 and 85 dB; it is of limited help when the threshold is greater than 85 dB.

Patients having sensori-neural loss of the sensory type may benefit from medical therapy when the causative factor is endolymphatic hydrops in the early stage of the disease. The eventual deterioration of hearing is delayed if exacerbations of hydrops are avoided. The distortion characteristic of end-organ loss of hearing limits benefits from amplification, but with auditory training and/or experience, amplification can be very useful in sensory-type sensori-neural hearing loss. These patients are largely dependent on speech reading for improvement in communication.

EVALUATING THE HEARING OF THE AGING

Audiometric techniques for testing the aged individual differ in some respects from standard testing patterns. The physical changes of old age often result in a slowing of reaction time, in muscular inefficiency, painful movement, and general debility. To compensate for the effects of these disabilities, adjustments must often be made in the testing procedures used. The following areas of test modifications may be used as required for any individual case.

1. Tone Presentation. Instead of the usual 2-sec. duration, it may be necessary to prolong the stimulus presentation as long as 5 sec., in order to give sufficient time for a response. Often the older person will respond only after the tone has been withdrawn, and this deviation can be accepted as a valid response so long as it is consistent.

2. Interval between Tones. The time between tone presentations may have to be lengthened, so that the patient can redirect his attention to the next tone. It may require 6 sec. or more between tones.

3. Behavioral Response. Many elderly people find it difficult to press a button or to raise a finger in response to the tone. A spoken "yes" or a nod of assent can be accepted as valid responses in such cases. It may be necessary sometimes to encourage a response with the question "Do you hear the tone? " This kind of leading question is not likely to produce a false-positive response in the older age group.

4. Use of Live Voice for Speech Reception. Live voice rather than recorded voice is preferred for speech-reception testing because it permits adjustments to the slower reaction time of the aging person. After a response has been given, 6 sec. or more may be required before the next word is presented. These longer intervals are not incorporated into recorded speech tests, and therefore standard tapes or recordings are impractical for older patients.

5. *Adaptation of Threshold Technique in Speech Reception.* The older person may have difficulty in understanding spondee words on first presentation, because of the problem of phonemic regression. It will be necessary then to familiarize him with the words, giving visual clues simultaneously with the speech, before the testing begins. In extreme cases a small number of spondees can be selected for thorough familiarity.

In rare instances an individual is found who cannot identify any of the spondee words, even after training. The tester must then settle for obtaining a threshold of awareness for speech rather than a threshold of perceptibility. The patient is instructed to respond by saying "yes" whenever he is aware of the examiner's voice. The tester then begins his voice up from inaudibility, in 2-dB steps, presenting random conversational speech or the question "Can you hear me now?" at each increase. The point of first response is the threshold of awareness. This kind of threshold does not yield the same information as that derived from the standard SRT technique, for the individual is responding to the lowest fundamental voice frequency, which may be 100 c/s. However, when it is necessary to compare different listening situations, such as performances with hearing aids, an awareness threshold allows one to make useful observations.

6. *Discrimination Test Modifications.* The standard PB lists may not be intelligible to the aging person because of his problem with phonemic regression. Easier tests may then be tried, such as the PBK-50, which was developed for children. The test may also be shortened by giving only 25 words, in order to forestall fatigue during a long test session.

If there is no understanding of any PB lists, another test procedure may be used to compare hearing efficiency under different conditions. Sets of balanced lip reading tests can be presented with both voice and visual clues, and the relative performance in each hearing situation scored. Such tests as the Utley lip-reading tests, the Lowell tests, and others can be used (17). Another test modification is to use lists of single words such as those compiled by Mason, Kelly, Moser, and others (17), and present them both visually and vocally.

When improvisations are made such as have been described, the tester must recognize that he has stepped beyond standardized procedures. However, it is more valuable to obtain some information about various listening conditions than none at all.

7. Modification for Tinnitus. The presence of ringing in the ear may cause the subject to confuse the pure tone with his own head noise. In such event a frequency-warbled tone can be used for the test stimulus rather than the usual pure tone. In addition, it is helpful to substitute an ascending-threshold technique for the standard combined procedure. The tone is brought up from inaudibility until the subject reports that it is heard, and that point is recorded as threshold. Several presentations of this ascending technique will fix a reliable threshold point.

8. Collapse of Ear Canal. A specific type of false test result is found rather consistently in the aging group. Some elderly patients have either extremely narrow external canals or flabby tissue at the outer portion of the canal. When an earphone is placed on such an ear, the pressure causes a complete closure of the ear canal, anywhere along the cartilaginous portion (18, 19). The result is an artifically induced air-conduction loss that can be 20 to 48 dB greater than the bone-conduction values. The error can be detected only if tuning-fork tests or free-field speech-reception tests are given. The tuning-fork tests will indicate a positive Rinné, in direct contradiction to the audiogram. The Weber test may or may not be illogical, but it often indicates a contradictory referral to the ear which has the lesser air-bone gap. If free-field speech-reception tests are given, the results will be much better than could be logically inferred from the audiogram. In order to obtain valid audiograms in such cases, it is necessary to place a firm, hollow tube into the ear canal to hold it open for the passage of sound from the earphone. A standard hearing-aid ear mold can be used for this purpose but may itself attenuate some frequencies. A second solution is to have an assistant pull the auricle firmly back at the helix, fit the earphone carefully over the ear, and continue the backward pull on the auricle during the test. It should be noted that an artificial air-bone gap of this type is occasionally found in the general adult population and even in children.

The modifications of test procedures which have been described represent solutions to the clinician's need to obtain information when he is confronted with deviations from classic behavioral responses. The persistent examiner will find that patient and sympathetic handling of the aging individuals will produce information that is well worth the extra time and ingenuity required.

REFERENCES

1. Ewing, I. R., and Ewing, A. W. G.: The ascertainment of deafness in infancy and early childhood. J. Laryng. & Otol., *59:* 309, 1944.
2. Cody, D. T. and Bickford, R. G.: Cortical audiometry. Proc. Staff Meet. Mayo Clin., *40:* 273, 1965.
3. House, H. P., and Glorig, A.: A new concept of auditory screening. Laryngoscope, *67:* 661, 1957.

4. Simonton, K. M., and Hedgecock, L. D.: Two frequency auditory screening: a clinical evaluation. Laryngoscope, *71:* 425, 1961.
5. Roach, R. E., and Carhart, R.: Clinical method for calibrating bone-conduction audiometer. A. M. A. Arch. Otolaryng., *63:* 270, 1956.
6. Jerger, J.: Bekesy audiometry. J. Speech & Hearing Res., *3:* 275, 1960.
7. Jerger, J., Shedd, J. H., and Harford, E.: On detection of extremely small changes in sound intensity. A. M. A. Arch. Otolaryng., *69:* 200, 1959.
8. Carhart, R.: "Bone conduction advances following fenestration surgery. Tr. Am. Acad. Ophth., *56:* 621, 1952.
9. Hallpike, C. S., and Cairns, H.: Observations on the pathology of Ménière's syndrome. J. Laryng. & Otol., *53:* 625, 1938.
10. Hallpike, C. S., and Wright, A. J.: On the histological changes in the temporal bones of a case of Ménière's disease. J. Laryng. & Otol., *55:* 59, 1940.
11. Lindsay, J. R.: Labyrinthine dropsy. Laryngoscope, *56:* 325, 1946.
12. Reudi, L.: Different types and degrees of acoustic trauma by experimental exposure of human and animal ear to pure tones and noise. Ann. Otol. Rhin. & Laryng., *63:* 702, 1954.
13. Schuknecht, H. F.: Presbycusis. Tr. Am. Laryng. Rhin. & Otol. Soc., 401, 1955.
14. Crowe, S. J., Guild, S. R., and Polvogt, L. M.: Observations on the pathology of high tone deafness. Bull. Johns Hopkins Hosp., *54:* 315, 1934.
15. Jerger, J.: Audiological manifestations of lesions in the auditory nervous system, Laryngoscope, *70:* 417, 1960.
16. Simonton, K. M., and Cody, D. T.: Unpublished data.
17. O'Neill, J., and Oyer, H.: *Visual Communication.* Prentice-Hall, Inc., New York, 1960.
18. Hildyard, V., and Valentine, M.: Collapse of the ear canal during audiometry—a further report. Arch. Otol, *75:* 422, 1962.
19. Ventry, I., Chaiklin, J., and Boyle, W.: Collapse of the ear canal during audiometry. Arch. Otolaryng., *73:* 6, 1961.

10

Evaluation of Hearing in Infants and Young Children

William G. Hardy, Ph.D.

Any attempt to evaluate the hearing of infants and young children is wisely based upon the premise that we do not know precisely how we hear, in terms of solid, demonstrable, neurophysiological fact. What must be accomplished, then, is an orderly interpretation of what a child does by way of responding to various kinds of acoustic stimuli, and what these responses may mean, or can mean to him.

THE DEVELOPMENTAL PROCESS

Birth to 10 Months. This is a *pre-language* state, and much of the baby's development depends on his learning to hear. In the course of early development, a child learns to be aware of sound, to pay particular attention to certain sounds, to perceive these sounds in foreground-background relationships, and eventually, to imitate them.

Ten to 24 Months. Later, meanings of sound in reference to objects and events begin to develop. This is a *pre-speech* state, quite variable in duration among a large group of normally developing infants. Vocal output by this time is jargonic but has freely variable pitch and inflection and some of the accents and stress patterns of connected discourse. At the end of this period, the child is talking in two- or three-word phrases, although with frequent jargonic interludes. A single verbal stimulus is ordinarily enough for him to learn a new word in appropriate reference.

Third and 4th Years. During this *pre-school* period the child's vocabulary grows rapidly. He learns to monitor his own speech output by paying attention to the details of what he hears and to compare this with what he hears himself say. He begins to articulate with attention to the details of phonetic utterance and to talk in the local dialect. The learning, the differentiating, and the production of language and speech involve a complex relationship among auditory, visual, and muscular stimuli and responses, and between peripheral and central mechanisms.

Provided that his hearing is reasonably normal, the growing child learns to reproduce the phonetic values and the meanings of his native community. With adequate self-monitoring in terms of auditory discrimination and auditory memory, he reproduces local speech patterns with considerable fidelity by the age of 4 years.

Deviations from Normal Development

Any serious disorder of the hearing system or the listening system directly interferes with the development of language, the development of speech, and the child's ability and willingness to respond to his environment within conventional behavior limits. The careful measurement of auditory function is in order when a child does not seem to react to sounds that are expected to interest him, does not seem to understand simple verbal references, does not talk at an age when most children do, or when his speech remains an unintelligible jargon. Such measurement is often a difficult task at best, for one must assess not only the child's reception of sound as this is expressed in some function of responsive behavior, but also his perception of sound. The reception of sound involves the peripheral auditory mechanism. The perception of sound involves refined descrimination and differentiation. The total process is one whereby the physical events of sound (reception, transduction, and transmission) and the psychological events (interpretation, memory, significance, and recall) are translated into operational experiences.

Very little is really known about sensory deprivation as it affects the hearing of the individual child, because hearing is much more than an appropriate response; and a lack of appropriate response may reflect much more than lack of audition. There are many kinds of deprivation or dysfunction which might account for lack of appropriate responses, for example, intellectual incapacity, inability to remember, inhibition, or poor co-ordination. Rarely can a diagnosis of impaired hearing be based upon a hearing test alone. All other aspects of diagnostic analysis (otological, pediatric, neurological, psychological, and sociological) must be considered. In the hands of an expert clinician, much can be learned from a baby's responses to a 512-double vibration (d.v.) tuning fork, but nobody would accept such responses, or lack of responses, as a *definitive* description of his auditory function. Auditory appraisal at the diagnostic level, therefore, must begin with a thorough medical and developmental history.

STEPS IN DIFFERENTIATION

For a differential diagnosis there are at least five basic questions to be answered: (1) What is the developmental history? (2) Is hearing involved? (3) If so, how much does the child hear? (4) How does he hear? and (5) What course of treatment or management is indicated? A sizable proportion of pre-school children have problems that are quite complex; these are multiple-handicapped children, whose difficulties may include several different aspects of behavior, of learning, and of communication. The answer to possible causative factors lies in an interpretation of each child's medical history. The answers to hearing involvement will be derived, not from any single or specific audiometric procedure, but from a battery of careful measurements and observations. The course of treatment will be indicated by a thorough assessment of the child—pediatric, otological, audiological, and psychological.

The Developmental Picture

Of particular importance is the child's developmental history, with special emphasis on the communicative aspects of social and intellectual maturity. Here is a rich source of fact on which to base impressions and judgments about hearing. It is most important to be able to relate parental reports of their observation of the child in the ordinary circumstances of daily living to the professional clinical observations. One would be well advised not to ask parents about the child's hearing or deafness, but rather to find out what they have seen the child do in the presence of specific auditory stimuli—voices, the sound of a doorbell, telephone bell, radio, or car horn, the bark of a dog, and the like. There are children who respond clearly once, but only once, to each of a series of sound stimuli; children who consistently respond to stimuli of moderate intensity, but without a vestige of localization; children who clearly respond to "little" sounds—squeaky toys, a modulated voice, a spoken *st-st-st*—but not to intense sounds; children who do not react to a loud call, but go to Mother with a hand out for money when the tinkle of the ice cream man's bell comes from two blocks away; children who pay no attention to a shout or a doorbell, but are curious about the twittering of the birds on a branch out of sight from the window.

All such children may present one aspect or another of auditory impairment, but rarely are they classically deaf in the sense of hearing nothing. A child's response to the sounds of free play, then to the controlled sound field of testing, may provide startling contrasts. Within the restricted situation, a child may localize a source of sound, as he apparently does not do in a freer situation. Some may receive sound but cannot perceive it. They may be alerted by sound, without being able to discriminate among different sounds. They may perceive differences in loudness, without being able to differentiate pitch. Not being able to differentiate sound, they may inhibit and learn to ignore it. Such details of auditory behavior may be revealed through careful questioning of parents.

Several other aspects of normal development may furnish useful clues to the status of the deviant child. The average child uses seven to 10 speech sounds by the time he is 6 months old and then moves into a pre-language jargon, with ready imitative inflection and stress. This does not typically continue without self-hearing in some degree. Yet when he cannot learn meaning references in terms of natural language development because of difficulties with attention, storage, and recall, he may well inhibit sound. Not being able to learn from speech stimulus, he learns to ignore sound. Many such children appear to be functionally deaf by the age of 18 months. Still others have a relatively unimpaired hearing system for receiving sound, but cannot listen without being alerted by loud sound. They cannot pay attention to the typical array of environmental sounds from which most children learn.

Parental observations and reports rarely provide a crystal-clear picture. However, many leads may be established if definite questions are asked and if parents are admitted as creditable reporters. Rarely will a young child be seen who is totally deaf in the sense that nothing is received or perceived. When this does happen, there is usually good etiological evidence in the medical history. Moreover, in the severely involved child, one is often dealing with a central pathway impairment, which may exist with or without causally concurrent problems of memory, recall, foreground-background perception, etc.

If hearing disability is a principal part of a particular child's problem, one must try to ascertain *how much* he hears, that is, what he apparently responds to in his normal environment. If the problem is other than a peripheral loss of sensitivity, however, attention must be directed toward *how* he hears. For this latter purpose, standard decibel notation is an inadequate description. Many children have central nervous system interferences; they may experience variable, undifferentiated events of sound without being able to distinguish or remember them. Do such children hear? This is a matter of definition. Some can learn to interpret sound usefully; some cannot. The task in testing their hearing is to try to discern whether more than the peripheral part of the auditory system is involved, and what capacities may possibly be developed by appropriate stimulus and training. No item of information about the child's communicative awareness can be ignored. The responsibility of the clinical audiologist is to describe the child and his hearing potential as thoroughly as possible.

Assessment of Hearing

There are many different tools, techniques, and procedures available for this assessment, ranging from common-sense interpretations of the simplest sort to highly complex interpretations of second- and third-order responses conveyed through complicated electrophysiological instrumentation. The inquiry into a child's auditory function should vary according to his developmental level. It is useful, therefore, to consider hearing tests for children in at least four ranks: (1) pre-language and (2) pre-speech in infancy; (3) pre-school; and (4) early school age.

The Level of Pre-Language (Readiness to Listen). Not much is known about the *details* of how a child learns to hear. That learning is involved is apparent, and therefore a relationship of stimulus and response exists. Because of this, the infant's social environment is important. If nobody pays attention to the child, his sensory learning will probably be retarded or deviant, as in cases involving brain injury or maldevelopment. Babies who are ignored do not usually learn to hear normally.

Several tools are at hand for the task of eliciting and evaluating infantile responses. Several observations can be made during the first 4 days of life. In a current study, a simple wooden clacker is employed, emitting a brief, sharp sound lasting approximately $\frac{1}{10}$ sec. Its balanced frequency range exceeds 8000 c/s and, at a distance of 12 ft., has an intensity value of 62 dB (re 0.0002 microbar). An observer faces the child, who is being held over an attendant's shoulder, and activates the sound source, which is behind the child. Various responses are elicited. These range from a quasi-Moro reaction* (total bodily response to sound) to several kinds of acousto-palpebral (eye blink, eye rollings, etc.) reactions and demonstrate that something is happening through the auditory mechanism. Few of the neonates respond with a cry. Interestingly enough, a 3-inch electric bell or a whistle with the same value of intensity but of much longer duration elicits few responses from this group of children. Similar observations have been made in the regular and premature nurseries.

It is important in the assessment of tiny infants to understand exactly what is being attempted. The tester is not trying to diagnose deafness. He is presenting certain stimuli and observing the responses. Either the baby responds in a way that observers can see and agree on, or he does not. Some responses are repeatable, others are not. If a baby does not respond, one cannot conclude that he does not *hear;* only that he does not *respond.*

This kind of sensory detection (true of most screening tests carried out early in life) is only an index, a means to divide subjects into two groups: those who react normally, and those who do not. Within the following 3 months of infancy, several things may be expected to happen develop-

---

* Moro was the name of a German pediatrician who first described this reflex.

mentally which broaden the range of inquiry. Within 2 months, under normal social circumstances, the baby begins to inhibit these overt responses to sharp sounds. Presumably he is beginning to learn what is not important in his environment. By 8 to 12 weeks, he pays more attention to the human voice than to casual environmental noises. He has begun to discriminate and to direct his attention. Certain kinds of sounds—familiar toys in the crib, mother's voice, the noises of food preparation—center and hold his attention. He listens to them and usually responds.

Accordingly, an important item in the clinical history is the presence or absence of an auditory orienting reflex. A 3-month-old who is developing normally can usually be awakened by mother's voice. He turns his eyes (often his head) toward the familiar sound of a rattle, the movement of wooden beads, and the like. This becomes a structured situation of hearing and listening which can be duplicated in the physician's office or in the well-baby clinic.

As the baby matures to approximately 20 weeks, muscular co-ordination and visual experience enhance his world. He learns to turn over and struggle to a sitting position. His auditory horizons are enlarged, and a dozen different sound sources may elicit as many as 14 or 15 different kinds of responses.

The Ewings of Manchester University, England, have been pioneers in the development of early screening tests of hearing, and several of their books give full accounts of the necessary tools and the way to use them. The basic idea is that the sound of familiar objects, of known intensities and frequency characteristics, can be employed in carefully structured situations. One person handles the sound sources, out of the baby's visual field, while another observes and evaluates the child's reactions.

The expressed aim of this approach to infantile screening tests is the evolution of a general screening test that could become a standard procedure in well-baby clinics. There is great merit in this idea, for it would serve not only as an early index of auditory responses, but also as an indicator of intellectually incapable or possible brain-damaged children with problems of sensory integration, co-ordination, and memory.

An important aspect of testing at the pre-language level can be related to auditory experiences. Infantile babble is a normal developmental phase. When this does not occur by 6 months of age, one has a reason to be suspicious. Many "good, quiet babies" are so because of sensory or intellectual deficiencies. Babble is a pleasurable experience of self-expression at first; later it becomes imitative and jargonic in quality. Baby learns to listen and to monitor himself; in a way, to appreciate his own vocal utterances. As this goes on through the course of development from 6 to 12 months, he begins to relate some of his sounds to certain events, and to relate other sounds that he hears to the same events. This sort of learning underlies what may be called *communicative awareness*, the dawning understanding by the baby that verbal exchange is important, something to pay attention to, something to participate in. Few children develop language and speech until this awareness of communicative interchange comes into being. For those with some serious auditory disability, the period of jargonic communication is far prolonged. The clinical determination of the stage of development of communicative awareness is important.

Aside from the information gleaned from parents, there are three kinds of reactions which can be observed at the level of pre-language development: (1) reactions (to noises and vocal stimuli) in a play situation; (2) responses (with particular attention to localization) to carefully controlled stimuli—toy sounds, voice, whistles, bells, masking noise, and the like—in a highly structured situation in a controlled sound field; and (3) responses to electrophysiological tests, that is, the conditioned responses of galvanic (or electrodermal) audiometry.

The first of these are commonly seen in the physician's office. They are common sense observations. What does the child do in the presence of a given stimulus? Does he turn his eyes, his head, stop his activity, or ignore the sound? Interpretation under these circumstances depends upon the variables of attention, interest, familiarity with the sound, and a number of psychological and social conditions. Two things are important: (1) that the quality of the sound is known by the tester, in terms of intensity and frequency, and (2) that lack of response is not confused with lack of hearing. Much more detailed verification is needed than such testing can offer. This kind of inquiry is at best a screening test. The lack of response is simply an index of behavior, which emphasizes the need for further inquiry.

The second situation requires special equipment and, preferably, a two-room situation, with one observer at the controls and another with the child. Both should have learned to observe and interpret with care. Sometimes responses are repeatable; sometimes they are not. Often there may be clear reactions (a turn of the eyes or the head, or a cessation of activity) to each *new* sound, but not to repeated presentations. Some children react more obviously to the cessation than to the onset of the stimulus. In many circumstances it is wise to explore with quiet sounds, rather than to continue for a long period with loud stimuli. A loud sound may elicit a Moro reaction, or some other form of a startle reaction, and a disturbed cry is evoked. It becomes important, then, to determine whether a softer stimulus will also evoke a cry. The ramifications of this kind of situation are endless, and it should be kept in mind that many times a presumed response will only be an occurrence of chance. A highly significant observation is one wherein the child more or less consistently localizes the source of sound, particularly when he is attending to some visual stimulus. This usually indicates auditory perception.

The third test situation—galvanic or electrodermal audiometry—requires a very special situation and had better be left to highly qualified personnel. Galvanic skin resistance (GSR) audiometry with infants is at best a difficult procedure, and many qualifications in the management of the child and in the interpretation of the responses must be maintained. In clinical practice, much more information than is shown in actual galvanic responses may be obtained.

The Level of Pre-Speech (Readiness to Talk). By and large, the procedures advocated for the infant in a pre-language state are applicable in the next developmental stage, that of pre-speech. As the 1st year of life may be described as a period of readiness to listen, the 2nd year involves readiness to talk. The time of word-onset is quite variable, but most children of reasonable intelligence who are developing normally have a few words (exclusive of *ma-ma* and *da-da*) at 12 to 14 months. There are many exceptions, which can be judged only in terms of the prenatal, perinatal, and developmental history.

A relatively mild conductive hearing problem can be a serious deterrent for the 16-month-old infant, whereas it may not be for the 3-year-old child. Most parents begin to worry about their child when he does not begin to talk in the latter half of the 2nd year. Both the child and parents would benefit greatly if a potential problem were detected much earlier. This is the rationale for an infant screening test in well-baby clinics within the first 6 to 10 months of each child's life.

If a baby is using approximately six to 20 words by the age of 18 months, is aware of verbal communication as a mode of social exchange, and employs a tuneful jargon, one may be reasonably certain that no serious hearing problem is involved. If he does not do these things, there may be a hearing deficit, a language-learning deficit, or a variety of other conditions. Many seriously retarded children do not begin to respond to minimal values of acoustic stimuli before the 4th year.

The tests previously described may be used with the child in the pre-speech or early speech period. Some estimate may also be made of the child's verbal linguistic intake. The 2-year old who hears should be able to follow a fair variety of verbal directions, and give good evidence of awareness of verbal meanings that are reasonable for him to know.

The Level of Pre-School. Past the age of 30 months, a child should be amenable to a wider variety of procedures for appraisal. He should draw a circle freely and do the formboard in reverse. He should communicate quite freely in phrases (or sentences). If he has only a peripheral hearing impairment, he should be able to lip-read many common social phrases. If these things are not happening, an investigation of hearing is in order.

Gross responses to sounds in a play situation should be observed, as well as reactions in a controlled sound field. Electrodermal response (EDR) audiometry can well be employed but cannot usually be carried out as a standard office procedure.

By 30 to 36 months of age, the so-called peep show and similar forms of conditioned audiometry are available. The idea of these audiometric procedures is basically the same, regardless of variations. One is dealing with an operational response: the child learns to do something in association with a sound. Naturally, he must perceive the sound in order to make the necessary association. With the peep show he must learn that when he hears the sound (usually a pure tone delivered in a sound field, although this test could be done monaurally with earphones), he presses a button to illuminate a picture which interests him enough so that he wants to keep on playing the game. Access to the correct button is controlled by the presentation of the test tone; if a tone is not presented, the picture cannot be displayed.

A variation of this procedure utilizes a set of pop-up toys. Still another has to do with the child's learning to move a block or a bead each time the test tone is sounded and perceived. Obviously, there are various factors of attention, intelligence, interest, capacity to listen, and the like involved in such a situation. A child who is deviant in other things than hearing can scarcely be expected to be co-operative or responsive, until or unless he has enough language to understand the meaning of the situation, and the social maturity to take part in it.

With this kind of operational conditioning, several training sessions are usually required. This is one feature of such testing that is not always clearly understood. The evocation of a consistent set of responses under these circumstances is very much a function of perception, memory, and learning, and cannot be taken for granted. By its very nature, operational conditioning in the testing of hearing in young children cannot help an observer to distinguish between a peripheral and a central impairment.

Special Techniques

Galvanic Audiometry (EDR—Electrodermal Response). As a means of observing responses to acoustic stimuli, galvanic skin-resistance audiometry was originally developed around a modified Pavlovian conditioned response. By pairing of a pure-tone stimulus (CS—the conditioned stimulus) with a shock (UCS—the unconditioned stimulus), in due time the tone alone is expected to produce the same kind of galvanic response that is typically produced by the shock. The tone acts as a warning, or alerting, signal. The establishment of the reflex depends upon this recurrent tone-shock sequence. When this warning relationship has been established, the shock is employed only as a reinforcing agent to offset inhibition or adaptation. Under ordinary circumstances, a 40% reinforcement is adequate; that is, with any 10 presentations of the tone, four are followed by shock.

Reliable EDR audiometry is not a simple matter. It is a procedure which requires appropriate equipment, a knowledge of routine audiometry, some acquaintance with the psychophysiology of audition, and experience with a varied array of subjects, ranging from the normal to the profoundly damaged child. As with most techniques of behavioral observation, both art and skill are involved; and due regard should be paid to the environment of the test.

In the selection of suitable equipment, one should keep in mind what it is that he is observing. The galvanic skin (or electrodermal) response is a function of the sympathetic nervous system. A minute current is applied via electrodes to the surface of the skin; a tone and shock evokes a response through the sympathetic nervous system; this response is mediated through the sweat glands, resulting in a lowering of the resistance of the skin to the current. The reaction is registered on a voltmeter as a wave response. Optimal responses may be expected when the interval between tone and shock does not exceed 0.5 sec.

Once a galvanic response has been established, the procedure is that of standard pure-tone audiometry. A combination of ascending-descending techniques is useful, with minimal acuity defined as the intensity level which evokes a response three times when the tone is increased in intensity from below the hearing threshold.

Infants in arms are tested with the mother holding the baby. The shock electrodes are placed on the calf of one leg, approximately 1 inch apart. The signal is presented monaurally, usually with the mother holding the earphone. The pick-up electrodes are placed on the soles of the feet, or on the two surfaces of one foot. The services of a colleague are often most useful in attracting the baby's attention to an interesting toy, but it is routine to test the tiny infant with mother (or nurse, with a hospital inpatient) as the only attendant. EDR audiometry is much easier with the child under 12 months of age than with the 3- or 4-year-old, but still it is not necessarily reliable as a definitive measure.

Occasionally, there will be a child in whom the galvanic response is inadequate. There are several possible reasons for this: an inhibited or otherwise inadequate sudomotor system; an unmyelinized or otherwise undeveloped sympathetic nervous system; a biochemical imbalance which interferes with psychophysiological relations of perception; etc. It has been demonstrated that there are four major sites of inhibition of the galvanic skin reflex, ranging from the frontal cortex, through the midbrain, to the internuncial pool. Various brain-injured or maldeveloped children may show the effects of inhibition. These are all operational factors, primarily physiological, which may interfere with sensory function; and the effect of most of them may be observed quite readily by the integrity of instrumental responses. In gross diagnostic terms, these things may be associated with various kinds of central nervous system maldevelopment or injury, or to a specific sensory deficit, like an undeveloped or damaged perceptive auditory system.

The facts of inadequate conditioning may be observed from various details. They may involve variations of CS-UCS time intervals, the nature of the CS itself (there are many observable differences with a given subject in the use of steady-state, pulsed, or warbled tone), time lag, extinction, adaptation, fatigue, etc. These facts can often be related to different causal or developmental features of a communicative problem. Many premature children, for instance, develop slowly in most regards, and this tendency can be seen in the detail of the galvanic pattern of some of these children. Many motor-palsied children produce a picture of galvanic responses clearly relatable to the muscular status, and one must offer the test stimuli in between times, so to speak. Children with disorders in learning language often ignore minimal sounds, and the galvanic test becomes a painstaking process of disinhibition.

The lack of a conditioned response in EDR audiometry does not necessarily mean "no hearing." If one looks, not for evidence of auditory response dependent upon conditioning, but rather for variability in the subject's auditory behavior, the lack of a conditioned response in the presence of sporadic or occasional responses is not a deterrent but becomes an indicative and useful finding. One is not measuring responses in terms of intensity and frequency; one is observing responses wherein the use of decibel notation is valueless. The point is to try to determine not how much the subject hears, but something about how he hears. Sometimes only pitch is involved; more often, only loudness; sometimes both.

Most children with peripheral impairments enjoy sound, are readily conditioned, and like the experience of listening. Most aphasoid children without impaired hearing seem to require much more time for conditioning but respond fairly consistently once the conditioning process has been accomplished. On the other hand, relatively few children with impairment of the high-central pathways (the cortico-thalamic tracts) can be satisfactorily conditioned. Many whose trouble apparently lies lower down in the brain stem can be. Those whose problems involve the organic listening circuit as well as the afferent pathways are indefinitely variable. There are many children with more diffuse disorders, involving a combination of central auditory distortion as well as aphasoid problems, who frequently demonstrate the variability of those who have only the central hearing problems and no basic language disorder.

When the problem is such that variability, in terms of frequency or intensity (or both) is involved, the basic stuff of which a conditioned reflex is made is missing. In these circumstances, one is looking for information about auditory function that is different from a classical measurement in decibel notation. A "normal" EDR audiogram is a common finding with a child who possibly has a central pathway impairment; yet he may be functionally deaf and unable to discriminate changes in pitch, loudness, or both.

When dealing with these children who have central disturbances, extensive consultation in pediatrics, neurology, psychiatry, and psychology is indicated. Lack of response to sound is *not* by itself an adequate description of the "deaf child."

Electroencephalographic (EEG) Audiometry. EEG audiometry has been carried out successfully with 2- and 3-year-old children. Unlike EDR measurements, EEG audiometry does not require the establishment of a conditioned response. It is a highly specialized technique and not freely available. Neither EDR nor EEG audiometry is a routine office examination. Both belong in special clinical procedures and should properly be left to highly experienced personnel in audiological centers where the findings may be useful as part of a battery of tests. As with all so-called "objective" measurements of audition, an appraisal of physiological events is needed. The point of all such audiometry is not to find out how much a subject hears, but how his auditory system works. This difference is not always clearly understood. A person may perceive an event as sound without being able to discriminate the acoustic details. Does he hear? In a way he does; yet, if he does not discriminate and understand, he may not react appropriately. We may perceive the acoustic events from the speaker of a foreign language with no awareness of meaning, and therefore no capacity for appropriate response. Unless the meaning of the language can be learned, one remains in this state of inappropriate or negative response. This is the situation with many aphasoid children who hear, but can neither understand nor remember. For others, the acoustic event happens, but it is gobbledygook.

Although known since 1939, EEG responses to acoustic stimuli have only recently received the attention of systematic study. The method has been used in sleep and in repose (with young children light sleep is usually a requirement). It describes central nervous system responses initiated at a level high up in the brain stem or thalamus. When these pathways are stimulated, they in turn activate the cortex. Four components of a total response have been described: (1) an on-effect, (2) a suppression of voltage, (3) frequent off-effects (K-formations), and (4) a delayed off-effect. Evidently the response in sleep and the suppression of the alpha rhythm in repose reflect an alerting function in audition and so must be interpreted as something other than a cortical synthesizing process. In this regard, the EEG and the EDR apparently report similar kinds of events. In terms of knowing what a sound means to the subject there is no adequate substitute for a consciously interpreted response, such as occurs in standard speech-hearing tests. These special electrophysiological tests are mainly useful under circumstances in which standard pure-tone and speech audiometry are impossible or impractical to use.

Picture-Show Techniques. There are several variations of "the peep show." All are based on a common principle. The child is rewarded when he hears, and he is not rewarded when he does not hear, or when he makes a false response when there has not been a signal. It has been demonstrated that with children of 3 to 5 years, this technique is superior in some ways to the procedure which requires that a hand be raised when the tone is perceived. The children under test prefer the picture presentation, and differences between the two procedures are negligible in determining acuity. Unfortunately one is not justified in expecting children with impaired hearing to act like children with normal hearing, and no such technique is useful for an affected child under the age of 2½ to 3 years.

Play-Conditioned Audiometry with Children. As early as 3 years of age, many children with considerable residual hearing are able to give voluntary, play-conditioned responses to pure-tone audiometry. The success of this technique depends largely on the ability of the examiner to interest the child and to hold his attention. An attitude of confidence is essential, for a child will usually respond best to the person who signifies that he expects him to co-operate. One should never ask, "Will you please do this for me? " but rather announce pleasantly but confidently, "Now we're going to do this."

The technique of play conditioning must be indefinitely variable. Adaptations to the needs of the individual child should be immediately available to the examiner. It requires abundant insight into the attention span of the particular child to determine when to vary the procedure. Among the toys that should be at hand are the following: (1) a set of a dozen plain, unornamented blocks, 2 by 2 inches; (2) a set of graduated colored rings on a large wooden peg; (3) a peg board with colored pegs; (4) marbles and marble board with depressions or a box, bottle, or other container in which to place the marbles; (5) a series of small animals that can be placed in a farmyard, or small cars to go in a parking lot; (6) toy airplanes, cars, animals and dolls; and (7) a set of noisemakers including rubber squeeze toys, wooden and metal clackers, small and large bells, soft and loud horns.

Prior to audiometric testing, it is extremely useful to obtain a gross estimate of the child's hearing level, with noisemakers and with speech audiometry. The estimated level will give the examiner an indication of the intensity level that will be required for the child to hear the pure tones with certainty.

The child's responses to various noisemakers should first be observed. He must be occupied in play with some quiet toys before the noises are presented. The examiner should then go behind the child to one side, well out of his visual field, and operate the noisemakers, alternating sides. A head-turning response, to the side of the noise, can be expected if the child hears on that side. If he continually turns only to one side, or seems confused as to where the sound originated, he may have a unilateral hearing difficulty. If he responds only to the louder of the noises, he may have a moderate hearing loss; if he does not respond at all, various problems should be suspected.

A speech-reception test can often be given to the child as young as 2 years. Toys representing the children's version of so-called spondee words should be available: a toy *airplane;* a *baseball;* a toy train (*railroad*); a doll's *armchair;* a *cupcake;* a toy *cowboy* doll; a *toothbrush;* some toy *playground* equipment. These lend themselves most easily to recognition. If these words are too difficult, more simple toy names may be used: a *car*, a *baby* doll, a *ball*, a *doggy*, a *kitty*. Such words can be used with the understanding that they are improvisations and do not represent standardized lists. The child is addressed through the loudspeaker or earphones and may be asked to point to the toy that is named, or to pick it up and hand it to the parent. It is sometimes useful to give the instructing phrase "Pick up the" at a higher level and then to switch the attenuator to the level to be tested when the key word is given. This method mobilizes the child's attention to the test word. Beginning at comfortably loud levels, the tester asks the child to pick up the toys. The intensity of the speech is gradually attenuated with each presentation and the lowest response level recorded.

If the child is not able to identify words and toys, a simple awareness level for speech can be obtained. With the child occupied in play, the examiner should call his name through the loudspeaker, beginning at below-threshold levels and gradually increasing the intensity until the child becomes aware of the speech or localizes the speaker. Various noises or filtered sounds can also be used to obtain this awareness level. From the results of this testing the examiner can estimate a comfortable level at which to initiate the pure-tone test.

All audiometric play stimulation should first be demonstrated by the examiner in an interesting manner. He may show the earphones to the child and put them on his own head, saying, "Hello, hello, this is a telephone, just like the one you have at home." He may then simulate the test conditions, picking up the block or peg and holding it to one ear, listen, and then say animatedly, "Oh, I hear it," and place the toy in the proper place. After a few demonstrations by the examiner and even by the parent, the earphones should be placed confidently on the child's head and the block or toy given to him immediately. The examiner or the parent may then hold the child's hand with the block close to one ear, and when the tone is presented, guide the child's hand to the spot where the block is to be placed. This should be repeated until the child is able to make the proper manipulation himself whenever he hears the tone. Care must be taken to choose the orienting tone so that it is loud enough to be heard, but not too loud to disturb him. If the child refuses the head-set, one earphone may be removed and held to the child's ear by the parent. Once the responses to loud tones have been established, the intensity of the tone is decreased in successive steps until the child no longer responds. The first response in an ascending series can then be recorded as threshold.

Although children vary in their ability to respond, in general the younger the child, the more simple should be the play stimulation. Following are listed the play stimulations which might be most applicable at various ages:

2 to 2½ years: Build a tower with plain blocks, or place marbles in a bottle.

2½ to 3 years: Place marbles in a marble board or drop them into a bottle or box.

3 to 3½ years: Place pegs in a peg borad, "building a fence" for a horse in the middle of the board, or for a car; or place rings on a peg.

3½ to 5 years: Peg board as above, or place farm animals in a farm-yard, or cars in a parking lot.

Whenever the child's attention lags, a quick switch to another technique will bring him back to the task. Sometimes the only indication of flagging attention will be his failure to respond at a level to which he previously responded well. One must watch closely for such signs and change techniques immediately.

Even beyond the age of 5 years, some children attend to the listening task better if play techniques are used. The mentally retarded child will respond to the techniques suited to his mental age level rather than to his chronological age level. It will therefore be useful to use play-conditioning techniques with many retarded children.

Imagination, sensitivity, and understanding are requisite to successful play audiometry. In addition, the examiner must provide an animated, attention-getting experience for the child. Obviously, the procedures described in this section obtain only when the child has a considerable amount of useful hearing and language understanding.

SUGGESTED ADDITIONAL READINGS

1. Barr, B.: Pure tone audiometry for preschool children. Acta oto-laryng., Suppl. 121, 1955.
2. Boies, L. R., Canfield, N., Carhart, R., and Keaster, J.: Hearing loss in preschool children; a guide for diagnosis and treatment. Tr. Am. Acad. Ophth., *56:* 835, 1952.
3. Bloomer, H.: A simple method for testing the hearing of young children. J. Speech & Hearing Disorders, *7:* 311, 1942.
4. Bordley, J. E., and Hardy, W. G.: A study in objective audiometry with the use of psychogalvanometric response. Ann. Otol. Rhin. & Laryng., *58:* 751, 1949.
5. Bordley, J. E., Hardy, W. G., and Hardy, M. P.: Pediatric audiology. Pediatric Clinics North America, *9:* 1147, 1962.
6. Derbyshire, A. J., and Farley, J. C.: Sampling auditory responses at the cortical level. Ann. Otol. Rhin. & Laryng., *68:* 675, 1959.
7. Derbyshire, A. J., and McDermott, M.: Further contributions to the E.E.G. method of evaluating auditory function. Laryngoscope, *56:* 558, 1958.
8. Derbyshire, A. J., Fraser, A. A., Bridge, M., and Bridge, A.: Audiometric measurements by electroencephalography. Electroencephalography & Clinical Neurophysiology J., *8:* 467, 1956.
9. Dix, M., and Halpike, C.: The peep show, a new technique for pure-tone audiometry in young children. Brit. M. J., *2:* 719, 1947.
10. Ewing, I. R., and Ewing, A. W. G.: The ascertainment of deafness in infancy and early childhood. J. Laryng., *59:* 309, 1944.
11. Ewing, I. R., and Ewing, A. W. G.: *Opportunity and the Deaf Child.* University of London Press, London, 1947.
12. Froeschels, E.: Testing of hearing of young children. Arch. Otolaryng., *43:* 93, 1946.
13. Goldstein, R., Ludwig, E., and Naunton, R. F.: Difficulty in conditioning galvanic skin responses: its possible significance in clinical audiometry. Acta oto-laryng., *44:* 67, 1954.
14. Goodhill, V., Rehman, I., and Brockman, S.: Objective skin resistance audiometry. Tr. Pacific Coast Oto-Ophth. Soc., *34:* 215, 1953.
15. Grings, W. W., Lowell, E. L., and Honnard, R. R.: Electrodermal responses of deaf children. J. Speech & Hearing Res., *3:* 120, 1960.
16. Grings, W. W., Lowell, E. L., and Rushford, G. M.: Role of conditioning in GSR audiometry with children. J. Speech & Hearing Disorders, *24:* 380, 1959.
17. Hardy, J. B., Dougherty, A., and Hardy, W. G.: Hearing responses and audiologic screening in infants. J. Pediat., *55:* 382, 1959.
18. Hardy, W. G.: Problems of audition, perception, and understanding. Volta Rev., *58:* 289, 1956.
19. Hardy, W. G., and Bordley, J. E.: Special techniques in the testing of children. J. Speech & Hearing Disorders, *16:* 122, 1951.
20. Hardy, W. G., and Pauls, M. P.: Significance of problems of conditioning in GSR audiometry. J. Speech & Hearing Disorders, *24:* 123, 1959.
21. Hardy, W. G., Hardy, J. B., Brinker, C. H., Frazier, T. M., and Dougherty, A.: Auditory screening of infants. Ann. Oto. Rhin. & Laryng., *71:* 759, 1962.
22. Goldstein, R., Hardy, W. G., Myklebust, H. R., Tenque, L., and Silverman, S. R. (chairman): Hearing in children—panel discussion. Laryngoscope, *68:* 218, 1957.
23. Hirsh, I.: *The Measurement of Hearing,* Ch. 10 & 11. McGraw-Hill Book Company, Inc., New York, 1952.

24. Jerger, J. (ed.): *Modern Developments in Audiology*, Ch. 4 & 5. Academic Press, New York and London, 1963.

25. Keaster, J. A.: A quantitative method of testing the hearing of young children. J. Speech & Hearing Disorders, *12:* 159, 1947.

26. Lowell, E., Rushford, G., Hoversten, G., and Stoner, M.: Evaluation of pure tone audiometry with pre-school children. J. Speech & Hearing Disorders, *21:* 292, 1956.

27. Marcus, R. E., Gibbs, E. L., and Gibbs, F. A.: Electroencephalography in diagnosis of hearing loss in the very young child. Dis. Nerv. System, *10:* 170, 1949.

28. Macfarlan, D.: Hearing-testing of little children. Hearing News, *26:* 9, 1941.

29. Utley, J.: Suggestive procedures for determining auditory acuity in very young acoustically handicapped children. E.E.N.T. Monthly, *27:* 590, 1949.

30. Waldrop, W.: A puppet show hearing test. Volta Rev., *55,* 488, 1953.

31. Winthro, F. B., Jr., and Goldstein, R.: An electrophysiologic procedure for determination of auditory threshold in children. Laryngoscope, *68:* 1674, 1958.

32. Darley, F. L. (ed): Identification audiometry—committee report monograph. J. Speech & Hearing Disorders, Suppl. 9, 1961.

11

Industrial Audiometry

Meyer S. Fox, M.D.

At one time hearing testing in industry was performed chiefly by the use of conversational and whispered voice, tuning-fork, and watch-tick tests, all of which gave a cursory estimate of an individual's hearing ability. The need for accurate quantitative measurements of hearing was not appreciated until 1947, when a large numer of industrial compensation claims for alleged loss of hearing due to occupational noise exposure were filed in the state of New York. Shortly thereafter many similar claims were filed in New Jersey and Wisconsin. While industrial compensation laws of the various states recognized loss of hearing resulting by accidental means, hearing loss as the result of working in noisy areas was more or less taken for granted, both by industry and its employees. In spite of the facts that industry was expanding, production was increasing, and machines and working conditions were becoming noisier, industry made no attempt to measure the worker's hearing quantitatively, or to follow his hearing status during the course of his employment. The combination of increased noise exposure and the admissibility of compensation claims emphasized the need for accurate quantitative hearing tests. For, in the absence of hearing records, it was impossible to determine the status of an employee's hearing prior to or during his employment.

Much of the material presented in this chapter and many of the recommendations are taken from the *Guide for Conservation of Hearing in Noise* (1). The recommendations set forth in the *Guide* are based upon laboratory and industrial experience.

In a very general sense, industrial audiometry is the discipline that organizes the effective administration of hearing-test procedures in industry and adequately monitors them. This chapter is a discussion of practical hearing-test procedures readily adaptable to any industry.

At the outset it is necessary to consider the responsibilities of the program. The cause of the hearing loss may include many precipitating factors; therefore the direct responsibility of the program should be under medical supervision. The physician who had interested himself in, *and acquainted himself with*, the various aspects of occupational hearing loss can qualify to supervise this industrial program. This supervision includes the ability to make the proper recommendations and disposition of cases on the basis of his interpretation of the audiometric data available.

Numerous industries purchase audiometers and merely turn them over to nurses or safety personnel with instructions to "make hearing tests." These records are frequently filed away to be used only in the event that some claim should arise at a later date. No provisions are made for medical supervision of the program, adequate training for the audiometrist, or interpretation of the results. Such an approach is not consistent with good medical practice, nor can training be considered adequate with a few simple instructions provided by the audiometer salesman. Furthermore, the low reliability and validity of records so obtained make them practically useless. The mere manipulation of dials and recording of numbers, without proper training and supervision, leads to inaccurate records and waste of time and money; and results of such testing are unscientific and misleading. (A recommended minimal training program is described later in this chapter.)

WHO SHOULD RECEIVE HEARING TESTS IN INDUSTRY

A general statement of policy regarding the extent of the industrial testing program is necessary. *All employees should receive a pre-employment reference audiogram.* This reference audiogram will serve as a base record of the employee's threshold hearing level against which any future change in hearing can be compared. The audiogram may serve as a significant and important consideration in job placement when given the proper interpretation by the medical supervisor. Also it will be available for medico-legal purposes if necessary. This recommendation is similar to the common practice in industry of making visual tests, blood tests, and other general pre-employment medical studies considered essential for the health and welfare of the workers.

TESTING ENVIRONMENT

Industrial plants, because of their high noise levels, need special areas or rooms for the performance of hearing tests. These special provisions for noise-controlled areas are necessary to prevent ambient noise from masking out the audiometric tone, thus changing the hearing level measurement.

Table 11.1 gives suggested maximal levels of background noise allowable when testing at various frequencies. Occasionally an area can be found in a plant which is sufficiently quiet to meet these specifications. This however,

TABLE 11.1*

Suggested allowable background noise levels for hearing conservation audiometry rooms

Octave band (c/s).........	300–600	600–1200	1200–2400	2400–4800	4800–9600
Level in dB (C scale) re 0.0002 dyne/cm.²........	40	40	47	57	62

It is assumed that (1) no frequencies below 500 c/s will be measured, and (2) well-fitted binaural earphones will be worn. No levels have been set for the octave bands, 37.5 to 75, 75 to 150, or 150 to 300 c/s. The noise in these bands has little or no effect at the *recommended* audiometric test frequencies.

* From the *Guide for Conservation of Hearing in Noise.* edited by Aram Glorig, M. D., p. 28. Supplement to Tr. Am. Acad. Ophth., revised 1964.

is extremely rare in most industrial environments because of the nature of their operational procedures.

It has been found to be more practical, and frequently less costly, to purchase a pre-fabricated, commercially available, audiometric booth, rather than to construct a suitable audiometric testing room locally. The performance of these booths has been found adequate in intensive field testing, and they provide a consistent, reliable measurement.*

The importance of proper test environment cannot be over-emphasized. Improper environment can and does produce inaccurate records of an individual's hearing level, resulting in an apparent reduction of hearing acuity because of the masking phenomenon. These records may be improperly interpreted and result in an erroneous judgment regarding an individual's employability, placement, or eligibility for compensation.

AUDIOMETRIC EQUIPMENT

The equipment to be used in the testing environment should be selected carefully. For industrial hearing-testing programs, a simple, but properly calibrated and maintained, discrete air-conduction audiometer is all that is essential.

Self-Recording Audiometry. This type of audiometry (formerly called "automatic") has been advocated for industrial hearing-testing programs, its purpose being to save time, personnel, and expense. Self-recording audiometry allows the subject to control the test instrument and make his own hearing-threshold determinations. Practical experience with self-recording audiometers has shown that the initial expense of the machine is greater, a suitable testing environment is needed for the performance of the test, and the time actually required is about the same as for manual audiometry. Some form of supervision is still required; otherwise subjects have difficulty in understanding and responding properly.

* Such pre-fabricated testing rooms are manufactured by Industrial Acoustics Company, Inc., 380 Southern Boulevard, Bronx 54, New York.

Self-recording audiometry has its greatest usefulness in large industrial plants where a great number of workers are to be tested at the same time and several machines could be used, there by allowing one technician to supervise the entire operation. Group testing, using a single audiometer with multiple earphones, which allows several subjects to be tested simultaneously, is not practical and should not be considered when discussing threshold audiometry in industry.

PERSONNEL REQUIREMENTS

Duties and Training of Industrial Audiometric Technicians

The person selected for the performance of industrial hearing tests should be an intelligent, interested, and well-motivated individual. This person, often referred to as an audiometric technician, can be selected from the first-aid, safety, or personnel departments. Usually nurses or female employees are selected for this assignment. However, because of rapid turnover of female employees, it may be practical and desirable to train one or more men to perform these duties.

Several attempts have been made to describe the audiometric technician. Perhaps the best definition can be derived from the description of the duties of this individual as recommended by the Subcommittee on Noise of the American Academy of Opthalmology and Otolaryngology, and the American Speech and Hearing Association. These committees agree that it would be desirable for audiometric testing to be done by an audiometrist, a person who meets the American Speech and Hearing Association requirements. However, certain duties may be delegated to an audiometric technician. This technician *can* conduct a *pure-tone screening test* and establish *air-conduction thresholds*, but these test results should be reviewed and evaluated by an otologist or an audiologist.

It is emphasized that the audiometric technician *should not* perform the following tests: (1) pure-tone air-conduction tests requiring masking; (2) pure-tone bone-conduction testing; (3) speech audiometry; (4) electrodermal response audiometry (EDR) (also referred to as galvanic skin response (GSR)); and (5) tests for malingering and psychogenic deafness.

Administrative decisions and decisions on the procedure to be employed regarding such things as screening levels, frequencies to be tested, techniques to be used, criteria for failure, interpretation of hearing tests, and follow-up recommendations should be made by the otologist or audiologist who is administering the testing program.

Suggestions have also been made for the minimal requirements for a short training course of an audiometric technician. Included in this minimal requirement is a supervised clinical practice. This requires that at least 10 supervised air-conduction audiograms be administered by each trainee.

The second recommendation of the joint committees is that the length of the course should be sufficiently long to present the lecture material, allow the student to assimilate the material presented, complete supplementary readings, and fulfill the clinical practice requirements. Another recommendation is that the course be presented over a period of several weeks.

With the limitations of duties of the technician outlined above, a discussion of some of the personal qualifications considered essential is now presented. It has been found that the task requires a great deal of personal motivation and interest before the technician will produce consistent, reliable audiograms.

Motivation will usually be influenced by the trainee's background and training. The training of audiometric technicians should include some basic knowledge in each of the following areas: fundamentals of sound, anatomy and physiology of the ear, nomenclature of the audiometer, and the points where failure of that instrument might occur.

The general rules for day-to-day maintenance of the equipment, and an awareness of the importance of the test environment in the proper assessment of the hearing level of the individual, should be studied. The well trained technician will understand what is meant by "industrial hearing loss" and "noise exposure." In addition, a comprehension of the extent of the problem, the objectives of a hearing-conservation program, and the proper use of ear-protection measures are essential knowledge.

The understanding of the responsibility and significance of the numbers recorded on each employee's record will frequently instill greater motivation in the average technician to secure the best possible data.

TESTING PROCEDURE

There are many different clinical audiometric testing techniques used in the performance of hearing tests. Variations in technique, however, can result in differences in hearing levels. The frequencies to be tested as recommended by the *Guide* (1) are 500, 1000, 2000, 3000, 4000, and 6000 c/s. Any additional frequencies may be added by the medical supervisor, either for diagnostic purposes or where local needs require them. The important frequencies are those which represent the necessary frequencies for the understanding of ordinary speech—namely 500, 1000, and 2000 c/s.

Records

Once the threshold for a specific frequency has been established, the technician must record the reading on a chart or record. The results obtained from a discrete frequency audiometric examination are known as an audiogram. Audiogram cards and charts are usually supplied by the manufacturer for recording data in a graphic form. This graphic representation places the hearing level in decibels in the vertical plane and the discrete frequencies in the horizontal plane, as illustrated in Figure 11.1.

This graphic representation is not flexible enough to be used effectively in the field of industrial audiometry. Audiogram blanks do not provide space for recording such items as past noise exposure, history of previous ear disease, military service, age, and use of ear-protection devices. Furthermore, they do not permit the recording of more than one test. A series of cards or charts are required for recording periodic examinations. This makes comparisons between tests difficult and leads to the accumulation of bulky files which may become lost or misplaced.

Figure 11.2 is a sample form recommended by the Research Center, Subcommittee on Noise (1), for use in industrial audiometry. It illustrates the type of record that will allow necessary test data to be entered on an efficient summary sheet. The back of the chart can be used for recording periodic follow-up tests making recommendations and other notes. The technician should be trained to complete the records accurately, so that all of the basic information will be provided.

Periodic Follow-up Testing

The initial pre-placement threshold hearing level which was referred to as a reference audiogram will serve as a base line from which the hearing

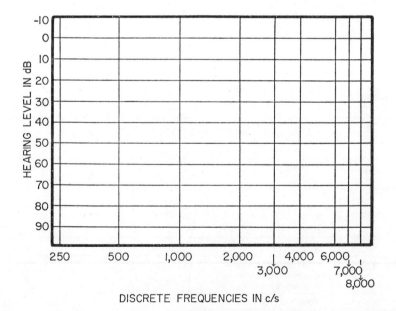

Fig. 11.1. Sample audiogram chart. It is important that all audiograms be properly identified as to whether they were made on the basis of the American Standards Association Audiometric Zero Reference Level of 1951 or the International Standards Reference Level of 1964.

		TYPE OF AUDIOGRAM	REFERENCE AND/OR PRE-EMPLOYMENT ☐
HEARING CONSERVATION DATA CARD NO._____			RECHECK ☐
			OTHER_____

A. IDENTIFICATION

LAST NAME	MIDDLE	FIRST	SEX	DATE OF BIRTH		
			MALE	DAY	MO.	YR.
			FEMALE			

SOCIAL SECURITY NUMBER	COMPANY NUMBER

B. CURRENT NOISE-EXPOSURE

JOB TITLE OR NUMBER	DEPARTMENT OR LOCATION	TIME IN JOB		
		NONE	MOS.	YRS.

NOISE-EXPOSURE			EMPLOYEES ESTIMATE OF OWN HEARING
STEADY NOISE	IMPULSE NOISE	PER CENT TIME NOISE ON	GOOD
CONTINUOUS ☐	CONTINUOUS ☐	10 20 30 40 50	FAIR
INTERMITTENT ☐	INTERMITTENT ☐	60 70 80 90 100	POOR

C. AUDIOGRAM

TIME SINCE MOST RECENT NOISE-EXPOSURE	DURATION OF MOST RECENT NOISE-EXPOSURE
0-20 MIN 1 HR 4-7 HRS 1 DA	0-20 MIN 1 HR 4-7 HRS
21-50 MIN 2-3 HRS 8-16 HRS 2-3 DAS	21-50 MIN 2-3 HRS 7+ HRS
4+ DAS	

AGE	DATE OF AUDIOGRAM	DAY OF WEEK	TIME OF DAY	EAR PROTECTION
				WAS EAR PROTECTION WORN? YES NO

RIGHT EAR								LEFT EAR							
250	500	1000	1500	2000	3000	4000	6000	250	500	1000	1500	2000	3000	4000	6000

D. PREVIOUS NOISE-EXPOSURE AND MEDICAL HISTORY

PREVIOUS EMPLOYMENT (LAST 3 JOBS)

TYPE OF WORK	FOR WHOM	HOW LONG

HISTORY	RECORD ANY COMMENTS SUBJECT MAKES ABOUT HEARING
HEAD INJURY (WITH UNCONSCIOUSNESS) ☐	
HEARING LOSS IN FAMILY (BEFORE AGE 50) ☐	
TINNITUS FOLLOWING NOISE-EXPOSURE R L	
STATUS	
PERFORATIONS OF DRUMHEAD R L	TECHNICIAN_____
DRAINAGE FROM EAR R L	
MALFORMATION OF EAR R L	PHYSICIAN_____

Fig. 11.2. Sample form for recording results of industrial audiometry

AUDIOGRAM

TIME SINCE MOST RECENT NOISE-EXPOSURE				DURATION OF MOST RECENT NOISE-EXPOSURE		
0-20 MIN	1 HR	4-7 HRS	1 DA	0-20 MIN	1 HR	4-7 HRS
21-50 MIN	2-3 HRS	8-16 HRS	2-3 DAS	21-50 MIN	2-3 HRS	7+ HRS
			4+ DAS			

AGE	DATE OF AUDIOGRAM	DAY OF WEEK	TIME OF DAY	EAR PROTECTION
				WAS EAR PROTECTION WORN? YES NO

RIGHT EAR								LEFT EAR							
250	500	1000	1500	2000	3000	4000	6000	250	500	1000	1500	2000	3000	4000	6000

AUDIOGRAM

TIME SINCE MOST RECENT NOISE-EXPOSURE				DURATION OF MOST RECENT NOISE-EXPOSURE		
0-20 MIN	1 HR	4-7 HRS	1 DA	0-20 MIN	1 HR	4-7 HRS
21-50 MIN	2-3 HRS	8-16 HRS	2-3 DAS	21-50 MIN	2-3 HRS	7+ HRS
			4+ DAS			

AGE	DATE OF AUDIOGRAM	DAY OF WEEK	TIME OF DAY	EAR PROTECTION
				WAS EAR PROTECTION WORN? YES NO

RIGHT EAR								LEFT EAR							
250	500	1000	1500	2000	3000	4000	6000	250	500	1000	1500	2000	3000	4000	6000

AUDIOGRAM

TIME SINCE MOST RECENT NOISE-EXPOSURE				DURATION OF MOST RECENT NOISE-EXPOSURE		
0-20 MIN	1 HR	4-7 HRS	1 DA	0-20 MIN	1 HR	4-7 HRS
21-50 MIN	2-3 HRS	8-16 HRS	2-3 DAS	21-50 MIN	2-3 HRS	7+ HRS
			4+ DAS			

AGE	DATE OF AUDIOGRAM	DAY OF WEEK	TIME OF DAY	EAR PROTECTION
				WAS EAR PROTECTION WORN? YES NO

RIGHT EAR								LEFT EAR							
250	500	1000	1500	2000	3000	4000	6000	250	500	1000	1500	2000	3000	4000	6000

AUDIOGRAM

TIME SINCE MOST RECENT NOISE-EXPOSURE				DURATION OF MOST RECENT NOISE-EXPOSURE		
0-20 MIN	1 HR	4-7 HRS	1 DA	0-20 MIN	1 HR	4-7 HRS
21-50 MIN	2-3 HRS	8-16 HRS	2-3 DAS	21-50 MIN	2-3 HRS	7+ HRS
			4+ DAS			

AGE	DATE OF AUDIOGRAM	DAY OF WEEK	TIME OF DAY	EAR PROTECTION
				WAS EAR PROTECTION WORN? YES NO

RIGHT EAR								LEFT EAR							
250	500	1000	1500	2000	3000	4000	6000	250	500	1000	1500	2000	3000	4000	6000

FIG. 11.2 (continued)

status of the worker can be followed and compared throughout the course of his employment. This is accomplished by means of periodic re-checks, screening tests, and/or threshold audiograms. The frequency of these tests will depend upon such factors as the initial audiogram, the age of the worker, the noise exposure, whether or not ear protection has been used, and the possible complaints of hearing or ear symptoms by the worker.

Periodic follow-up examinations are necessary where the worker is exposed to potentially hazardous noise levels. The first follow-up test should be made approximately 9 to 12 months after job placement unless an earlier test is indicated by long continuous exposure to noise levels greater than 100 dB average octave band levels at 300 to 600, 600 to 1200, and 1200 to 2400 c/s, complaints of severe tinnitus, excessive temporary hearing loss, or excessively prolonged recovery from temporary threshold shifts. All follow-up tests should be made after as long a period of absence from noise as is practical (but at least 16 hours) to allow for as much recovery as possible from temporary threshold shift (temporary change in hearing level) produced during the previous work day.

Properly designed screening tests are satisfactory follow-up measurements. These tests may be divided into two main types. One specifies the presentation of all of the previously recommended discrete frequencies at a predetermined intensity level of 15, 20, or 25 dB. These tests do not establish the subject's hearing level but indicate only that his hearing level is at least as good as the levels set. If the level is worse than the screening level established for any one of the six frequencies, a threshold audiogram at that frequency should be made to establish the magnitude of the change before any further recommendations can be made.

The other type of screening method that has been successfully used in industry is the single-frequency screening technique. Since the initial shift in an individual's hearing level as a result of noise usually will occur (and is greatest at) the 4000 c/s tone, the single-frequency test employing this tone has proved effective. The tone presented at pre-determined intensity is easy to administer, requires very little time, and can be used in areas where the ambient noise levels are high. When the subject fails the screening test as compared to his original audiogram, a complete threshold audiogram to measure the magnitude of the change should be made.

From a practical standpoint, if there is no greater change than 10 dB between the pre-employment reference audiogram and the initial follow-up test, subsequent tests may be given at approximately annual intervals, unless otherwise indicated. In ordinary noise-exposure conditions, retests of hearing at yearly intervals have proven to be most practical and effective. Unnecessarily frequent testing of hearing which reveals no change in the subject's hearing level is not warranted, and it involves added expense and time.

TABLE 11.2

Occupational hearing loss

Cause of Hearing Loss	Location of Damage to Ear	Type of Hearing Loss	Medical Name	Legal Name	Suggested Names	
					Agent-identifying	Damage-identifying
Continuous noise exposure	Inner ear structures	Inner ear loss	Noise-induced hearing loss, occupational hearing loss, or acoustic trauma	Occupational hearing loss	Noise-induced hearing loss	Auditory trauma (due to long continued noise exposure)
Sudden explosive blasts	Inner ear and/or middle ear structures	Conductive, inner ear, or mixed loss	Acoustic trauma	Acoustic trauma	Acoustic trauma (to the ear)	Auditory trauma (due to sudden noise)
Mechanical blows to the head and/or ear	Inner ear and/or middle ear or external canal	Conductive, inner ear, or mixed loss	Acoustic trauma	Acoustic trauma	Mechanical trauma (to the ear)	Auditory trauma (due to blows to head)
Barometric pressure changes	Middle ear and/or inner ear	Conductive, inner ear, or mixed loss	Aerotitis barotrauma or Caissons disease		Aerotitis barotrauma (to the ear)	Auditory trauma (due to sudden pressure changes)
Burns (heat as opposed to chemicals)	Middle ear and/or inner ear	Conductive, inner ear, or mixed loss			Thermal trauma (to the ear)	Auditory trauma (due to heat burns)

REFERRALS AND DISPOSITION

If the pre-employment reference audiogram shows an average hearing loss of more than 15 dB in the speech frequencies 500, 1000, and 2000 c/s, the employee should be referred for an otological and audiological examination, as well as a placement evaluation, before assignment to a job. Such referral is also advised for employees whose audiograms show any unusual irregularity, particularly in an abrupt loss beginning at 2000 c/s. A pre-employment audiogram showing loss, however, should not be used as a determining factor in rejecting a prospective employee, unless such a loss would seriously interfere with a job requiring speech communication.

An effective program of industrial audiometry as described is contingent upon the understanding and co-operation of all who participate, and are effected by its scope.

REFERENCE

1. Glorig, A. (ed.): *Guide for Conservation of Hearing in Noise.* Supplement to Tr. Am. Acad. Ophth., revised 1964 (A.A.O.O., 15 Second Street, S.W., Rochester, Minn.).

SUGGESTED ADDITIONAL READINGS

1. Davis, H. (ed.), and Silverman, S. R. (co-ed.): *Hearing and Deafness.* Holt, Rinehart, and Winston, Inc., New York, 1960.
2. Glorig, A.: *Noise and Your Ear.* Grune & Stratton, Inc., New York and London, 1958.

12

Evaluation of Non-Organic Hearing Loss

Aram Glorig, M.D.

Malingering, by definition, originally meant "feigning illness in order to avoid duty—as a soldier or sailor." This definition was expanded to mean the willful imitation of illness, or its severity, or a deliberate simulation, usually for purposes of *monetary* gain. The currently accepted meaning of malingering is willful feigning of a disorder for gain (whether it be immediate monetary gain or a remote intangible satisfaction).

The tendency to "play sick" is deeply rooted in both the animal and human world. It ranges from the sly "play sleep" of the cat intent on fooling mice to the convenient "headaches" of the matron facing an unpleasant social obligation. Probably everyone at one time or another has indulged in some sort of malingering. It was not until a strong motivation in the form of monetary compensation was introduced that malingering became a serious social and economic problem.

True malingering is intimately related to a reward of some kind, usually military retirement benefits or workmen's compensation. It does not exist without some motivation. In the military services, for example, feigning illness could lead to exclusion from distasteful or hazardous duties, or a medical retirement benefit, with the result that 25 to 30% of all military hearing-loss cases must be treated as suspected malingerers.

In civilian life, workmen's compensation payments or insurance settlements make it quite worthwhile to pretend a hearing loss. (It has been-estimated that of all industrial claims for damage, 90% are possible malingerers and 20% are obvious malingerers (1).)

A major problem exists in that malingering is not a simple behavior pattern. The malingerer could perhaps be classed as a person with a character disorder—one who shirks his social responsibility and refuses to maintain a strictly honest attitude, and who *consciously* feigns illness. On the other hand, an individual with a psychogenic hearing loss is simulating illness *subconsciously* and is no longer dishonest nor deliberate, and thereby cannot really be classed as a malingerer.

The practice of labeling a person simulating an illness as a malingerer is being discouraged by many examiners. They point out that inasmuch as simulation of an illness may be either conscious or unconscious, it is wise to be extremely careful before terming a patient a malingerer. Actually, in diagnosis, malingering is a most serious charge and is seldom proved without an actual admission by the patient of intent to defraud.

A committee studying the problem (1) preferred to classify these types of simulation under the name "non-organic hearing impairment." They state:

> Non-organic hearing impairment designates auditory dysfunction for which no plausible anatomical or chemical basis can be found. The term includes auditory disorders ranging from conscious, purposeful malingering to non-conscious, apparently purposeless disorders variously called hysterical deafness, psychogenic deafness, and the like. Conditions existing outside the auditory system, such as mental deficiency, senility, and brain injury, which tend to affect hearing adversely, constitute a separate problem. However, these conditions must be identified and excluded in order to establish a diagnosis of non-organic deafness or hearing loss.
>
> The specification of types of non-organic hearing impairment at present rests on no precise terminological framework. Description tends to depend on factors such as motivation, causation, and degree of impairment. For example, the factor of motive may be regarded as extending from deliberate seeking of tangible reward to unconscious avoidance of unpleasant circumstances. In the individual case, unfortunately, motive is more easily inferred than specified with any degree of assurance. The extent of conscious volition is difficult to determine short of a frank confession. The causes of non-organic hearing impairment are not known, although plausible contributing factors occasionally can be discerned. At the present time, only the presence of non-organic auditory disorders can be determined with reasonable assurance. The amount of non-organic hearing loss may be measured only with difficulty if at all.

TESTS

One fact which must always be kept in mind when testing is that only a few methods can measure non-organic hearing impairment even approximately, and then only under favorable conditions. The problem facing the examiner is not just to determine the presence of non-organic hearing loss —which is relatively easy—but to determine whether this loss is conscious or unconscious simulation.

The techniques available to the examiner fall into four general classifications: informal procedures, routine tests, tests of control of auditory response, and so-called "objective" tests.

Informal Procedures

The *patient interview* is extremely important, for an intelligent and experienced observer can frequently expose a malingerer quickly at this time. Obvious discrepancies in auditory behavior that do not correlate with the test performance may be noticed. The patient's attitude toward his hearing, as revealed in the interview, supplies the examiner with an important clue. The person with a true hearing loss is usually worried and shows it. The malingerer, however, displays a more nonchalant attitude and appears quite unconcerned. It is in the interview also that motivation for simulation may be revealed, perhaps accidentally. Hardly any individual malingers without a motive, and when the motive is discovered and removed, the problem often disappears.

Routine Tests

Two routine tests are the *repeat pure-tone thresholds* and *repeat speech-reception thresholds*. In the pure-tone test, which is a standard pure-tone threshold test administered via audiometer, the inexpert listener will usually have difficulty duplicating his threshold on a repeat test unless he has a true hearing loss. However, the expert malingerer (a person simulating a hearing loss who has considerable experience with such tests) can duplicate pure-tone thresholds quite easily. He does this by mentally establishing a loudness level well above threshold and waiting until that level is reached before responding.

False *speech-reception thresholds*, on the other hand, are difficult to duplicate. Speech is a transient signal with a temporal pattern, and differences will occur when repeat tests are made if the alleged threshold is spurious.

Inconsistent thresholds, therefore, either pure-tone or speech, suggest non-organic hearing loss, and further testing is necessary. A consistent threshold, however, is no guarantee that the problem is *not* non-organic hearing loss.

Tests of Control of Auditory Response

The techniques designed to interfere with willful attempts to control the response to auditory signal are pure tone-speech relation, Doerfler-Stewart (DS), Lombard, Stenger, swinging story, delayed playback, and motor response to auditory feedback.

Pure Tone-Speech Relation. In this technique the routine pure-tone and speech reception test thresholds are compared. The basis of this comparison rests on the discovery that, in general, the average of the pure-tone thresholds at 500, 1000, and 2000 c/s agrees with the speech-reception threshold as obtained with the spondee test lists, within 10 or 12 dB or better, in all valid hearing tests. Therefore, if the average of the pure-tone thresholds at these three frequencies disagrees by more that 10 to 15 dB with the SRT (as obtained with spondee words), then non-organic hearing loss should be suspected. The disagreement usually shows the pure-tone threshold to be higher, for control of response to pure tones is easier than that to speech signals.

Doefler-Stewart Test (DS). This is one of the best tests available, for it provides a qualitative and a quantitative estimate of impairment. The equipment is easy to assemble, and the test has the effect of discouraging the potential malingerer. It depends upon the effect of variable masking with a tailored noise on the response to speech signals and is designed to break down the spurious loudness level. By varying the relationship between the two signals, the loudness-level "yardstick" is disturbed. An abnormal result, therefore, suggests non-organic hearing loss. Where some sort of "gain" is a motivating influence, the DS should be used routinely.

The Lombard Test. This is a classic procedure and can be quite useful if used properly—and at the right time. It is only a qualitative, not a quantitative indicator, however. Its results depend upon the effect of noise on the speech-auditory feedback system. If hearing is normal or nearly normal, the noise that is introduced into the alleged bad ear will produce an increase in voice level. The Lombard can be used in alleged unilateral hearing loss but it is better adapted to alleged bilateral hearing loss. Its great defect is its susceptibility to learning. Repetition and poor presentation reduce its effectiveness; it is more useful with naive than sophisticated individuals.

The Stenger Test. The Stenger is the best test available for unilateral hearing loss. It is based on the principle that when two tones of identical pitch are sounded simultaneously in each ear, if the two ears are normal, the tone will be heard exclusively in the one ear in which it is louder and cannot be heard in the other ear in which it is substantially weaker. Unilateral malingering, however, is not common, and the Stenger fails unless the instrumentation is precise and the technique standardized.

The Swinging Story Test. This test, in which a story is presented to the subject and the stimulus switched from ear to ear, is good only in unilateral simulated hearing loss. It has the same disadvantages as the Stenger and is not as sound psychoacoustically, although it has pointed a suspicious finger at many a unilateral malingerer.

The Delayed-Playback Test. The test is also called the "feedback" or "delayed side-tone effect" test, and has shown considerable promise as a measure of non-organic hearing loss. If done properly, it is very difficult for the subject to control his responses; thus good technique is extremely important. Inasmuch as speech is monitored by hearing, if the "auditory feedback circuit" is broken in any way, the monitor is no longer in control. This test is one way in which it is possible to break into a physiological "feedback" circuit. For example, if the test is applied to a person whose simulation is subconscious, the delayed speech should not confuse him; but, on the other hand, the malingerer should be confused because he is unable to control the effects of the delayed speech on his monitoring feedback circuit.

It has one important disadvantage. When there is a moderate organic loss with an overlay, the test is limited because of the need for high signal levels.

The Motor Response to Auditory Feedback. This technique is relatively new and requires considerable experimental work to determine its actual validity and reliability. Theoretically, however, it has promise. It is based on the relation between motor response and audition. For example, tasks which require rapid repeat motor activity, such as key tapping, show differences when the sound produced is fed back to the ear. These differences vary when the auditory sense is eliminated.

Objective Tests

The so-called objective tests of hearing focus on the measurement of the electrodermal response (EDR), the electroencephalographic record (EEG), and the eye-blink response.

The Electrodermal Response Measurement (EDR). Formerly called the psychogalvanic skin response, it is perhaps the most widely used of the "objective" techniques, particularly in the military services. It is a matter of opinion, however, as to whether it is either objective, or a test. An objective test, by definition, is one which requires no active, i.e., voluntary or conditioned, response. The EDR depends upon conditioning, which at times is difficult if not impossible, and the results must be interpreted by *trained* observers.

One area in which the EDR can be particularly useful, however, is in the effect it has on the individual. There is a certain awesome quality about attaching electrodes to the individual and informing him that his responses will be entirely automatic. This effect carries over so that frequently, regardless of the EDR findings, the subject will respond accurately to other tests following the EDR procedure.

Under any condition, however, the accuracy of the test is dependent upon the ability of the technician to condition his subject, and to interpret the results properly.

The Electroencephalograph (EEG). This technique has proved useful to a certain degree. It is severely limited, however, because of equipment needs and the fact that there is no specific and unique wave form peculiar to an auditory signal. There are changes, to be sure, in whatever wave form is present at the time the auditory stimulus is presented. These changes decrease rapidly, however, as the signal approaches threshold intensity, and disappear before absolute threshold is reached. A possibility exists that low-level outputs from the cortex can be averaged by computers so that cortical activity in response to auditory signals can be used as an indication that the auditory mechanism is intact. The expense of the equipment necessary for such a procedure at present prohibits its use as a routine measure.

The Eye-Blink Test. One of the most basic auditory reflexes is the startle response. One of the components of this response is the "eye blink." A measure of this response relative to auditory stimulus was developed, based on the knowledge that despite repeated exposure to varied stimuli, the reflex never really disappears. To date, the technique has been used primarily in research and thus far displays only limited value. The blink disappears as level is decreased to 10 to 15 dB above threshold and the procedure cannot be used except in centers where proper equipment is available.

These "objective" tests may be generally considered lower-order auditory tests; i.e., they test lower order neural mechanisms. If there is a positive result, neural activity which includes the auditory system from the standpoint of continuity of transmission of a sound stimulus is indicated. A negative result, however, does not specifically mean a break in the auditory system. The EDR and eye blink are reflex type mechanisms and may therefore be completed without the need of higher cerebral centers. Similarly the EEG indicates auditory activity by non-specific brain wave changes. So far none of these tests has denoted changes in responses which indicate a difference in neural activity between a conscious and subconscious block.

Narcosis and Hypnosis

These procedures are successful only in the hands of experienced psychiatrists and then only to a limited degree. They are used best with individuals who have suffered from sudden shock resulting in a sudden hearing loss. They serve little or no purpose in persons whose hearing loss has been present for several years.

SUMMARY

Conscious simulation of loss cannot be demonstrated by test alone. Each of the tests discussed will indicate the difference between a non-

TABLE 12.1

Test Classes	Specific Items	Equipment	Class of Results	Evaluation	Rating
Informal procedures	History & examination; Auditory difficulty with conversation Patient attitude Motivation Speech changes Lip reading	Intelligent, experienced observer	Indicative, qualitative	Patient interview very important. Experienced observer can make good estimate of auditory efficiency	Good to excellent
Routine	Pure tone	Standard pure-tone audiometer; standard speech audiometer	Indicative	Inconsistent multiple pure-tone tests are usually positive indication of non-organic hearing loss. Speech tests also may be used	Good
Tests of control of auditory response	1. Pure-tone speech relation	1. Pure-tone & speech audiometers	1. Indicative, qualitative	1. When SRT (speech reception threshold) and pure tone level at 1000 c/s are widely separated, non-organic hearing loss must be suspected	1. Good
	2. Doerfler Stewart (DS)	2. Two channel controlled noise and speech	2. Qualitative, quantitative	2. The DS should be routine in all cases where personal gain is motivation	2. Excellent
	3. Lombard	3. Controlled	3. Qualitative	3. Severely limited by learning	3. Fair
	4. Stenger	4. Matched controlled two-channel (pure-tone and/or speech)	4. Qualitative, quantitative	4. When properly done, impossible to beat in unilateral cases	4. Excellent
	5. Swinging story	5. Two-channel speech	5. Indicative	5. Positive results, meaningful; unilateral cases	5. Fair
	6. Delayed playback	6. Good quality tape recorder with delayed playback head	6. Indicative, quantitative	6. Positive results strongly indicative; needs more research	6. Good
	7. Motor response to auditory feedback	7. Key-tapping device	7. Indicative	7. Promising	7. Good
So-called objective	1. Electrodermal response (EDR)	1. EDR system (commercially available)	1. Qualitative	1. Difficult to interpret; pure-tone tests useful	1. Fair
	2. Electro-encephalograph	2. EEG equipment	2. Qualitative	2. EEG requires complex equipment. Interpretation of results is difficult	2. Fair
	3. Eye blink	3. Phonograph pick-up and oscilloscope or high-speed ink writer	3. Indicative	3. Special equipment—not dependable near threshold	3. Fair

241

organic and organic hearing loss, but none can sub-divide the non-organic hearing losses into conscious and subconscious simulation. In order to be absolutely certain that the non-organic hearing impairment is conscious simulation, one must obtain an admission to defraud. (Note: These tests are also discussed in the chapters on Pure-Tone Audiometry and Speech Audiometry.) (See Table 12.1.)

REFERENCE

1. Critical evaluation of methods for testing for non-organic hearing impairment. Minutes of the 2nd meeting of working group No. 36, Armed Forces National Research Council's Committee on Hearing & Bio-Acoustics, Washington, 1959.

SUGGESTED ADDITIONAL READINGS

1. Keschner, M.: Simulation (malingering) in relation to injuries of the skull, brain and spinal cord. In *Injuries of the Skull, Brain and Spinal Cord,* edited by Samuel Brock, p. 361. The Williams & Wilkins Company, Baltimore, 1940.
2. Doerfler, L. G., and Stewart, K.: Malingering and psychogenic deafness. J. Speech & Hearing Disorders, *11:* 181, 1946.
3. Bordley, J. E., Hardy, W. G., and Richter, G. P.: Audiometry with the use of galvanic skin resistance response: a preliminary report. Bull. Johns Hopkins Hosp., *82:* 569, 1948.
4. Galambos, R., Rosenberg, P. E., and Glorig, A.: The eyeblink response as a test for hearing. J. Speech & Hearing Disorders, *18:* 373, 1953.
5. Lee, B. S.: Effects of delayed speech feedback. J. Acoust. Soc. America, *22:* 824, 1950.
6. Lee, B. S.: Artificial stutter. J. Speech & Hearing Disorders, *16:* 53, 1951.

Appendix 1

The following is a glossary of some of the common terms used in audiometry. The expert engineer may notice some incompleteness and possibly some technical omissions. In the interest of the non-technical reader, the author takes full responsibility.

Absorption Coefficient—a number which signifies the fraction or portion of acoustical energy that is absorbed when sound strikes the surface of a given material. Theoretically, α (absorption coefficient is usually designated by the Greek letter *alpha*) may range from 0.00 (complete reflection) to 1.00 (complete absorption), but these extreme values are not readily obtained in practice. Materials do not absorb acoustical energy equally well throughout the audible frequency range; consequently, values of α are usually quoted for several different frequencies. A single number, the value of α for a frequency of 500 c/s (Hz), is sometimes quoted as an approximate absorption coefficient.

Acoustic Feedback—any repetitive process by which a portion of the acoustical output of a system is returned to the input and is thus recirculated through the system. Acoustical feedback causes the familiar "howl" which is produced when the microphone of a public address system is so placed that it can pick up sound radiated by the loudspeaker. Electrical "noise," generated in the electronic parts of the system, is converted by the loudspeaker into sound. Some of this sound feeds back into the nearby microphone, is amplified, feeds back from the speaker into the microphone again, and is reamplified, etc., finally building up into a loud howl.

Acoustic Trauma—generally refers to auditory damage from acoustic signals. However, because the damage varies according to the type of noise or sound, especially when the signal is steady or impulsive, "acoustical trauma" is preferred when the damage is produced by sudden explosive or impulsive sounds such as an explosion or a heavy impact. When the signal is steady and the damage is produced slowly over a period of time, it is preferable to use the term "noise-induced hearing loss."

Acoustical Pulse—a sound of limited time duration; one which begins and ends abruptly: a click, gunshot, burst of noise, etc.

Acoustics—of or pertaining to the ear or hearing and/or to sound or the science of sound.

Acuity—the sharpness, clearness, or distinctness with which one is able to hear a sound; hence, usually auditory acuity.

Air Conduction—a term used by clinicians to indicate the path through the air in the external ear canal and across the middle ear by which sound travels to the inner ear. A hearing test given with earphones is called an "air-conduction" hearing test. (See bone conduction.)

Ambient Noise—(background noise)—the total residual noise, exclusive of any intentional signal, in an electroacoustical system or in a physical environment such as a test room. These are examples of ambient noise: the hum in an amplifying system, noises generated in a room by the movement of persons or by equipment, noise transmitted into a room through walls, doors, windows, etc.

Amplification—(gain)—a number which indicates the relative magnitude of the output signal of a reproducing system, compared with the magnitude of the input signal. Amplification may be expressed as the direct ratio of output to input or as a logarithmic ratio of output to input, i.e., in decibels. If an amplified output signal has 1 million times more energy than the input signal has, the amplification is 1,000,000:1 or 1,000,000. This corresponds to an energy amplification of 60 dB.

Amplification, Selective—the amplification of sounds of certain frequency to a greater degree than, or to the exclusion of, sounds of other frequencies.

Amplifier—any device for intensifying sound waves. Amplifiers are of two general types: (1) those that capture more of the energy of a sound than is possible with the unaided ear and, by concentration of this energy, build up more intense sound waves; and (2) those that intensify sound waves by means of electrical circuits using transformers or vacuum tubes or both.

Amplitude—the range of movement of a vibrating body. Directly related to intensity.

Amplitude Distortion—see Electroacoustic Characteristics.

Anechoic (Echo-Free) Room—a specially designed and constructed sound-absorbing room. A very high percentage of the sound energy generated in an anechoic chamber is absorbed by the special covering of the walls, ceiling, and floor. The highly absorbent material which lines the interior of such chambers is usually in the shape of deep wedges: the thin edge of the wedges point into the room. The chamber is usually equipped with a wire mesh or sometimes a set of rails suspended above the bottom wedges so that equipment can be moved easily into or out of the room. Anechoic chambers are used whenever it is important to be able to generate sounds and make sound measurements without interference from reflections. These rooms must also provide a high degree of isolation from external sounds.

Articulation Test—any of several hearing tests designed to measure the intelligibility of speech or of speech sounds. There are vowel-articulation tests, consonant-articulation tests, word-articulation tests, sentence-articulation tests, etc.

Artificial Ear—see Coupler.

Attenuate—in acoustics, to reduce in intensity, as of tones or speech sounds. Attenuation may be effected mechanically through absorption of the energy of tones or sounds by the walls of the chamber through which they pass. With tones or sounds that are electrically transmitted, attenuation may be accomplished by a lowering of the sensitivity of a microphone, by moving the speaker (or source of sound) farther from the microphone, or by reducing the factor of amplification of a circuit into which a microphone or oscillator feeds. Ideally, electrical attenuation results in reduction of intensity only, without a change of overtone structure, of the tones or sounds transmitted; while mechanical attenuation usually results in, or is accompanied by, quality changes.

Audiogram—a record of hearing losses measured at several different, usually discrete, frequencies. Audiograms commonly include measurements of losses at 500, 1000, 2000, 3000, 4000, 6000 c/s (Hz). Diagnostic audiograms may include measurements at lower frequencies and at higher frequencies.

Audiometer, Continuous-Frequency—an audiometer whose output frequency may be changed in steps of 1 c/s throughout the entire frequency range of the instrument.

Audiometer, Discrete-Frequency—an audiometer whose output is limited to pure tones of pre-selected frequencies. The usual discrete frequency audiometer generates tones at 250, 500, 1000, 2000, 3000, 4000, 6000, and 8000 c/s (Hz).

Audiometry—the technique of measuring hearing. Measurements may be made of the auditory response to any of several auditory stimuli, but fixed-frequency pure tones and speech sounds are most commonly used.

Audiometry, Electrodermal—a method of measuring hearing by measuring changes in skin resistance that are associated with a conditioned auditory response.

Auditory—of or pertaining to the ear and/or hearing.

Auditory Memory Span—the ability to recall sounds, usually tested by presenting a series of unit vowel sounds spoken at the rate of 1 per sec.; at the conclusion of the series, the subject repeats the vowels in the order given.

Auditory Training—training designed to teach a person with impaired hearing how to make the best use of his residual hearing.

Auditory Threshold—the sound pressure level of the minimal acoustical signal that evokes an auditory sensation for a specified fraction of the number of times the signal is presented to the ear. The auditory threshold for spondaic words, for example, is defined as the minimal sound pressure level at which a subject can repeat correctly 50% of the words presented to him. Auditory thresholds are different for different stimuli, and the particular stimulus used must be identified.

Bel—the unit of intensity; a logarithmic unit expressing the ratio of two amounts of power (see Decibel).

Bone Conduction—a term used by clinicians to indicate the pathway through the cranial bones by which sound reaches the inner ear. (See Air Conduction.)

Binaural Alternate-Loudness Balance Test—a procedure for comparing judgments of loudness: sound is presented first to one ear, then to the other; the intensity of the sound presented to one ear is adjusted until the sounds in both ears are judged to be equally loud.

Cochlea—the auditory part of the internal ear, shaped like a shell, containing the basilar membrane upon which are distributed the end organs of the acoustical nerve.

Complex Tone—a sound wave composed of several frequencies (pure tones). If these frequencies can be expressed as small, whole-number multiples of the lowest frequency in the complex wave, the tone is said to be composed of a fundamental and harmonic overtones.

Conductive Loss—a hearing impairment due to failure of the mechanics of the middle ear, or from the failure of air vibrations to be transmitted into the inner ear.

Continuous-Frequency Audiometer—see Audiometer, Continuous-Frequency.

Coupler—a device used to "couple" an earphone with a microphone for purposes of measuring the acoustic output of the earphone. Couplers are often made in the form of hollow brass cylinders which are designed to present to the earphone the acoustic impedance of the average human ear.

Damping—decreasing the amplitude of vibrations of a sounding body due to the absorption of energy by the surrounding medium.

Dead Room—a room which provides an unusually large amount of sound absorption. The extreme dead room is the anechoic chamber.

Decibel—(written dB)—a dimensionless unit used to express a logarithmic ratio of two amounts of energy, power, intensity, voltage, pressure, etc. The ratio, in decibels, of two intensities, I_1 and I_2, is calculated as follows: (1) find the numerical value of the ratio $I_1:I_2$; (2) find the logarithm to the base 10 of this number; and (3) multiply the logarithm by 10. The resulting number is the intensity level in decibels of I_1 re I_2. For example: assume that I_1 is 100 times more intense than I_2, then (1) $I_1:I_2 = 100$; (2) $\log_{10} 100 = 2$; (3) $10 \times 2 = 20$, and the intensity level of I_1 is 20 dB re I_2. Note: When voltage level and pressure level are calculated, the logarithm is multiplied by *20* rather than by 10.

Difference Limen—(usually designated DL, also known as "just noticeable difference" or as "Differential Threshold")—the smallest change in a given physical property of stimuli that produces an observable change in sensation. For example, the smallest change in frequency (of an acoustical stimulus) that can be detected by the ear.

Diffraction—the scattering or bending of sound waves around small obstacles.

Diplacusis—means, literally, "double hearing." Generally applied to a condition which judges a single tone, presented alternately to the right and left ears, as having a different pitch in the two ears.

Disability—a physical or mental incapacity; one who has a disability is disabled, or unfit, or has a handicap. Because of variable legal provisions and court interpretations, this definition of disability should not be regarded as a legal definition. The physician may frequently be misunderstood, particularly within a legal framework, when he uses the term "disability" in the medical sense. The word "impairment" does not have specific legal interpretations, and is preferred for use in medicolegal contexts.

Discrete-Frequency Audiometer—see Audiometer, Discrete-Frequency.

Distortion—a change of an original sound wave pattern imposed by the response limits of the structure or media through which it passes. These changes may affect frequency, phase, and/or amplitude.

Distortion, Amplitude (or Non-Linear)—the inexact reproduction of an input signal. Amplitude distortion is present when the output of an electroacoustical system is not proportional to the input. It results in the production of extraneous frequencies (frequencies not present in the input) in the output, thus making the output wave form different from the input wave form.

Dyne—a unit of force; the force required to move a mass of 1 gram with a velocity of 1 cm. per sec.

Dyne/cm.²—the unit of measurement of sound pressure.

Earphone—an instrument (designed to be worn close to the ear) for converting electrical energy into acoustic energy; an electroacoustical transducer. All earphones are similar in that they contain a diaphragm which is set into motion by electrical or magnetic forces. The moving diaphragm sets air into motion and thus generates sound. The motion of the diaphragm corresponds to the pattern of the electrical current fed into the earphone; thus the acoustical output of the earphone is a reproduction of the electrical input. The name of the type of earphone usually indicates the source of the force that activates the diaphragm. For example, crystal earphones, dynamic or moving coil earphones, and magnetic earphones.

Electroacoustic Characteristics—the properties (frequency distortion, amplitude distortion, efficiency, etc.) of a device or system which converts electrical energy into acoustical energy or vice versa.

Electroencephalographic (EEG) Audiometry—a highly specialized testing technique which is sometimes used when standard pure-tone and speech audiometry are impossible or impractical to use. With this test, brain waves are measured to determine whether or not an auditory event has been perceived by the subject.

Equal-Loudness Contours—curves which show the relationship that must be maintained between sound pressure level and frequency if tones of various frequencies are to produce the same loudness sensation for "normal" listeners. Equal-loudness contours show clearly that all tones of the same sound-pressure level do not sound equally loud.

Free Field—a space filled with a homogeneous medium whose boundaries do not measurably affect the sound field within the space. An anechoic chamber is a good approximation to a free-field space.

Frequency—(of a phenomenon that occurs periodically or cyclicly in time)—the number of repetitions of a pattern or of an event that occur in unit time. Frequency usually is expressed in cycles per second, written in one of three ways; c/s, cps, or Hz (Hertz).

Distortion—non-uniform performance of a reproducing system characterized by lack of constancy of amplification of input signals of the same magnitude but of different frequency; selective amplification of tones of different frequency.

High—a vibratory rate of 2400 c/s (H_z) or higher, the range of pitch in which are located the characteristic sounds of sibilants and fricatives in speech.

Range—the extent of frequencies to which a system responds; for example, the "audible frequency range" of response of the young human ear includes the frequencies between 16 and 20,000 c/s (Hz). The frequency range of a loudspeaker may be 50 to 15,000 c/s (Hz).

Response—a quantitative description of the electrical or acoustical output of a system; the magnitude of the output is shown as a function of the frequency of the input signal.

Fundamental—the lowest component frequency of a periodic wave, the principal component of a sound wave; the component having the greatest wave length.

Gain—see Amplification.

Handicapped (Person)—one who is at a disadvantage in a social or an economic competition because of a physical or mental defect.

Harmonic Content—(of a complex sound)—the ratio of the acoustical power in all the higher harmonics to the acoustical power in the first harmonic (the fundamental).

Harmonics—those components of a complex tone whose frequencies are integral multiples of the fundamental frequency of the tone. The fundamental frequency is called the first harmonic; the second harmonic has twice the frequency of the fundamental, etc.

Hearing Level—see Levels, Hearing.

Hz—(Hertz)—International symbol for cycles per second.

Impedance—the opposition to the transmission of sound in a given medium. It is proportional to the density of and to the propagation velocity within that medium.

Impedance, Mechanical—the opposition of a given structure against a vibratory force attempting to set that structure into motion.

Industrial Hearing Loss—a hearing loss that is causally related to one's employment.

Intelligibility of Speech—the degree to which speech sounds can be heard and repeated correctly. Measures of intelligibility currently are expressed as the percentage of words a subject hears and repeats correctly when a special list of phonetically balanced (PB) words is presented to him orally.

Intensity of Sound—the amount of acoustical energy that passes through unit area in unit time. Since energy per unit time is defined as power, intensity may also be expressed as "sound power per unit area." The units commonly used are: houles per second per square centimeter, or watts per square centimeter. The intensity of the weakest audible sound has been estimated to be 10^{-16} watts per square centimeter.

Interrupter Switch—an audiometer control switch that permits the stimulus tone to be cut off from the earphones but leaves the audiometer circuits in operation, thus making it possible to change the frequency and/or the intensity level of the stimulus tone without communicating to the test subject the extraneous noise generated during the changes.

Lateralization Test—a diagnostic test used to determine whether the status of hearing is the same in both ears. The classic lateralization test is the Weber test, in which a vibrating tuning fork or the bone oscillator of an audiometer is placed in the center of the forehead. Differences in the response of the two ears to the tone thus generated may be used to help diagnose hearing loss.

Level—a particular convenient way of expressing how much a given amount of some physical property of sound exceeds a reference amount. Levels are commonly calculated from the logarithm of the ratio of the given amount to the reference amount. In acoustics, the unit of level is usually the decibel. More than one reference value may be used for a given physical property (reference sound pressures, for example, are 0.0002 dyne/cm.², 1 dyne/cm.², etc.), and it is absolutely necessary to identify the reference whenever values of level are quoted. A sound pressure level of 50 dB re 0.0002 dyne/cm.², for example, does not have the same sound pressure level as a sound of 50 dB re audiometric zero.

Level, Hearing—the number of dB re audiometric zero at a specified frequency.

Level, Loudness—the loudness level of a sound is numerically equal to the sound pressure level (in dB re 0.0002 dyne/cm.²) of a 1000-c/s (Hz) tone judged by a group of normal hearing listeners to be equally as loud as the sound in question. The unit of loudness level is the phon. There is no simple relation between loudness level—a physical quantity —and loudness—a psychological attribute of the auditory response.

Level, Sensation—the number of decibels that sound is above the threshold of audibility of a specific ear.

Level, Sound-Pressure—SPL—sound-pressure level (in decibels) is a logarithmic ratio of the existing sound pressure, p, and a reference sound pressure, p_0. A common reference pressure, p_0, is 0.0002 dyne/cm.². Sound pressure level in decibels may be found from the following formula:

$$SPL = 20 \times \log_{10} \frac{p}{p_0}$$

$$SPL \text{ (re 0.0002 dyne/cm.}^2\text{)} = 20 \log_{10} \frac{p}{0.0002 \text{ dyne/cm.}^2}$$

Limen—a threshold of sensation.

Lip Reading—see Speech Reading.

Localization—the determination, by auditory responses alone, of the direction from which sound comes to the ears. Under favorable circumstances man can determine the direction of sound paths to within a few degrees.

Logarithm—(to the base 10, usually written $\log_{10}$)—the $\log_{10}$ of a number is the power to which 10 must be raised to give that number. Consider the number 100: 10^2 (ten squared) $= 10 \times 10 = 100$. Therefore, since ten must be raised to the second power to give 100, the $\log_{10}$ of 100 is 2. Similarly $10^3 = 10 \times 10 \times 10 = 1000$; therefore, the $\log_{10}$ of 1000 is 3. All numbers between 100 and 1000 have $\log_{10}$ between 2 and 3. The $\log_{10}$ of 200 for example, is 2.30103; for 400 it is 2.60206, etc. Tables of logarithms to the base 10 are provided for quick reference and calculation. Bases other than 10 are sometimes used, for example $\log_2$ or $\log_e$ ($e = 2.718$), etc.

Loudness—the intensive attribute of an auditory sensation in terms of which sound may be ordered on a scale extending from loud to soft. Loudness is determined largely by the intensity of the sound stimulus, but it is also affected by frequency and by wave form. The unit of loudness is the sone.

Loudness Contour, Equal—see Equal Loudness Contours.

Loudness Contour, Monaural—equal loudness contours for loudness judgments obtained with right ears only or with left ears only, as opposed to binaural loudness contours.

Loudness Level—see Level, Loudness.

Malingerer—one who feigns illness or disability in order to gain an end.

Masking Noise—(as the term is used in audiometry)—sound used deliberately to raise the threshold of audibility for a stimulus signal.

Maximal Acoustical Output—the highest sound intensity a system is capable of generating within specified distortion limits.

Microphonics or Microphonic Effects—unwanted extraneous signals generated in an electrical circuit element by the vibratory motion of its normally non-moving parts.

Monitored Live Voice—a method for presenting speech sounds to subjects whose hearing is to be tested with speech. Words are spoken into a microphone by a tester who monitors the level of his spoken words by means of a meter which reads the average output level of the microphone. The speaker regulates his voice to keep this level as nearly constant as possible.

Moro's Response (Reflex)—(sometimes called "Moro's Embrase" after the initial description by the German pediatrician)—the tendency of a young infant to stiffen and throw out the arms following a sudden, sharp sound or sudden vibration.

Noise—any unwanted sound.

Noise, Broad-Band—a sound in which energy is present over a wide range of frequencies. Those frequencies close to the specific one being tested cause masking interference.

Noise, Narrow-Band—sound in which energy is concentrated within a small frequency interval.

Noise-Induced Hearing Loss—although any hearing loss caused by continuous noise or by sudden noise might be called a noise-induced hearing loss, the term is usually restricted to mean the slowly progressive inner ear hearing loss that results from exposure to continuous noise over a long period of time.

Non-Linear Distortion—(see Distortion, Amplitude).

Non-Organic Hearing Impairment—any auditory dysfunction for which no plausible anatomical or physiological basis can be found.

Occupational Hearing Loss—a hearing loss that is causally related to one's employment; in the legal sense, hearing loss, as defined by statute, that is causally related to one's occupation.

Ossicle—a small bone; any of the members of a chain of three bones, found in the middle ear, from the outer drum membrane of the tympanum to the membrane covering the oval window of the inner ear (malleus, incus, stapes).

PB (Phonetically Balanced) Word List—a group of single-syllable words so selected that the frequency of occurrence of speech sounds within the group is the same as the frequency of occurrence of the same sounds in an average vocabulary of conversational American English. PB words are used to determine discrimination scores for speech.

Peak Clipping—the non-uniform response of an electroacoustical system that effectively limits the magnitude of the output signal to some predetermined maximal level by not reproducing that portion of the signal which would otherwise exceed this level.

Pitch—that attribute of auditory sensation in terms of which sounds may be ordered on a scale extending from low to high such as a musical scale. Pitch is determined largely by the frequency of the stimulus, but it is also affected by intensity.

Psychoacoustics—the field of study that is concerned with man's responses to acoustic stimuli.

Pulse Generator—a device that produces pulsed signals; often an electronic instrument.

Pure Tone—a continuous sound of a single frequency; a tone not accompanied by overtones or by other sounds.

Random Noise—a complex sound wave in which the amplitudes of the component frequencies vary in time, but at any instant the amplitudes of the various frequencies are distributed according to a normal probability distribution.

Recruitment—a clinical term used to denote an auditory response characterized by an abnormal increase in loudness.

Refraction—the bending of sound waves around small objects.

Resonance—an intensification, at certain frequencies, of the output of a mechanical vibrating system, or of an electrical or acoustical oscillating system. Resonance occurs when the rate of oscillation of a force (or signal) applied to the system is the same as a natural frequency of vibration of the system. (A natural frequency of vibration is the rate at which a system vibrates when it is started in motion but is left to vibrate without interference or assistance from external forces.) Complex systems may have more than one natural frequency.

Reverberant Room—(also called a "live" room)—a room in which sounds persist for a relatively long period of time after they have left the source. This persistence of sound is due to multiple reflections (echoes) from highly reflecting room surfaces.

Reverberation—the persistence of sound at a point in space for a relatively long time after the direct sound from the source has reached and passed that point. Reverberation is caused by reflection from walls, baffles, etc.

Selective Amplifications—see Amplification, Selective.

Sensation Level—see Level, Sensation.

Sensation Unit—the smallest change of intensity that can be detected by the normal ear. It is approximately equal to 1 dB.

Signal to Noise Ratio—the ratio of the intensity of a signal to the intensity of the residual noise in the absence of the signal. To find this ratio in decibels, subtract the sound pressure level of the noise in decibels re 0.0002 dyne/cm.^{2} from the sound pressure level of the signal in decibels re 0.0002 dyne/cm.^{2}. The difference is the signal to noise ratio in decibels re 0.0002 dyne/cm.^{2}.

Sinusoidal Wave (Sine Wave)—a sound wave that forms a smooth and continuous outline which repeats itself in a cyclic manner. The wave pattern derives its name from the fact that it can be described mathematically by sine (or cosine) functions.

Sound Level Meter—an instrument consisting of a microphone, an amplifier, frequency-weighting circuits, and an output meter; used to measure sound levels in decibels re the standard reference sound pressure 0.0002 dyne/cm.^{2}.

Sound Pressure—Sound-induced alternations in pressure above and below the existing static pressure in a medium. Several different values of sound pressure at a point may be "measured." For example: instantaneous sound pressure, the sound pressure at a given instant in time; maximal sound pressure, the maximal value reached by varying instantaneous sound pressure; peak sound pressure, etc. The unit of sound pressure is usually the dyne per square centimeter or the microbar.

Sound-Pressure Level—see Level, Sound-Pressure.

Sound Treating—a method of building construction that minimizes both the amount of external ambient noise transmitted into the interior of the structure and the levels of ambient noise produced inside the structure.

Speech-Discrimination Test—a hearing test used to determine the subject's ability to hear and to repeat correctly the American English speech sounds represented in PB word lists.

Speech Reading—(also called Lip Reading or Visual Hearing)—interpreting the movements of the lips, face, head, and hands as an aid to communicating by speech.

Speech Reception Threshold (SRT)—the minimal sound pressure level at which 50% of the test words presented to the subject are repeated correctly. Spondaic words are commonly used to measure speech reception threshold.

Square Wave—a succession of identical acoustical or electrical rectangular pulses so spaced that the time duration of the pulse is just equal to the time period between successive pulses.

Standard Reference—an arbitrary amount of some physical property of sound such as frequency, voltage, etc., used as a base for comparison in determinations of intensity level, pressure level, frequency level, voltage level, etc. (See Levels.)

Standing Waves—a fixed or stationary wave pattern produced when particles in a medium are acted on by sound waves that have the same frequency and amplitude but are traveling in opposite directions. The standing wave pattern in a room is affected by the frequencies in the sound, the size and shape of the room, material on the walls, etc.

Temporary Threshold Shift—the decrease of sensitivity to sound after exposure to acoustical stimulation.

Threshold of Hearing—the minimal value of sound wave pressure which will produce a sensation of tone from a given frequency.

Threshold of Pain, Tickle, or Discomfort—the sound pressure level of the minimal acoustic stimulus that produces the pertinent auditory sensation for some specified fraction of the number of times the stimulus is presented to the ear.

Timbre—the overtone structure of a voice; that characteristic by which two tones of equal volume and pitch are distinguished from each other; resonance.

Tinnitus—a ringing or buzzing in the ear.

Tone—a sound wave capable of evoking an auditory sensation of definite pitch; may be a complex tone or a pure tone.

Tone Control—a control by which the frequency response of a system may be varied.

Transient—any acoustic signal of short duration.

Transducer—a device that converts electrical energy to sound energy or vice versa; for example: earphones, microphones, loudspeakers, etc.

Warble Tone—a sound whose frequency rises and falls within fixed limits around a mid-frequency. The region within the fixed limits is known as the warble band.

White Noise (Acoustic)—a sound whose frequency spectrum is continuous (no gaps or frequencies missing in the included frequency range) and uniform (all frequencies occurring with the same average intensity). White noise is not necessarily the same as random noise.

Vibration—A complete, rapid, back and forth motion of an object or medium.

VU Meter—(Volume-Unit Meter)—a meter that measures acoustical signal power on a decibel-type scale. The scale of the meter is labeled in volume units (VUs) and not in decibels. The reference power here is non-standard, and consequently zero on this scale does not correspond to zero on any of the standard decibel scales. (This meter reads zero when 1 milliwatt of power is generated in a 600-Ohm resistor across which the meter is connected.) VU meters are commonly used to monitor input signals to recording equipment or to broadcasting equipment.

Appendix 2

THE INTERNATIONAL STANDARD REFERENCE ZERO FOR PURE-TONE AUDIOMETERS AND ITS RELATION TO THE EVALUATION OF IMPAIRMENT OF HEARING

HALLOWELL DAVIS

Central Institute for the Deaf, St. Louis, Missouri

FRED W. KRANZ

Otarion Electronics, Inc., Ossining, New York

International reference zero levels for pure-tone audiometers have been agreed upon and recommended by the International Organization for Standardization (ISO) and are under consideration for inclusion in a new American Standard for Audiometers. The new ISO levels are desirable because (1) the shape of the threshold contour is more accurate, (2) the threshold levels are reproducible from laboratory to laboratory and from country to country, and (3) they represent the only apparent escape from permanent ambiguity and confusion in international exchange of audiometric information. The new ISO levels differ significantly from the American Standard values of 1951, in terms of which our present rules and laws for calculating percentage impairment of hearing for compensation purposes are written. The apparent difficulties arising from the numerical differences can be easily overcome, however, because it is possible to go from the 1964 ISO scale to the 1951 ASA scale by a simple subtraction before beginning such calculations. For the average of the three frequencies 500, 1000 and 2000 c/s the difference to be subtracted is 11 dB.

For many years leading otologists and audiologists, both in the United States and in Europe, have desired a set of international standards for audiometers. One reason for this is that the present American standard reference threshold levels, embodied in the 1951 specification for Audiometers for General Diagnostic Purposes,[a] differ significantly from the corresponding British standard levels. The British standard is now employed not only in Great Britain but in most European countries as well. The

Reprinted from the *Journal of Speech and Hearing Research*, March 1964, Vol. 7, No. 1.

[a] Z24.3-1951: American Standards Association, 10 East 40th Street, New York 16, New York.

American values are based on determinations of the threshold of hearing in "normal" ears made in the United States National Health Survey in 1937. The British values, sometimes referred to as a "standard of normal hearing," were developed from studies carried out in England in the early nineteen-fifties. The British determinations were made fifteen years later than the American, using more modern equipment, better acoustic conditions and improved psychoacoustic techniques and they differ by about 10 dB, on the average, from the corresponding 1951 American standard values.

The International Organization for Standardization took this situation under consideration in 1955. Its writing group examined carefully and critically all of the published data on the thresholds of normal hearing. In all, fifteen different studies were found, carried out in five different countries (almost half of the studies were done in the United States), which met modern criteria of acoustic surroundings and psychoacoustic procedures. The agreement among these studies was found to be quite good; and all of them differed clearly from the 1951 American standard. After several years of calculation and discussion these data were combined to form a truly international standard reference zero for the uniform calibration of pure-tone audiometers.[b] This standard was approved by the Council of the ISO in 1963 without a dissenting vote and the recommendation is being published in 1964.

In 1959, while discussions of the international zero reference level were still in progress, the Committee on Conservation of Hearing of the American Academy of Ophthalmology and Otolaryngology endorsed the principle of such an International Standard. The Committee recognized explicitly that the international standard would probably be quite close to the British standard and significantly different from the 1951 American standard. The American Academy of Ophthalmology and Otolaryngology as a whole endorsed and accepted this principle in 1960. Similar endorsements were also voted by the American Otological Society and by the American Speech and Hearing Association. Now, in 1963, the Committee on Conservation of Hearing has reaffirmed its earlier endorsement and it expresses the strong hope that a new American Standard for Audiometers including the international zero reference level will be approved and adopted in the near future. The committee intends in any case to employ the international zero level and hopes that it will soon come into general use.

During the same period, 1958 to 1963, a writing group of the American Standards Association prepared a new American Standard for Audiom-

---

[b] ISO Technical Committee 43—Acoustics, No. 554, "A Standard Reference Zero for the Calibration of Pure-Tone Audiometers," American Standards Association, 10 East 40th Street, New York, N. Y.

eters. This draft combines in a single document and brings up to date the current American Standards entitled *Audiometers for General Diagnostic Purposes (Z24.3-1959)*, *Specification for Pure-Tone Audiometers for Screening Purposes (Z24.12-1952)* and *Specification for Speech Audiometers (Z24.13-1953)*. Most of the changes in substance are technical modifications, usually in the direction of specifying somewhat closer tolerances or making more explicit the statements of objectives and procedures. A major change, however, is the incorporation of the new ISO set of zero reference levels.

The proposed new American Standard for Audiometers was circulated in 1963 to the appropriate committee members of the American Standards Association for letter ballot. The editorial reorganization and the technical modifications met with unanimous approval, but several negative votes were cast on the basis of difficulties that might arise from the adoption of the international reference zero levels. The letter ballot has therefore been withdrawn to allow time for further consideration and explanation of the international reference levels and their implications.

Advantages

The case for the international ISO reference zero levels rests upon two propositions: (1) the change from the present (1951) American Standard to the new international levels is desirable, and (2) the change, although it will entail some temporary inconvenience during a transition period, can be made without jeopardy of any vital legal or financial interests.

There are three major reasons why the change in the standard reference threshold level is desirable. First, a general requirement of a standard is that it be based on measurements that can be reproduced with reasonable accuracy. It is true that results resembling the present American Standard are often obtained in tests made rather casually under so-called "clinical conditions," but the values so obtained scatter rather widely. On the other hand, threshold values obtained in all of the careful studies made under fully specified and reproducible conditions have centered quite closely around the new ISO standard. The 1951 American Standard has therefore only a limited inherent prestige, and although it has served a useful purpose it cannot possibly compete with the ISO standard for world-wide adoption.

Not only are the 1951 American Standard levels higher by about 10 dB on the average but the shape of the 1951 threshold contour differs significantly from that of the ISO. All of the studies on which the ISO Standard is based and also widespread clinical experience indicate that the contour of the 1951 American Standard is wrong. Our subjects' hearing thresholds regularly appear to be *relatively too good* at 250 and 500 c/s and to be *im-*

paired at 4000 c/s. The so-called "4000 cycle notch" in audiograms has been recognized for many years and has led to considerable concern on the part of otologists. At least a part of the notch is due to the faulty shape of our standard reference contour. Actually, as a numerical comparison of the two standards shows, the 1951 American Standard is relatively too lenient by about 5 dB at 250 and 500 c/s and is too stringent by about 5 dB at 4000 c/s as compared with the middle and the two ends of the frequency scale. It is important for otologists and audiologists to correct this distortion because erroneous conclusions have been based on it in the past.

Finally, the use of a single international standard will terminate the confusion and ambiguity that now make it extremely difficult to compare audiometric measurements made in the United States with those made in Great Britain and Europe, where the British Standard is now employed. Practically speaking, it will soon be essential for any American otologist or audiologist writing for an international audience to employ the ISO Standard, and before many years the use of the ISO Standard will probably be required by most leading scientific journals.

Doubts and Difficulties

Some of the arguments against adopting the ISO Standard hinge on the trouble it will cause or else on the expense of replacing or recalibrating the audiometers now in use. These arguments can be dealt with directly and briefly. Another class of objections hinges on questions of the legal status of the new and the old standards during the transition period and on possible misinterpretations of the implications of the new standard for the calculation of "percentage impairment of hearing." These doubts deserve full and careful consideration.

There is no denying that there will be some trouble and some confusion during the transition period which will follow the introduction of the ISO Standard. The difference in decibels is significant, and otologists and audiologists will have to learn to readjust their mental standards of what is within normal limits, what constitutes a significant hearing loss, etc. For several years it will be extremely important that every audiogram be clearly labelled to indicate the scale according to which it is plotted. Such difficulties always attend any significant change in a scale or reference standard. However, if the change is accepted as ultimately desirable and inevitable, the total amount of confusion and relearning is least if the change is made immediately, before any more students and technicians learn the old standards and before any more data are recorded on the old scale. Prompt and unified action represents the quickest and easiest way to the ultimate goal.

Clearly there should be no need for immediate replacement of old audiometers with new ones or even of immediate recalibration of old instruments. Recalibration to the new standard should be perfectly practical whenever an audiometer is returned to the manufacturer for recalibration as it normally should be every year or two. Thus no great extra expense to users will be involved, nor will the facilities of the manufacturers of audiometers be taxed unduly.

The only valid reason for concern about the transition period, which will last for at least two or three years, is a doubt as to the legal status of records made during the transition period on old instruments that may not conform in all respects to the proposed new ASA Standard. To meet this difficulty, it should be easy to write into the standard itself an explicit statement concerning the transition period to the effect that, for all medico-legal purposes such as compensation, audiograms should be considered equally valid, regardless of the basis of the calibration of the audiometer, so long as the calibration is accurate by one scale or the other and provided it is clearly indicated on each audiogram *the scale according to which the hearing threshold levels are actually plotted.* As the relation between the 1951 American scale the ISO scale will be simply a matter of a difference of a few decibels at each frequency it will be easy to go from one scale to the other by simple additions or subtractions of these differences. A list of the differences and the rules for using them will be explicitly included as part of the next American Standard for Audiometers.

A Possible Misinterpretation and a Clarification

The most serious objection, which actually was the basis for most if not all of the negative votes cast against the new standard in the recent ballot of the American Standards Association, is the concern that a new zero reference level might establish automatically a new definition of "normal hearing"; and that consequently certain existing laws, rules and guides might be interpreted by lawyers or referees to mean that impairment of hearing would begin at the same number of decibels of "hearing loss" indicated on an audiometer calibrated to the new standard as it does on present audiometers. If this were done, however, the "percentage impairment" of a given listener would be significantly greater when measured with a new standard instrument than with present audiometers, and he would be entitled to greater compensation. This would be manifestly unfair and improper and would create an intolerable situation.

The term "percentage impairment of hearing" is used here, in accordance with AMA usage,[c] to designate the degree of handicap that is associated with a particular impairment of hearing. It implies a medical evaluation and is a percentage used in the calculation of compensation for industrial

[c] Committee on Medical Rating of Physical Impairment. Guides to the Evaluation of Permanent Impairment. *J. Am. Med. Assn.* 1958, 168: 475.

hearing loss. Different rules have been employed in different places and at different times to derive this "percentage impairment" from threshold measurements made with a pure-tone audiometer, but whatever rule is employed, it is perfectly obvious that the calculated percentage impairment of a listener's hearing must remain the same whether the audiometer is calibrated according to the old standard or a new one. Percentage impairment of hearing, i.e., hearing handicap, depends on a man's ability or inability to hear sounds of a certain physical intensity, but not on the scale used on the audiometer. *The proposed change in the audiometric reference zero must not be construed as altering in any way the evaluation of impairment of hearing. The only difference is to add one numerical detail of calculation.*

The American Standards Association is a voluntary organization and it has no legal authority to change, directly or indirectly, the amount of compensation that is related to a given degree of impairment. Neither can it decide what is "normal" in a medical or in a social sense. Too many shades of meaning are attached to the word "normal." We should think of a range of normal hearing, not of a single set of values. *The new reference zero levels are not designated as a "standard of normal hearing," either in the ISO recommendation or in the proposed American Standard.* For reference zero levels one particular set of values, one particular contour, must nevertheless be chosen. The zero contour must have the correct shape and lie at a well defined level. The ISO contour actually lies near one edge of the zone of normal hearing, and it is a more satisfactory base for audiometric measurements than the 1951 ASA levels. It is based on the hearing acuity of selected young individuals, tested by approved methods under perfect audiometric conditions.

What the adoption of the ISO standard will do is to establish a different relation between the number of decibels on the dial of an audiometer and the physical intensity of the sound that the instrument produces. But the percentage impairment of a listener must, of course, remain the same when his hearing is measured first on an audiometer with the old calibration and then on one with the new. A simple way to achieve this will be to subtract appropriate corrections, which will be given in the proposed new American Standard, from the readings made on the new scale.

The relation between the two audiometric scales and the relation of each to the range of normal hearing and to the scale of percentage impairment recommended by the American Academy of Ophthalmology and Otolaryngology (AAOO) are illustrated in the accompanying chart. Here the ISO scale is displaced upward relative to the 1951 ASA scale by 11 dB. The scale of percentage impairment may be entered from either of the audiometric scales. Note the wide range of normal hearing, which extends

HEARING LEVELS IN COMMON USE

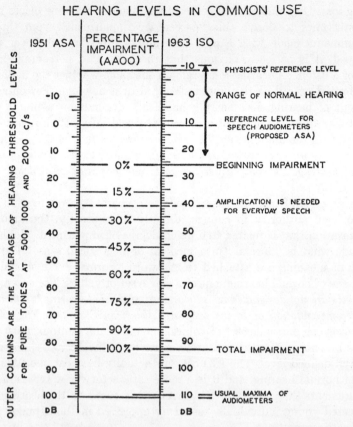

FIG. A2.1. Comparison of two audiometer scales and the AAOO percentage impairment scale. The center column represents percentage impairment of hearing, calculated according to the rule formulated by the Subcommittee on Noise in 1958 and adopted by the AAOO in 1959 for use in cases involving compensation. "1963 ISO" refers to the reference zero levels for pure-tone audiometers recommended by the International Organization for Standardization. (These levels were approved by that organization in 1963 but their publication will bear the date 1964.) "1951 ASA" refers to the audiometric scale defined in the American Standard for Audiometers for General Diagnostic Purposes, Z24.5-1951. The reference level for speech audiometers is the one written into the proposed (1963) revision of the American Standard for Audiometers, not yet approved. It differs by only 2 dB, however, from the present (1951) ASA standard. The reference level for speech audiometry is defined in terms of a 1000 c/s calibration tone and therefore its relation to the scales in the figure, which represent the averages of hearing levels for three frequencies, is not exact.

from the very best hearing threshold level measured under the best conditions to or nearly to the level at which impairment, in the sense of handicap, is considered to begin.

The rule for estimation of *percentage impairment* of hearing recommended by the AAOO in 1959[d] refers to the average of the audiometric measurements made at the three frequencies 500, 1000 and 2000 c/s. The average of the readings for these three frequencies will be 11 dB higher if the audiometer is calibrated to the 1964 ISO values than if it is calibrated to the 1951 ASA values. Thus the appropriate correction for this average is 11 dB. *The subtraction of this correction should be regarded as a necessary and sufficient step in the technical procedure of audiometry under the new standard if the purpose of the measurement is to calculate percentage impairment of hearing under rules that were written before 1964.*

If and when a new American Standard for Audiometers incorporating the ISO zero reference level of 1964 is issued, the AAOO recommendation of 1959 should be modified to read: "For every decibel that the estimated hearing level for speech exceeds 15 dB by the American Standard of 1951 or 26 dB by the American Standard of 196–, allow one-and-one-half per cent in impairment of hearing up to the maximum of 100 %. This maximum is reached at 82 dB by the American Standard of 1951 and at 93 dB by the American Standard of 196–." (The full titles of these standards are: "Audiometers for General Diagnostic Purposes," Z24.5-1951 and "American Standard Specifications for Audiometers," in preparation.) It will clarify the situation still further if the various states, organizations, and jurisdictions that have adopted similar rules make the corresponding amendments in due time.

During a transition period of several years many old audiometers already in use will still be calibrated according to the American Standard of 1951 while new instruments will be calibrated according to the proposed new standard. The basis of calibration will, of course, be clearly marked on each new instrument. "Hearing threshold level," not "hearing loss," will be the designation on the intensity dials of the new audiometers. But on each audiogram that is recorded during the transition period, it will be absolutely essential to indicate whether the hearing levels are expressed in terms of the 1951 ASA or the 1964 ISO values. Boxes for checking one or the other or an explicit statement will be printed on every audiogram blank.

Pertinent Excerpts from the Proposed New American Standard

The proposed new American Standard for Audiometers includes a list of the exact differences in decibels at each frequency between the 1951 ASA and the 1964 ISO reference threshold levels, and also several statements which are pertinent to the problem of estimating percentage impairment of hearing. They read as follows:

---

[d] Report of the Committee on Conservation of Hearing. D. M. Lierle Chairman. Guide for the Evaluation of Hearing Impairment. *Trans Amer. Acad. Ophthal. Otolaryngol.*, 1959, 63: 238.

Transition to Hearing Threshold Level

"The standard reference threshold levels given in Table 2 of this standard are those adopted by the International Organization for Standardization (ISO). These values differ considerably from those which have been in use in the U.S.A. since 1939, officially adopted in 1951 and given in Table 2 of the American Standard Specification for Audiometers for General Diagnostic Purposes, Z24.5-1951. The latter may conveniently be termed the 1951 ASA values.

"The following table gives these two sets of reference threshold values, in terms of the Western Electric 705-A earphone and the 9-A coupler. The numerical values given in the 1951 specification have been shifted by 74 dB to put them on the basis of 0.0002 microbar, and have been rounded off to the nearest 0.5 dB to accord with the ISO method of presentation.

Frequency	Reference Threshold Levels		
	1951 ASA	1964 ISO	Differences
125	54.5 dB	45.5 dB	9 dB
250	39.5	24.5	15
500	25	11	14
1000	16.5	6.5	10
1500	(16.5)	6.5	(10)
2000	17	8.5	8.5
3000	(16.)	7.5	(8.5)
4000	15	9.	6.
6000	(17.5)	8.	(9.5)
8000	21	9.5	11.5

The figures in parentheses are interpolations.

"There will inevitably be a period of time during which there are in use some audiometers calibrated to the 1951 ASA threshold levels and some calibrated to the 1964 ISO threshold levels. In order to facilitate the orderly transition from the use of the one set of reference levels to the other, it is strongly recommended that the following procedures be adopted.

1. Audiometers calibrated to the 1964 ISO values are to be identified by the designation 'Hearing Threshold Level—ISO 1964' for the attenuator dial.

2. On an audiogram form, the vertical scale is to be designated 'Hearing Threshold Level in db.' During the transition period, the horizontal scale is to be labeled as follows:

Frequency, c/s

	125	250	500	1000	1500	2000	3000	4000	6000	8000
Difference in dB (1964 vs. 1951)	9	15	14	10	10	8.5	8.5	6.0	9.5	11.5

3. The audiogram form is to include the following notations:

This audiogram is plotted on the basis of:

☐ 1964 ISO reference thresholds

☐ 1951 ASA reference thresholds

(Check one of these squares)

Readings obtained on an audiometer calibrated to the 1951 ASA thresholds may be converted to, and plotted as, 'Hearing Threshold Levels' based on the 1964 ISO reference thresholds by *adding* the appropriate 'Difference in dB' at each frequency. To convert readings based on the 1964 ISO reference thresholds to readings based on the 1951 ASA reference thresholds, *subtract* the 'Difference in dB.'

4. On the audiogram form, the line of 'Difference in dB' may be in smaller type than the 'Frequency' line. Also the last two sentences of 3 may be so located on the audiogram that their reproduction in a journal may be conveniently optional.

Percentage Impairment of Hearing

"In adopting the ISO reference levels in place of the reference levels of Z24.5-1951, the American Standards Association does not intend or imply that any change should be made in other standards or rules based on the 1951 levels. In particular, *until the rules for compensation purposes have been modified by the appropriate organizations or jurisdictions to recognize specifically the new reference levels, all measurements of hearing threshold level made according to the ISO scale shall be converted to 1951 ASA values before the calculations for compensation purposes are made.* In accordance with Appendix (C), this conversion is made by subtracting the 'dB Differences' there given from the values of hearing threshold level measured with an audiometer calibrated to the 1964 ISO values.

Relation to other Standards

"Similar conversions to 1951 ASA values shall be made before applying the specifications as to hearing loss mentioned in American Standard Method for the Measurement of Real-Ear Attenuation of Ear Protectors at Threshold, Z24.22-1957.

"The American Standard Criteria for Background Noise in Audiometer Rooms, S1.3-1960, is only indirectly involved. Its specifications are not sufficiently stringent to ensure measurement at ISO hearing threshold levels at all frequencies. The standard remains unaffected, however, until its next revision. Where reference is made therein to the zero hearing threshold level of American Standard audiometers, it shall be clearly understood that it still means the American Standards of 1951 and 1952."

Approval by the Committee on Conservation of Hearing

As noted above, the 1963 ISO reference zero levels for pure-tone audiometers are more reproducible as to level and more accurate as to the shape of their contour than the (1951) American Standard levels. For these reasons, and in the interest of international standardization, the Committee on Conservation of Hearing of the American Academy of Ophthalmology and Otolaryngology voted, on 8 December 1963, to adopt for its own use the new ISO standard values, as of 1 January 1965. The Committee expresses the hope that the proposed revised American Standard for Audiometers, incorporating the ISO reference zero levels, will soon be approved and brought into general use.

This article was prepared for and approved by the Subcommittee on Noise, and approved in principle on 8 December 1963 by the Committee on Conservation of Hearing of the American Academy of Opthalmology and Otolaryngology. The senior author is a member of the Subcommittee on Noise of the Committee on Conservation of Hearing of the American Academy of Opthalmology and Otolaryngology. The co-author is chairman of the Writing Group on Audiometers of the American Standards Association.

Preparation of this article was supported by Public Health Service Program Project Grant, No. B-3856, from the National Institute of Neurological Diseases and Blindness to Central Institute for the Deaf.

Index

Electroencephalographic audiometry, 218, 240
Environment
  audiometric, 97–106
  conditions required, 100–106
  industrial audiometry, 225
  noise, 97–100
    broad-band, 98
    measurement, 99
    narrow-band, 98
    vibration, 99
  prefabricated audiometric rooms, 103
Equal loudness level test, 137–141
Equipment, audiometric, 188–191
Eye-blink test, 240

Fowler, E. P., 8
Frequency theory, 4
Functional hearing loss (see also Non-organic hearing loss), 193

Galvanic audiometry, 194, 215–218, 239
Glorig, A., automatic group screening audiometer, 172
Glossary, 243
Goldstein, M., 9
Group screening tests (see Screening tests)

Hartmann, A., 5
Hearing
  atypical phenomena, 64–69
    diplacusis, 68
    perstimulatory fatigue, 64
    recruitment, 66
    temporary threshold shift, 64–66
    tinnitus, 67
Hearing-conservation program, 178–183
Hearing evaluation in children
  developmental process, 207–210
    deviations from normal, 208
  differential diagnosis, 209–221
    developmental picture, 209
    electrodermal response audiometry, 215–218
    electroencephalographic audiometry, 218
    galvanic audiometry, 215–218
    picture-show techniques, 219
    play-conditioned audiometry, 219–221
Hearing level, 52–54
Hearing loss
  conductive, 194, 198
  evaluation of non-organic (see Non-organic hearing loss evaluation)

functional, 193
non-organic (see Non-organic hearing loss evaluation)
sensori-neural, 195–201
Hughes, D. E., 6
Hypnosis, 240

Incus, anatomy, 2
Industrial audiometry, 224–234
  equipment, 226
  personnel requirements, 227
  procedure, 228–234
  testing environment, 225
Infants, evaluation of hearing in (see Hearing evaluation in children)
Instruments for monitoring live voice, 163
International standard reference zero, 256–266
Intertone, 23
Inverse-square law, 31

Jones, I. H., 10

Lombard test, 160, 193, 238
Loudness
  equal-loudness contours, 56
  level in phons, 55
  level in sones, 55
  sensation level, 55
Loudness-balance test, 135–137

Malingering, 193, 235–242
  delayed-speech feedback test, 161
  Lombard test, 160
Malleus, anatomy, 2
Management of patient, 201–203
Masking, 61–64, 115–118, 122–124
Measurement
  levels
    interval scales, 80
    nominal scales, 78
    ordinal scales, 79
    ratio scales, 80
  nature of mathematics, 73
  numbers in, 74–78
  principles, 72
  recent developments in theory, 82–84
  transformations, 81
Measurement of sound (see Sound wave, measurement)
Method of adjustment, 49
Method of limits, 49
Middle ear, 2
Mistuned consonances, 23